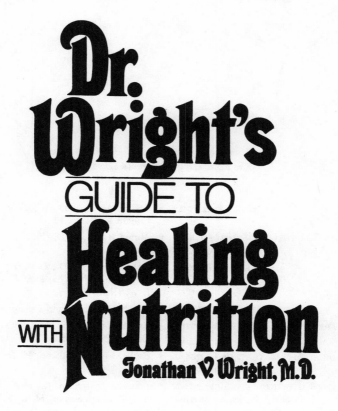

# Dr. Wright's GUIDE TO Healing with Nutrition

### Jonathan V. Wright, M.D.

*The Keats Health Reference Library*

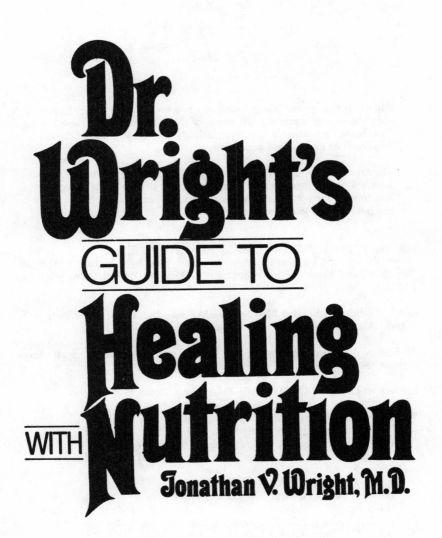

# Dr. Wright's GUIDE TO Healing Nutrition
## WITH

### Jonathan V. Wright, M.D.

Keats Publishing, Inc., New Canaan, Connecticut

## For Holly

Although the author has exhaustively researched all sources to ensure the accuracy and completeness of the information contained in this book, we assume no responsibility for errors, inaccuracies, omissions or any inconsistency herein.

The treatment of illness must be supervised by a physician or other licensed health professional. The information presented in this book is intended for education only and does not contain treatment recommendations for the public.

Library of Congress Cataloging-in-Publication Data:

Wright, Jonathan V.
    [Guide to healing with nutrition]
    Dr. Wright's Guide to healing with nutrition / by Jonathan
  V. Wright ; including an appendix on nutrients and bone health by
  Dr. Wright and Alan R. Gaby. — Rev. ed.
      p.    cm.
    Includes bibliographical references and index.
    ISBN 0-87983-530-3
    1. Diet therapy.  2. Nutrition.  3. Health.  I. Gaby, Alan.
II. Title.  III. Title: Doctor Wright's Guide to healing with
nutrition.  IV. Title: Guide to healing with nutrition.
RM216.W87   1990                                        90-5036
615.8′54—dc20                                            CIP


Printed in the United States of America

Published by Keats Publishing, Inc.
27 Pine Street (Box 876)
New Canaan, Connecticut 08640

9th printing—January 1995

# NOTICE

The information presented here is intended to be informative, and to provide some insight into nutrition as a means of achieving the best health possible. It is meant to complement the advice of your physician, not replace it.

As you read through the many cases, keep in mind that although they appear similar to your own, they may not be. Everyone has different needs depending on age, sex, health, current diet, family background, and lifestyle. You may be quite different, so following the same treatment path could cause problems.

Remember, it's your responsibility to be informed about your health, but it's also your responsibility to inform. So don't be afraid to discuss this information with your physician.

# CONTENTS

# PROLOGUE

The hunter stalked his prey through the awakening forest. As the early rays of the sun filtered through the branches overhead, he moved noiselessly from tree to tree. Finally halting, he quickly but carefully fitted an arrow to his bowstring, aimed, and let fly. This time he hit his mark; he was glad, because he had not eaten since the previous day. He walked to where his arrow had fallen, carefully removed the chocolate-covered jelly doughnut, and walked away, eating his breakfast.

The four women had wandered far to find food for the mid-day meal. Finally the oldest, wise in the ways of their tribe, saw a familiar plant. She'd seen it only once as a girl, but had remembered it. From it they gathered the cans of spaghetti and meatballs, and started home.

The children, thirsty again, ran to the tree they knew well. At this time of year, it provided the most delicious orange-fla-

*vored fruit drink, with 50 percent more vitamin C than the competing tree on the other side of their village.*

Does all that sound a bit ridiculous? I'm sure you'll agree it does, but there's an extremely serious point: we probably have the same bodies, physically and biochemically, that the primitive hunter, the prehistoric-women, and their children had thousands, tens of thousands, a million years ago. Certainly there are individual differences, but the overall human plan has been the same, as far as scientists can tell, for roughly three to four million years.

For all but the last 10 to 12 thousand of those years, or 99½ percent of the known time that man has been on earth, the food eaten by our ancestors has been what they could hunt, fish, gather, or dig. Even agriculture and large-scale domestication of cows, pigs, chickens, and other food animals is (relatively speaking) in its infancy in the whole history of man, having been practiced for only ½ percent of the time span of our race.

The instant in time occupied by widespread use of refined flours, refined sugars, and synthetic food chemicals is barely one hundred years long.

Simply put, your body and mind are suited to (scientists sometimes say adapted to) the types of foods that people have eaten for hundreds of thousands of years. They aren't suited to the radical dietary changes of the last one hundred years. No wonder so much of the illness of our century is due to what we eat. Our bodies are trying to tell us something is wrong.

The changes produced in the way we live by science and its technology are at once a blessing and a curse. Some of these changes are highly desirable; other changes, particularly in our food, are like trying to fit a horse and buggy with rockets and send it to the moon.

In the long run, it won't fly. It's time to return to the food our bodies are best suited to.

Now let's look at one more scene. This time, we see a

conscientious mother, trying to care for her family by preparing for them the best foods she knows how. She's serving a good cut of beef, vegetables fresh from the store, milk for the children, whole-grain bread, and fruit. She's proud of herself; what could be a better balanced meal?

Actually, she's done well, and better nutritionally than many. Many dietitians would be pleased; governmental authorities would proclaim that such healthful fare needs no supplementation: "Everything needed is in the food."

But the beef has antibiotic residues, and is much more fatty that it should be, as the animals were force-fed grains, and inactive.

Some of the vegetables were grown in zinc-deficient soil, in one of the 32 states reported deficient by the United States Department of Agriculture in 1961. Others are lacking manganese and selenium. They're all minus considerable B vitamins and vitamin C, lost in transportation and storage. Naturally, they all have small quantities of pesticide residue.

The milk, high in calcium and protein, is also high in cadmium and lead, as the cows were pastured near a busy freeway, a few miles downwind from a large industrial factory. The factory's met antipollution requirements, mostly, for the last 3 years . . . but what it dispersed into the soils from the air over the previous 30 years won't ever be fully known.

The unblemished fruit was kept that way with the help of insecticides, which also penetrated into the fruit itself to a small degree, after helping to kill the bugs. Of course since the fruit was grown thousands of miles away, some of it was picked green, and gas-ripened.

No, this isn't a scare story. It's a for-real description of many an average meal. If it hasn't made you want to stop eating, it hopefully will help you to understand why, in our century, even the best diet isn't good enough, if we want to stay as healthy as we can.

As you proceed through this book, keep in mind the long history of our species, and the changes of our century. I hope this perspective will help you to understand the "how" and—more important—the "why" of nutritional therapy, preventive medicine, and nutritional biochemistry.

# INTRODUCTION: PREVENTION HAS COME OF AGE

We have the world's best "crisis care" system. We expect to be in a well-equipped modern hospital if we need a life-saving operation. We all cheer the latest medical advances and cures. Rarely do we read anymore about heart and kidney transplants. Now only the artificial heart, combining technological marvel, surgical skill, and individual courage, captivates us on the 11 o'clock news. But, as much as we admire those modern medical miracles, each of us hopes never to experience them personally. Keeping the heart, liver, and kidneys we started with seems much more desirable than replacing them—and certainly considerably cheaper.

Many of us are now beginning to take back responsibilities for our own health care. We're tired of medical costs running away with our hard-earned dollars. And we're beginning to recognize that a healthier, longer-lasting life is part of the bargain.

One of the most dramatic changes of this decade has been a significant reduction in the numbers of illnesses and deaths from heart disease, much of which was attributed to an increased public awareness, and a change in exercise and dietary habits.

Advertising, too, reflects our increased interest in staying healthy and preventing illness. "Sugar-free," "no preservatives," "low-salt," "all natural," "no caffeine," and similar phrases are plastered across labels and billboards with greater frequency than just a few years ago. Supermarkets have opened health-food sections to promote nutrition awareness. And the world's largest pharmaceutical manufacturer advertises vitamins regularly in publications for both physicians and consumers.

Many employers have joined the trend. They're providing running tracks and athletic facilities and featuring salad bars in their company cafeterias. Programs on stress reduction, aerobics, and diet are also becoming increasingly available to employees.

Universities and even a few medical schools are taking a much harder look at disease *prevention* rather than treatment. A continuing medical education course I attended last year had presentations on essential fatty acids; nutrition and platelet function; and the influence of diet on autoimmunity, cancer, heart disease, and other diseases of aging. And in 1982, the Massachusetts Institute of Technology held its *first* scientific conference regarding the effects of nutrition on behavior.

The Bob Hope International Heart Research Institute in Seattle announced its emphasis on the prevention of heart disease. Lester Sauvage, M.D., head of the Reconstructive Cardiovascular Division there, has been quoted in local newspapers—recommending good diet and suggesting that vitamins $B_6$ and E might be helpful.

The National Cancer Institute also has followed the trend towards disease prevention, commissioning a study on the relationship of diet and nutrition to cancer. Released in 1982, the report concluded that there's a "growing accumulation" of evidence that leafy green and yellow vegetables might protect against cancer; that vitamin C "is associated with a lower risk of cancer, particularly gastric and esophageal cancer"; that there is "limited evidence that vitamin E may inhibit tumorigenesis [formation of tumors]"; and that "increasing the intake of total fat increases the incidence of cancer at certain sites, particularly the breast and colon."

Yes, times really are changing. After seven rejections, Linus Pauling, Nobel Prize winner in chemistry, finally got a government research grant to investigate nutrition and cancer.

It's one of the premises of this and my last book that diet and dietary supplementation play a major role in preventing illness and achieving optimum health. And that by ending the radical dietary experimentation of the last century, and returning to a "new traditional" diet along with intelligent supplementation, each of us can stay much healthier and prevent considerable illness.

The second premise of these volumes is that diet and carefully chosen supplementation will successfully help many problems usually treated with drugs or surgery. The more conservative diet and nutrient approach, based on principles of human physiology, biochemistry, and research published in medical journals, can't cure everything—but can make more radical intervention a necessity much less often.

The first few chapters are organized in the same systematic way I approach nutritional medicine. Vitamin A for this, zinc for that, tyrosine for something else.... They're all important, but only as final steps in the nutritional-biochemical approach. A proper foundation must be established for their use. A whole-food, unchemicalized diet is step one. Steps two and three are making sure the diet is digested and absorbed, and that there's no food intolerance. Often an individual's health problems can be more than half solved with just steps one through three. While the case studies illustrate the use of vitamins, minerals, and other dietary supplements in effective illness treatment, basic diet is always more important, and should never be overlooked.

Although major change is underway in medicine, you're unlikely to find a system of prevention or treatment at your family doctor's office. Resistance tags along with change, so any medical metamorphosis will take time. Nutritionally oriented health care isn't yet accepted or taught in medical schools. But it's on its way.

Meanwhile, there's a great deal you can do on your own.

While health-care professionals debate the issues, we're all getting older. We may as well be as healthy as we possibly can along the way. It's my hope that what I've written will provide you with information on staying healthy in the best possible way on your journey through life.

# Addendum to the 1990 Edition

Happily (and healthfully) for all of us, the trends noted so optimistically in 1984 have not only continued but accelerated. Last year, two pharmaceutical firms (one a "major" company) introduced "drugs" to help reverse macular degeneration (deterioration of the retina of the eye with loss of vision, previously thought to be "due to age"). These "drugs" turned out to be simply combinations of nutrients! Hopefully, these will be only the first of many such "drugs," although admitting that they're nutrients will probably be much longer in coming.

Macular degeneration is the topic of one of the eight new chapters added for this Keats paperback edition. As can be seen by comparing the "drugs" noted above with this new chapter, the drug companies got the ingredients right . . . but still would likely not have helped the problem. Unfortunately, even the correct nutrients won't help if they're not being absorbed, a theme that recurs often in this book, as well as in my other collection of cases, "Book of Nutritional Therapy," published in 1979.

It might be assumed that aside from the eight "new" cases, most of the rest of this book is "getting out of date," and that the 1984 collection must be. Fortunately, it's not so: folks are finding the descriptions and treatments just as relevant now as when they were "new." Why? The secret is, they're not new, they're as "old as the hills."

Or at least as old as the human race. If we make the (probably) safe assumption that human bodies have had the same requirements for the same range of essential nutrients ever since human bodies first existed . . . then zinc to help heal chronic ulceration, or vitamin A to relieve heavy menstrual bleeding aren't "old" or "new" . . . they simply "are," and very likely have "always been." It's only that we all didn't know these details until lately!

Likewise, all the health problems caused by poor digestion/assimilation of nutrients or by food allergies mentioned in these books have been there all along, and likely "always" will be there, until or unless we get entirely "new-model" bodies with entirely different inner workings.

In case this appears too "know it all", I'll say right now for the record that my knowledge of nutritional therapeutics is woefully incomplete! What I can share with you now is (hopefully) less than 1% of everything there is to know about the subject. Despite all the progress of the past few years, there's still not enough money and effort being devoted to nutritional and nutrient research, and there are still those who say it's nonsense, quackery, and actively oppose its practice. But their numbers are shrinking.

What I do hope to help make "out-of-date" and "obsolete" are the health problems described in this book, and perhaps others in the future. If you'll read 'em, I'll write 'em, and we can get it done together.

*J. V. Wright*

# ACKNOWLEDGMENTS

The author thanks Nathan Keats for making this edition possible; Alan Gaby, M.D. for his contribution of Appendix C, for his dedication to research, teaching and practice of nutritionally oriented medicine, and most especially for his partnershipin our seminars for physicians; and is grateful to all of themostly-ignored researchers and practitioners listed in the references. Without thier work, this book would not have been possible.

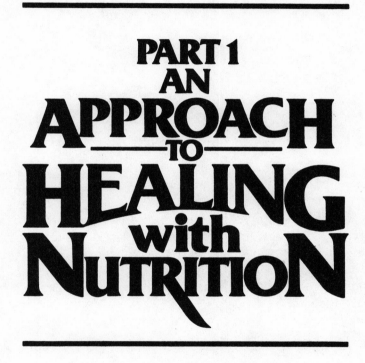

PART 1
AN
APPROACH
TO
HEALING
with
NUTRITION

# SATISFACTIONS AND FRUSTRATIONS OF NUTRITIONAL MEDICINE

1

Why do men and women choose to spend a major portion of their lives as physicians? The answer would seem obvious: to aid in healing the sick, to restore the injured, and, insofar as possible, to provide guidance in the prevention of illness. There are always other reasons, as individual for each physician as the rest of his or her own personality, but for myself and nearly every physician and medical student I've known those are the primary reasons.

"I should hope so," you may say. "Who'd want to see a doctor who didn't have those goals in mind?" More experienced (some might say cynical) readers might be prompted to observe, "Watch out—when he starts out with high-sounding phrases he's trying to sell us something."

In the long run, I am. I'm trying to "sell" you on the concept of good health, but not as something to be "bought" from doctors or anyone else. Good health is usually within your reach and capabilities if you want it, and are willing to plan and work for it. You may need to work only a little, or perhaps a lot, but the control of the effort and its outcome is determined mostly by you.

The greatest satisfaction of therapeutic medical practice is in successfully helping a "not-well" person become well. In the preventive parts of my own practice, I derive at least an equal if not greater satisfaction from helping to prevent illness before it occurs.

In nutritional-biochemical practice and holistic practice in general there is particular satisfaction in achieving and maintaining health through means in tune with nature and our beings, as part of an overall, interconnected, universal pattern.

## Tangible Results

It's particularly satisfying to me to observe anginal pain recede then disappear with diet, exercise, and vitamins; to watch a literally blue-black foot and lower leg, threatened with amputation, become pink and healthy again; to hear that osteoarthritis pain is gone or gallbladder attacks have ceased as food sensitivities and allergies are avoided. I've observed the disappearance of chronic fatigue, depression, prostate problems, bursitis, eczema, acne, kidney stones, cystic mastitis, menstrual pain, headache, and many other problems outlined in this and my previous book. One of my greatest satisfactions is in helping children who've been chronically ill with one infection after another for years become well again.

Being able to provide guidance for a diversity of problems without resorting to potentially toxic drugs, surgery, or other means "not natural to the body" is an added dimension of satisfaction in nutritional-biochemical practice, even though that's never possible 100 percent of the time.

Which brings us to a source of frustration: not being able to help everyone with nutritional-biochemical or (through referral) other holistic means. Sometimes toxic chemicals, surgery, or even radiation has to be employed. Even more frustrating, sometimes nothing works, nothing is possible, holistic or otherwise, and health cannot be restored. That's a great frustration for me or any physician, but it's bound to happen. (Even though I'm noting this frustration, there's no plea for sympathy; that should be reserved for the patient who can't be helped.)

Well, that's all nice, too, you may be thinking. So far you've shared with us that you're satisfied, even pleased when people get better through natural, holistic means, and frustrated when they don't. For this, you needed all those words? There must be something else.

There is. One of my greatest frustrations in nutritional-biochemical practice is knowing that there are many serious illnesses that could be helped or even prevented, right now, by nutritional, biochemical, and other holistic means. But it isn't being done.

Cancer can sometimes be helped or cured through nutrition, biochemistry, and autosuggestion. Multiple sclerosis can be helped with diet and other holistic means. Proven cases of lupus erythematosus have been helped by Philippine faith healers. Many birth defects are preventable. Heart attacks and strokes are preventable. The list of problems that nutritional-biochemical and other holistic practitioners could help—now—is a very long one. As noted before, 100 percent success can never be attained, but great progress could be made . . . not years from now, but now. It's very frustrating to know this for sure and yet not be able to do anything about it.

"Wait a minute, here," you might ask. "Aren't you the same writer who once said it wasn't reasonable to expect nutrition and/or biochemistry to cure cancer? Or multiple sclerosis? Now you're saying it can be done, at least sometimes. So why aren't you doing it?"

## Health Freedom Curtailed

Put very bluntly, nutritional, biochemical, and holistic cures of cancer and other very serious illnesses are entirely possible, but not reasonable to expect unless you think it reasonable to ask your doctor to risk a jail sentence for trying.

In the United States of America, there is no liberty for each of us to take care of our own health in whatever manner we see fit. It's your body, your health, but if it's your own personal preference not to be cut open, drugged, or radiated for cancer, call your travel agent.

Americans have given up the freedom to take care of themselves in favor of the dubious security of supposed protection from "quackery," "unscientific," and "ineffective" medicine.

Strong language? Not at all. A congressional report concludes that only 10 to 20 percent of present-day "scientific" medical procedures has been shown to be of benefit by controlled clinical trial. One possible interpretation of this congressional document is that 80 to 90 percent of modern scientific medicine has no better scientific proof behind it than snake oil.

It's very frustrating for me to know that there is so much more that could be done in health care, so much more that I personally could do. Because I did go into medicine with a primary goal of aiding the sick, helping to restore the injured, and above all preventing illness in the first place. Naively, like any medical student, I expected to be able to carry out those goals limited only by my lack of knowledge. Instead, I'm forced to practice medicine with one hand tied behind my back.

Enough of philosophy, my frustrations, and satisfactions. It is my hope that citizens of these United States will recapture their freedom in matters of health care before many more celebrations of America's freedom have passed.

# REFERENCES

**Cancer**
Satillaro, Anthony J. *Recalled by Life*. Houghton Mifflin, 1982.

**Lupus Erythematosus**
Kirkpatrick, Richard A. "Witchcraft and Lupus." *Journal of the American Medical Association*, January 8, 1982, p. 176.
——. "Witchcraft and Lupus Erythematosus." *Journal of the American Medical Association*, May 15, 1981, pp. 1937–1938.

**Medical Technology**
Office of Technology Assessment, U.S. Congress. *Assessing the Efficacy and Safety of Medical Technologies*. U.S. Government Printing Office, 1978, p. 7.

**Multiple Sclerosis**

Swank, Roy L. *A Biochemical Basis of Multiple Sclerosis.* Charles C Thomas, 1961.

Swank, Roy L., and Pullen, Mary-Helen. *The Multiple Sclerosis Diet Book: A Low-Fat Diet for the Treatment of M.S., Heart Disease and Stroke.* Doubleday, 1977.

# 2 THE NUTRITIONAL-BIOCHEMICAL CHECKUP

*"Will nutritional biochemistry help me? . . . What is it, anyway? . . . How can I tell if a doctor who takes the nutritional-biochemical approach could do anything for me?"*

"Nutritional biochemistry" is a term I often use to describe the kind of medicine I practice. Simply put, it means preventing and treating illness, and maintaining health and well-being by using substances natural to our bodies—food, water, vitamins, minerals, amino acids, hormones, and other molecules. Doctors who work with nutritional biochemistry employ drugs or surgery if absolutely necessary; when a more natural approach doesn't work; or in emergencies, when there's little time. Fortunately, by taking the nutritional-biochemical route, they prescribe drugs and surgery in only a small minority of cases.

In this chapter, you'll learn about three important topics nutritionally oriented doctors explore that are rarely addressed in a standard medical history, even a "complete" one. Then we'll do an imaginary checkup, with emphasis on clues to nutritional status.

Medical students are taught to take a health history in a standard way. First, the "chief complaint," the main problem or problems are covered. Then comes a symptom review of each bodily system, such as cardiovascular, gastrointestinal, and respiratory. Next is the "past medical history," which lists hospitalizations, operations, medications, allergies, childhood illnesses, and accidents. "Family history" follows, with records of any known ailments of blood relatives, and "social history" completes the interview with questions about occupation, hobbies, alcohol and other nonprescription drug use, as well as exercise. Some details may vary from school to school, but that is the *standard* general format memorized by generations of medical students.

In addition to the standard medical history, I emphasize questions that yield information about these three key areas:

- "What food are you eating?"
- "Is it being digested and absorbed?"
- "Are you sensitive or allergic to the food you eat?"

Although it's hard to understand, even today most medical students aren't taught to make a complete record of a person's diet. Without such a record, the topics of digestion/absorption and food sensitivity can't even be considered.

Now let's do that imaginary checkup. It'll actually be a "combined" checkup, using observations made on children and adults, women and men. Obviously, all of these findings wouldn't coexist in the same individual. But they briefly summarize some of the points I make to the many medical students who visit my office to find out what nutritional biochemistry is all about.

Our imaginary checkup will focus mostly on clues to nutritional status, as that's what this book's about. I won't attempt to include the physical signs of all the diseases discussed in a textbook of medicine. A real checkup by myself or any other nutritionally oriented doctor, however, always includes inspection for signs of those diseases, too.

Many of the observations which follow aren't original with me. They've been noted, mostly one at a time, by practicing physicians. In order not to break the flow of the discussion, references are listed at the end of this chapter.

Combined here are the physical signs I've found most reliable as basis for further investigation or treatment. But remember, 100 percent accuracy of any single observation isn't likely; it's always best to gather as much evidence as possible from health history, physical exam, and laboratory analysis before making decisions. Please keep in mind that self-diagnosis can be tricky and deceptive. Any serious symptoms deserve medical attention. What follows are some of the thoughts that might occur during the course of a physical exam, and some of the comments I might make to the imaginary person being examined, or to a medical student.

# An Imaginary Checkup and the Clues I Look For

Let's start with the scalp. That's a really terrible case of dandruff, flakes all over. This person is eating too much refined sugar; eliminating it would improve the dandruff a lot. Probably has insufficient essential fatty acids, too. Keep in mind B complex with emphasis on $B_6$ and selenium.

This lady's hair is thinning out too much. It could be the estrogen she's taking. B complex, especially $B_6$ and folate may help, but she might need to stop the hormones. She's not taking hormones? Then check to see if she has hypochlorhydria (low stomach acidity). If she does, her protein won't digest as well, and many minerals won't be absorbed efficiently, so her hair falls. This doesn't apply to "male-pattern baldness" or alopecia.

There's redness to this man's forehead, particularly in the central part. His skin looks shiny and scaly, with a slightly yellowish, greasy appearance. It's especially bad in the eyebrows, and extends down the nose. He has it on his cheeks, and even his chest. A bad case of seborrheic dermatitis. Think of B vitamins again, especially para-aminobenzoic acid and B$_6$. Also, essential fatty acids. In this case, the type in primrose oil is frequently preferable. However, occasionally all of this isn't helpful, and vitamin B$_6$ in a topical cream is best. (Oddly, with the topical cream, it frequently worsens for a few days before improving.)

Let's look in the ears. A chronic problem with excess earwax. Probably not enough essential fatty acids again. Lack of them surfaces in a number of skin conditions.

Behind the ears, the skin is cracked. That's usually a zinc problem. Patience: It frequently takes weeks for zinc to help, even when it's well absorbed.

See the diagonal crease across the earlobe? It may be a sign of increased susceptibility to cardiovascular disease. Best to check closely for cardiovascular risk factors and maybe have a treadmill electrocardiogram done.

Speaking of creases, I think we missed something on this man's forehead. Ask him to frown. See? There are those maybe four vertical creases within about half an inch of the midline of his forehead when he frowns. If he has upper abdominal pain, too, better check for duodenal ulcer.

Back to the ears. Another child with fluid behind the eardrums. Wouldn't be surprised if she gets ear infections easily. Test for allergies, using the RAST (radioallergosorbent test). No point in letting it go until tubes are needed in her ears.

Oh, a cloudy appearance to the lens of the eye. Cataract. Fortunately, not far gone. Have a glucose-insulin tolerance test done for blood sugar or insulin abnormalities. Eliminate any refined sugar. There's a chance this person doesn't metabolize lactose (milk sugar) well. Consider eliminating all sources of it.

Bioflavonoids inhibit an enzyme, aldose reductase, that's reported overactive in the lens of diabetics, leading to cataracts. Think of riboflavin (vitamin B$_2$), vitamin A, and vitamin C also. Before leaving the diabetic eye, remember bioflavonoids to slow down leaking of the retinal vessels. Magnesium is important, too. Be cautious with vitamin E unless you're positive vitamin K is normal.

"Floaters" or blood spots in a nondiabetic eye? Think of bioflavonoids again, but also choline, inositol, and vitamin K.

The white of one eye has turned all red suddenly on one side.

Check blood pressure . . . it's usually normal, but it's best to be sure. This scleral hemorrhage isn't dangerous, just the result of a broken blood vessel. If it wasn't trauma, consider bioflavonoids and vitamin K, once more.

This child has had enough sleep, hasn't been crying lately, and still has those dark circles beneath the eyes. He has horizontal creases in the lower lids. Sometimes those dark circles are called "allergic shiners"; the lines are called Dennie's lines. Along with puffiness in the lower eyelids, these signs usually mean allergy. Although adults have dark circles beneath the eyes during pregnancy, hormone treatment, and when fatigued, such circles frequently indicate allergy, also.

Speaking of allergy: Here's a child less than two years old whose pupils are often dilated to nearly one-quarter inch or more. Allergy, especially milk allergy, is again suspected.

Check the nose. Polyps inside? Not only allergy probable here, but salicylate sensitivity. This person should be wary of aspirin as well as artificial food additives, many of which are salicylate based, and foods containing naturally occurring salicylate.

Now an adult, with many dilated capillaries in the cheeks and perhaps on the nose, could be overconsuming alcohol. But if not, our lab shows a frequent correlation with low stomach acidity. The correlation is even stronger when the dilated capillaries are accompanied by a general reddening of the facial skin, most pronounced in the cheeks and forehead, and scattered medium to large acnelike pimples, a condition called rosacea.

Acne itself, from a mild case of scattered pimples to deep cysts, is over the face and back. Very likely eating and sensitive to sugar and other refined, processed food, and not getting enough zinc or the right types of essential fatty acids. In a bad case, there's usually allergic involvement. An adult past 25 with acne almost always has food allergy.

Now, here's an older person with a slightly yellow cast to the facial skin, no red tones at all. It certainly could be jaundice, on a rare occasion, but that's usually a deeper orange-yellow. Much more often, there's a lack of vitamin $B_{12}$, usually due to a degree of low stomach acidity and vitamin $B_{12}$ malabsorption. Sometimes there's a problem with absorption of other B vitamins as well. Pink-red tones return to the skin with $B_{12}$ injections; the faint yellow tinges fade, often disappear.

# The Tongue Gives Clues to Vitamin B Deficiencies

Please stick out your tongue. There, see how it's smoothed out in some areas, rough in others? Almost like a contour map. Cracks and grooves scattered throughout. Very occasionally, such tongue appearance is inborn and unchangeable, but often there's a shift toward a more normal appearance with adequate B vitamins, sometimes swallowed, sometimes injected. A persistent crack at either corner of the mouth, termed angular cheilosis, also signifies a lack of B vitamins, with emphasis on riboflavin. When there's a very pale tongue, accompanied by paleness of the inner surface of the lower eyelids (easily seen when pulled down), you should check for anemia. If anemia's present, it's most often iron deficiency, but it can be a lack of other nutrients, too, as well as nonnutritional causes like internal bleeding.

Inside the mouth again: canker sores. They keep coming back? Most often, allergies to foods. Overly large tonsils, frequently infected, or a tongue "scalloped" around the edges by pressure from the teeth should touch off a search for allergies.

Now, down to the neck. Intermittently swollen lymph glands, persistent at times? Especially with large tonsils, too. The odds favor food allergies once more. Just to be sure, check for serious disease, but it's usually not present.

Look at the "skin tags" scattered on the neck. Sometimes they're quite numerous. They often appear under the arms, or elsewhere. All locations indicate the same thing. Test for blood sugar abnormality.

Moving over to the shoulder, we find a sore, tender-to-pressure spot right at the side, where it slopes into the arm. Bursitis. $B_{12}$ is the related nutrient. A series of injections frequently does a lot of good. Sometimes swallowing a large quantity helps, too, but injection is more reliable.

Further down, on the side and back of the upper arm there are numerous small bumps in the skin. These usually go away with vitamin A; at times, however, B complex and essential fatty acids are needed as well. Occasionally, when the bumps are especially numerous, pancreatic enzymes are helpful, probably by promoting the absorption of vitamin A and essential fatty acids.

On to the hands. The nails are breaking, chipping, splitting, won't grow. Look for hypochlorhydria (low stomach acidity). Nearly every time, it's present. Keep calcium, zinc, essential fatty acids, and thyroid in mind, but always look for low stomach acid first.

Here's a teenager with white spots all over the fingernails. Zinc. Even when zinc measurements on hair, blood, or urine are reported "normal," white spots disappear almost every time when extra zinc is included. Although teenagers have the greatest frequency of white-spotted nails, their appearance at any age usually indicates the same thing.

Think zinc when cracks occur in the skin of the fingertips. Cracks heal with zinc, as do tiny blisters which appear, sometimes in rows, along the margins between the tops and sides of the fingers.

"Knots" starting to appear on the end joints of the fingers? Keep vitamin $B_6$ in mind, and niacinamide, too. The "middle" joints getting a little puffy, swollen, and tender? Niacinamide (an active form of niacin) is the most important nutrient to remember. However, the amounts needed are often large, and laboratory monitoring is advisable.

Both these types of joint problems are usually termed "degenerative arthritis" or "osteoarthritis." If the diagnosis is positive for rheumatoid arthritis, niacinamide helps a little, but most often isn't a complete control, as it is frequently in osteoarthritis (given an adequate and monitored intake).

For an individual with osteoarthritis in the hands as well as elsewhere, keep two other things in mind: the "nightshade" food family sensitivity, and allergy to nearly any food or foods. Food allergy testing should be done, and a trial of "no-nightshade" diet (avoiding potatoes, tomatoes, peppers, eggplant, and tobacco) is important.

Now look at the backs of the hands. If you can't see the tendons clearly and the fingers look a little puffy there may be a need for extra vitamin $B_6$. Try this please: Hold the hands out, fingers straight. Keeping the joints where the fingers join the palm straight, flex the fingers at the last two joints. Bring the tips of the fingers down to touch the palm, all the while keeping the first (palm-to-finger) joints unflexed and straight. Looks like this person can't do it. Add $B_6$ to his list.

Turn his hand over. There's a thickening of the tissues in the palm along the course of the tendon to the fourth finger. If it gets bad, it pulls the finger over. Might need surgery at that point. Lots of vitamin E is indicated. Make sure to monitor blood pressure with this quantity, although it's rarely a problem. Just as important, do a glucose-insulin tolerance test soon. Such tissue thickening, called a Dupuytren's contracture, has been identified as another warning sign for blood sugar disorders.

Look at this child with red, scaly, sometimes cracked and oozing skin on the hands. Particularly between the fingers, at the wrists, in front of the elbows, and, when bad, capable of covering the rest of the skin between. It's behind the knees, too, a little at the ankles, and in spots all over sometimes. It's called eczema, of course. Think of food allergy, usually multiple foods. Extremely helpful nutrients to keep in mind include zinc, essential fatty acids, and vitamin C. Secondarily, vitamins A and E, as long as they're from nonallergenic sources.

Over to the spine. First, see if the head can be rotated equally to both sides without moving the shoulders. If there's greater rotation to one side than the other, a trip to a competent chiropractic or osteopathic practitioner is indicated. Secondly, exert equal and moderately forceful pressure (stopping immediately if it hurts) on each and every vertebral spine from the base of the skull to the tailbone. The vertebral spines surface as that row of hard bumps down the middle of the back. Press straight inward on them.

If one or more hurt with pressure, or feels more tender than the rest, there's a problem best solved by manipulative means. Using very gentle pressure, you can frequently feel a very slight swelling over the vertebral spines most tender to forceful pressure.

# Caffeine Sensitivity: A Likely Cause of Breast Lumps

Let's move around from the back to the breasts. This woman has nodular areas scattered through both breasts, sometimes tender before periods, occasionally tender all the time. We've already excluded the possibility of cancer; she's probably had mammography done. Usually multiple, benign nodules are fibrocystic disease, sometimes called cystic mastitis. She's quite likely caffeine sensitive. Ask her to eliminate coffee, tea, chocolate, cocoa, cola drinks, and over-the-counter caffeine-containing medications. Next, think of vitamin E. She probably needs iodine, too. Other nutrients to keep in mind include $B_6$, essential fatty acids, and magnesium.

Just where each rib joins the breastbone, particularly on the left, it's quite tender to pressure. Several rib breastbone junctions are involved, but the third through sixth ribs seem worst. Women have this problem much more often than men; that's one clue to which nutrient to consider. $B_6$, of course.

Here's a finding which may be an important clue to nutritional status, but may mean one or several things: an abdomen full of gas. (Unless of course it's the result of a recent giant dish of beans or too much vitamin C.) Look for stomach acidity or insufficient pancreatic enzymes. Either or both may lead to poor digestion of foods, and consequent excess gas formation. Frequently, excess gas is a result of allergy or sensitivity to foods. Don't forget lactose intolerance (inability to digest milk sugar). Sometimes it's a combination of these factors. Food-allergic individuals are often hypochlorhydric; cow-milk-allergic people often are lactose intolerant.

Certainly nonnutritionally related problems can lead to "a belly of wind," but the above are important considerations.

Next, legs and feet. Scattered, small, pimplelike red spots at the base of hair follicles on the front of the thighs often fade away with a little more vitamin A, as do the "bumps" on the upper arms previously mentioned.

Sore knees in this past-45 person; one's a little swollen. When the kneecap is compressed and the knee is flexed, extended, and flexed again, grating can be felt within the joints. Tests have been negative for rheumatoid arthritis. It's been termed osteoarthritis, degenerative arthritis, or sometimes cartilage deterioration. Niacinamide indicated here, with precautions.

Now a young knee, 13 years old or so. There's a greater than usual prominence where the tendon from the kneecap joins the main bone of the lower leg. It's very tender when pushed on; it hurts so much it's keeping its owner out of sports this year. Selenium needed here, along with vitamin E. If this knee responds as do most similarly affected knees, its Osgood-Schlatter disease should be gone in a month or two.

The skin on the front of the lower legs is very dry, flaky. Insufficient essential fatty acids again. In this same area, patches of skin are an irregularly mottled brownish-yellowish color. One thing to keep in mind is potential blood sugar difficulty.

Now press over the long bone of the lower leg. Moderate pressure. It's sore. Consider calcium, of course. But oddly enough, niacinamide also.

Puffiness and swelling is in the tissues of the lower legs and ankles. Once heart, kidney, and liver diseases are excluded, allergy to foods and blood sugar difficulties are common causes.

Here's swelling in the lower legs again, this time in a pregnant woman in her last few months. The swelling is slowly getting worse. Her blood pressure's starting to rise, and there may be protein starting to show in the urine. Definitely not enough good quality protein in her diet. Vitamin $B_6$ and magnesium are urgently needed, and should be started as soon as possible. There's no need at all for this early case of toxemia to get worse or, for that matter, to occur in the first place.

Another case of varicose veins. Sure, it "runs in the family," but likely there's not been enough dietary fiber in the past, allowing pressure buildup in the abdomen, in turn creating back pressure on the veins from the legs and dilating them. Remember vitamin E, bioflavonoids, and magnesium, too.

Finally, to the feet. There's a thick ridge of callus along the inner surface of the heel that tapers off towards the back of the arch. There's not enough vitamin A here. It'll take several months of an adequate intake to nearly eliminate such callus.

Here's an older person's feet. Check for the pulse on the back of the foot, and behind the prominence of the ankle bone on the inner side. Can't find a pulse anywhere, or only a weak one? Maybe one foot's a lot better than the other? Could be a sign of atherosclerosis in the artery of the leg.

## Physical Signs Are Important Clues

That's the end of our nutritionally related checkup for now. The observations noted do not constitute anything close to all of those made during a complete checkup—just the nutritional-biochemical additions, and a few other matters I find important.

Please understand that these observations are ones I find most useful in practice, as do many doctors who take a nutritional-biochemical approach. And remember, this is still a minority viewpoint. Many times, when individuals with whom I've worked discuss it with other doctors, they're told it's a lot of nonsense. Certainly these doctors are as entitled to their opinions as I am. In a free society, results will speak for themselves.

It's important to understand that there isn't a 100 percent "cause-and-effect" relationship between each physical finding and the nutrient(s) mentioned along with it. These are associations I've found reliable in a high percentage of cases. But, even though the nutrients should be thought of (and in most cases, used) to alleviate the abnormality mentioned, it doesn't necessarily mean that a relative lack of a certain nutrient or nutrients is the cause. Maybe it is, but perhaps the nutrients help overcome a problem with a different cause.

Let's take eczema as an example. Zinc, essential fatty acids, vitamin C, and, secondarily, vitamins A and E will clear up most cases of eczema when used in adequate quantities. But many cases of eczema don't happen and don't need clearing up if allergenic foods are kept away.

Specific quantities of various nutrients were purposely omitted, since the intent of our "nutritionally related checkup" is to discuss physical clues to nutritional-biochemical status, and to illustrate part of this approach in health care. More exact detail about many of the conditions mentioned, along with guidelines to nutritional therapy, can be found in the case studies in this and my previous book.

Following a physical exam, laboratory evaluation is done, general and specific. This will be the subject of the chapter "ABCs of Nutritional Testing." But for now, let's go back to those three important questions mentioned a few pages back. "What food are you eating?" "Is it being digested and absorbed?" "Are you sensitive or allergic to the food you eat?" They'll be the subject of the next three chapters.

## REFERENCES

**Allergy**

Breneman, J. C. *Basics of Food Allergy*. Charles C Thomas, 1978, pp. 225–226.

## Diabetes

Margolis, Jack, and Margolis, Lawrence S. "Skin Tags—A Frequent Sign of Diabetes Mellitus." *New England Journal of Medicine*, May 20, 1976, p. 1184.

Spring, Maxwell, and Cohen, Berton D. "Dupuytren's Contracture: Warning of Diabetes." *New York State Journal of Medicine*, May 1, 1970, p. 1037.

## Eyes

Liu, Hsi-Yen; Giday, Zs.; and Moore, B. F. "Certain Bovine Milk Protein Inducible Eye Signs in Patients with Allergic Malabsorption." *Journal of Pediatric Ophthalmology*, vol. 10, no. 1, 1973, pp. 7–11.

## Gastrointestinal

Gerrard, John W., ed. "Disorders of the Gastrointestinal Tract and Autonomic Nervous System in Allergic Patients." In *Food Allergy: New Perspectives*. Charles C Thomas, 1980, pp. 44–84.

## Skin

Trujillo, Nelson P., and Warthin, Thomas A. "The Frowning Sign Multiple Forehead Furrows in Peptic Ulcer." *Journal of the American Medical Association*, August 5, 1983, p. 218.

Wyre, H. W., Jr. "The Diagonal Earlobe Crease: A Cutaneous Manifestation of Coronary Artery Disease." *Cutis*, March, 1979, pp. 328–331.

# 3 THE CASE FOR A "NEW TRADITIONAL" DIET

Imagine that the number of diabetics in your community triples in only ten years . . . five times as many men over 40 develop diseases of the arteries . . . a once rare operation is now performed frequently . . . your teenagers and their friends begin suffering from a skin disease unknown when you were young . . . and worst of all—a new type of cancer appears among the women of your community.

Now imagine that this disease epidemic spreads across the entire United States. Newspaper headlines would blare, "Epidemic Spreads." Researchers would dive for their laboratories. Medical journals would publish worried editorials. Public health officials would knit their brows. And politicians would demand a congressional investigation.

Seem too unreal even for your imagination? Surprisingly enough, exactly these events have occurred right here in North America. What's even more astounding is that the culprit is known. So why haven't you heard about it?

Perhaps because the victims are Eskimos of northern Canada and we rarely get much news from the far north. In fact, most of us probably know more about Sergeant Preston of the Yukon than about our northern neighbors. The more likely reason, though, is the identity of the culprit. Even though it's been responsible for problems all over the world—among Polynesians, blacks, Caucasians, Orientals, and American Indians—it's nothing foreign or exotic. In fact, it's so familiar to most of us that it's become invisible.

What is the hidden force believed to be the cause of so many problems in so short a time?

Civilization. More specifically, "civilized" diet. That, according to Otto Schaefer, M.D., an internal medicine specialist who has investigated and actually documented the Eskimos' move into a new life.

Although the Eskimos in Alaska and Greenland have had ever-increasing contact with Europeans since the late 1700s, Canadian Eskimos, particularly those living inland, have only had close contact with outsiders since the mid-1940s. Dramatic changes in the way of life for most Eskimos started in the mid-1950s, following the construction of military and civilian airports along radar stations across the Canadian Arctic. By 1971, according to Dr. Schaefer, only a "dozen or so" Eskimo families across the entire north of Canada maintained a nomadic, "precivilized" life. In less than one generation, nearly the entire population changed from a native way of life to midtwentieth-century modern.

Before the 1950s, Canadian Eskimos lived in large groups in hunting camps, migrating with the food supply and season. Their homes were made of skin or canvas tents, or snow houses in some areas. The protein in their diet came mostly from fish, caribou, fowl, musk ox, polar bear, rabbit, and fox. Vegetable foods, scarce and variable according to season, included roots, leafy greens, seaweed, and occasionally berries.

By the mid-1960s, the old ways changed drastically. The typical Eskimo family now lived in a house at an airstrip or defense installation. Food and clothing were bought from stores. Men worked at the base, eating their three meals a day at the cafeteria, which soon showed in their bulging bellies. And the women stayed home, no longer gathering roots, seaweed, and berries, whiling away their time chewing on chocolates instead of animal skins and drinking sugary soda pop.

The whole composition of their diet changed, says Dr. Schaefer. The amount of protein foods they ate each day dropped to less than half of what it was, from a little over 11 ounces to 3½. The decrease in protein food made more room for other foods, so that now *half* of all their calories came from carbohydrates.

More important than the amount of carbohydrates, however, was the kind. They changed from whole, unrefined, and unprocessed to just the opposite—highly processed and refined— becoming especially rich in sugar.

In fact, what Dr. Schaefer found by searching through trading-post food records was that within one decade the Eskimos *quadrupled* their former sugar intake.

Looking again at the total carbohydrate picture, complex carbohydrates (from vegetables and grains) fell from 82 percent to less than 50—a figure interestingly similar to the U.S. and other westernized countries.

That change in refined carbohydrates, or as Dr. Schaefer called them "rapidly absorbable carbohydrates," is believed to be related to the Eskimos' rise in diabetes. In a series of tests, Dr. Schaefer found that the Eskimos had problems keeping their blood sugar levels stable after eating a lot of sugar. They began to experience a seesawing of their blood sugar levels because their bodies weren't used to such a flood of sugar.

So it's not surprising then that diabetes tripled in ten years. Dr. Schaefer notes that his group "discovered more new cases of diabetes in one group of Eskimos living in the Canadian Western Arctic than occurred in Eskimos in *all* of Canada a few years ago!"

Diabetes wasn't the only problem brought on by such a newly found lifestyle. Diseases of the arteries among men over 40 increased fivefold. These findings are actually confirmed by x-ray evidence of calcification of the leg arteries of men aged 40 to 69 who had lived in the new settlements ten years or more.

The rare operation that became commonplace was gallbladder surgery. In fact, in the ten years prior to the late 1950s there was no gallbladder surgery at all at the hospital to which all Eskimos were taken. In that hospital and two new ones which have opened subsequently, gallbladder surgery is now routine.

And the unknown skin disease that became common among the young was acne. That's right. Acne was previously unknown to Canadian Eskimos before the mid-1950s. No need for pimple creams, blemish hiders, antibiotics, or the latest wonder drug. With a "civilized" diet, high in sugar and refined carbohydrates, acne became common. According to Dr. Schaefer, "Many Eskimos themselves blame their pimples on the 'pop, chocolate, and candies' the youngsters consume as if addicted. One wonders what these people and other old northerners would think if they were to read some recent medical publications, in which dermatologists belittle or deny the role of dietary factors in the pathogenesis [cause] of acne vulgaris."

Unfortunately, that's not all. The growth of Eskimo children has been unnaturally accelerated. Both height and weight are greater than preceding generations. Puberty is occurring earlier than ever before. All that despite over two-thirds less average daily protein. It's my conclusion after reviewing the data from both human and animal studies that the earlier puberty and greater height and weight of twentieth-century children is a distinctly unhealthy development, largely attributable to an inferior diet, *not* an "improved" one.

Lastly, reports Dr. Schaefer, "In both Alaska and Greenland, breast cancer has been found only recently among native people. It was not seen in earlier times."

Certainly, other factors affect the health of the Eskimos— their more sedentary lifestyle and their move from the outdoors, with its fresh air and natural lighting, to indoor, oil-heated, and artificially lit surroundings. But the greatest share of blame for the Eskimos' sudden epidemic of ill health is squarely placed by Dr. Schaefer on their modern "civilized" diet.

# The Civilized Diet to Blame for Poor Health

Unfortunately, the appearance of new diseases among the Eskimos along with a sudden increase in other problems are not isolated events. The replacement of traditional whole-food diets with "civilized," processed-food diets—high in sugar and salt and low in fiber—has been associated with an increase in similar diseases all around the world.

The Maoris, for example, who migrated from far-scattered islands in the eastern Pacific to New Zealand, have succumbed to a "civilized" diet similar to the Eskimos. "The more an Islander takes on the ways of the West, the more prone he is to succumb to our degenerative diseases," says Ian Prior, M.D., a cardiologist and director of the epidemiology unit at the Wellington Hospital in New Zealand, who led an expedition to study these people. "In fact," he continues, "it does not seem too much to say our evidence now shows that the further the Pacific natives move from the quiet, carefree life of their ancestors, the closer they come to gout, diabetes, atherosclerosis, obesity, and hypertension."

Dr. Prior and his team chose to study three groups of Maoris, who could be characterized as "native," "westernized," and halfway between. These Polynesian people are thought to have migrated southwestward across the ocean in their canoes, leaving settlements behind, making it quite convenient to compare different groups of the same people.

The "native" group live on Pukapuka, a remote island 300 miles northeast of Samoa. They eat fish; taro (a starchy root vegetable); coconut; limited quantities of rice, flour, and sugar; and no salt.

The "halfway" Maori live on Rarotonga, a somewhat larger island several hundred miles southeast of Samoa. The group chosen had lived in town for ten years or more, with ready access to shops and "European-style" food. Their diet includes canned meat, canned fish, bread, taro, rice, bananas, cabbage, onions, tomatoes, coconut, and higher quantities of both salt and sugar.

The "westernized" Maori live in New Zealand, following a way of life and eating similar to the population of European origin.

The difference in both diet and disease pattern is most quickly summarized in the accompanying illustration of Dr. Prior's report.

The trend is absolutely clear: In almost every comparison, the more civilized the diet the greater the incidence of disease.

The New Zealand Maoris who have been exposed longer to European lifestyles "have arrived," says Dr. Prior. "In fact, it appears they have surpassed their European neighbors in the frequency with which they become victims of and die [of hypertension, atherosclerosis, and similar diseases]."

Again, diet isn't the only factor influencing disease patterns. Like the "westernized" Eskimo, the New Zealand Maoris live in modern homes, get less fresh air, and probably less exercise (Dr. Prior notes that on Rarotonga "the women exercise very little, if at all"). It's not my intention to say that 100 percent of the increase in illness is due to diet. However, both Dr. Schaefer and Dr. Prior indicate clearly and emphatically that dietary change is the *major* factor. Based on their evidence and other similar observations from around the world, I can only agree.

Another native-to-civilized diet change accompanied by disease can be seen in Yemenite Jews. A. M. Cohen, M.D., a specialist in internal medicine from the Rothschild Hadassah University in Jerusalem, along with two other researchers, studied Israelis originally from Yemen—a country south of Saudi Arabia. One group had lived in Israel for more than 25 years, and ate a "civilized" diet like most Israelis. The other group, of the same ages, had lived in Israel for ten years or less. This second group had lived in Yemen most of their lives, eating the types of foods common there at the time, a diet much closer to the traditional human pattern.

The recent immigrants were found to have significantly less diabetes mellitus, atherosclerotic heart disease, and high blood pressure than the older immigrants, suggesting a protective effect from their previous traditional diet.

# *The Road to*

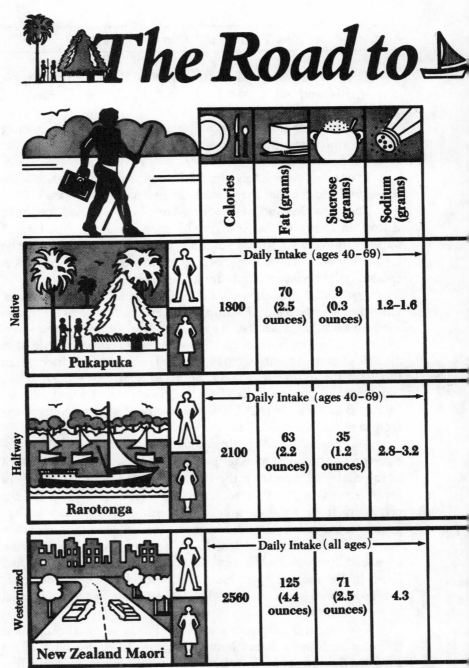

|  |  | Calories | Fat (grams) | Sucrose (grams) | Sodium (grams) |
|---|---|---|---|---|---|
| **Native** | **Pukapuka** | Daily Intake (ages 40–69) | | | |
| | | 1800 | 70 (2.5 ounces) | 9 (0.3 ounces) | 1.2–1.6 |
| **Halfway** | **Rarotonga** | Daily Intake (ages 40–69) | | | |
| | | 2100 | 63 (2.2 ounces) | 35 (1.2 ounces) | 2.8–3.2 |
| **Westernized** | **New Zealand Maori** | Daily Intake (all ages) | | | |
| | | 2560 | 125 (4.4 ounces) | 71 (2.5 ounces) | 4.3 |

*Adapted with permission of* Nutrition Today *magazine, P.O. Box 1829, Annapolis, Maryland 21404. July/August, 1971.*

# Civilization

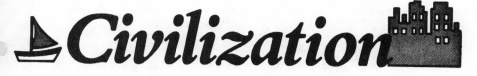

| Cholesterol (mg/100 ml) (ages 50–59) | Obesity | Gross Obesity | Gout | Diabetes | High Blood Pressure | Ischemic Heart Disease |
|---|---|---|---|---|---|---|
| | ←————— Percent of Population (age 30 and older) —————→ | | | | | |
| 187 | 7 | 0.7 | 7 | 2 | 2 | 2 |
| 200 | 21 | 2.2 | 0 | 4.4 | 4.4 | 1.4 |
| 212 | 8 | 3.7 | 3.7 | 6.2 | 21 | 4.3 |
| 235 | 22 | 25 | 0 | 9.5 | 36 | 5.5 |
| 232 | 18.6 | 9.1 | 13.3 | 11.9 | 16.9 | 4.9 |
| 225 | 21.8 | 21.4 | 2.5 | 9.3 | 25 | 8.9 |

*Illustration by Leslie Flts*

And although the food eaten in both Yemen and Israel contained about the same quantity of protein, the Israeli diet contained more calories and fat. The Israelis, in fact, carried around an average of 22 pounds more than the recent immigrants from Yemen.

As among the Eskimos, though, the largest difference was in the type of carbohydrate consumed. "The carbohydrates consumed in Yemen were mainly or solely starch," report the researchers. "Almost no sugar was consumed. In Israel, there is a striking increase in sugar consumption, though little increase in total carbohydrates." The sucrose (sugar) eaten was found to be 0.23 ounces daily in Yemen, but 2.2 ounces daily in Israel—nearly a tenfold increase!

The researchers conclude in part: "If a nutrient is an etiological [causative] factor in . . . heart disease or diabetes, the increased consumption of sucrose *might* be responsible, directly or indirectly, for the higher prevalence of those diseases in those Yemenites who have lived for years in Israel."

A greatly increased intake of sugar is a common thread in Dr. Schaefer's study of the Eskimos, Dr. Prior's work among the Maoris, and in Dr. Cohen's work with the Yemenites.

Others, too, have noticed that connection, most notably Denis P. Burkitt, the famed British fiber expert. Although many physicians and almost all food companies and their advertisers have recognized that restoring fiber to a refined-food diet (or better still, not removing it in the first place) is good for the health, getting rid of refined sugar is not yet recognized as an equally important goal. Yet in his own observations Dr. Burkitt has found that "the first change in traditional food is usually the addition of sugar. This is followed by substituting white bread for part of the less processed cereals customarily eaten."

Even though the great increase in refined sugar and the processing away of fiber is very important in explaining some of the difference in disease patterns between groups following "native" and "westernized" diets, trying to blame the presence or absence of one or two components of the diet for the entire difference is frequently futile, confusing, and even counterpro-

ductive. Researchers have also pointed a finger at the pasteuriza-
tion of milk; the relative lack of zinc, chromium, magnesium, and
other minerals; deficiencies of B vitamins, vitamin A, beta-
carotene, and other vitamins; the intentional addition of food
chemicals; and even the unintentional addition of insecticides,
pesticides, industrial chemicals, and toxic minerals as the cause of
much disease in "civilized" areas of the world.

Far too much paper, ink, and energy has been wasted on
attempts to blame or exonerate various parts of the Western diet as
the cause of one or more of our modern diseases, or of the increase
in their incidence. It's far more productive, I think, to look at the
overall change in diet from traditional to civilized, admitting that
we may never be able to prove to the last degree the exact effects
of every item noted above on each individual person. We're on
much more solid ground trying to identify the cumulative effects
of diet change as seen in groups of people.

Unfortunately, recent generations of scientists have been
thoroughly stuck in a molecule-by-molecule debate over the
effects of diet on health, while literally millions of people living in
civilized nations have become unnecessarily ill from preventable
illnesses whose causes could probably be identified by the same
Eskimos who saw the obvious connection between diet and their
children's health.

You don't need to let preventable illness happen to you or
your family. While the experts endlessly debate details, you can
take a lesson from the Eskimos, the Maoris, and the Yemenite
immigrants to Israel.

About this time you might be thinking (and reasonably so)
that's all very fine, but the world's people aren't going to move
back to native villages and start living on wild game, fish, roots,
leaves, nuts, berries, or whatever they can grow themselves. I
agree. If for no other reason, there are too many of us. Besides, I
like hot and cold running water (distilled or filtered before
drinking, of course), books, magazines, television occasionally, and
not having to walk 30 miles each way to a symphony or department store. Not much opportunity for that in the average native
village. There must be another alternative.

# Eat Whole Foods As Fresh As Possible

There is. And you can start by simply evaluating your own diet. Gradually make your food as similar to the ancient human pattern as presently possible. That means not only the actual food eaten, but every step from the soil in which it's grown to the way it's cooked. Avoid salt, refined sugar, and white flour. Eat whole foods—fruits, vegetables, and grains—as fresh as possible. And stay away from additional synthetic chemicals.

Encourage others to follow your healthy attitude. Begin with your family and friends, then take your concerns to the marketplace.

What you buy at the store and what you eat control what food is brought to market. You've seen the increase in advertising for sugar-free foods, foods with "no preservatives," and no-sugar, no-salt baby foods. These products generally won't be offered for sale if there's no one to buy. But by becoming more aware of the effect of food on health, ignoring nutrient-poor *non*traditional foods, and buying more and more nutrient-rich whole traditional foods, at least some of us have persuaded food suppliers to begin the long trip back toward a health-promoting diet.

Of course it will take a while. Minds and markets rarely change overnight. Many consumers and food marketers don't yet realize that healthful food is not drab, dry, and lifeless, but more rich, varied, flavorful, and attractive than anything ever achieved with sugar, salt, and artificial chemicals.

If we *all* persist with ourselves, our families, and our markets and supermarkets, the change will come. It may take until our grandchildren's day, but they and future generations will be grateful—and more healthy. Through the use of a "new traditional" diet many more of us can complete our days as strong and healthy as age allows.

## REFERENCES

**Africans**

Hill, Peter, and Wynder, Ernst L. "Plasma Hormone Levels in Pre and Post Menopausal Vegetarian Women Fed a Western Diet." *Federation Proceedings*, abstract no. 3357, March 1, 1979.

**Eskimos**

Schaefer, Otto. "When the Eskimo Comes to Town." *Nutrition Today,* November/December, 1971, pp. 8–16.

**General**

Burkitt, Denis P. "Some Diseases Characteristic of Modern Western Civilization." *British Medical Journal,* February 3, 1973, pp. 274–278.

Campbell, G. D. "Diabetes in Asians and Africans In and Around Durban." *South African Medical Journal,* November 30. 1963, pp. 1195–1208.

Foster, George M. *Traditional Cultures: and the Impact of Technological Change.* Harper & Row, 1962, p. 38.

Trowell, H. C., and Burkitt, D. P. *Western Diseases: Their Emergence and Prevention.* Harvard University Press, 1981.

Van Rensburg, Schalk J. "Epidemiologic and Dietary Evidence for a Specific Nutritional Predisposition to Esophageal Cancer." *Journal of the National Cancer Institute,* August, 1981, pp. 143–251.

**Japanese**

Suzuki, K., and Mitsuoka, T. "Increase in Faecal Nitrosamines in Japanese Individuals Given a Western Diet." *International Cancer Research Data Bank,* March, 1982, p. 2.

**Jews**

Cohen, A. M.; Bavly, Sara; and Poznanski, Rachel. "Change of Diet of Yemenite Jews in Relation to Diabetes and Ischaemic Heart-Disease." *Lancet,* December 23, 1961, pp. 1399–1401.

**Micronesians**

Prior, Ian A. M. "The Price of Civilization." *Nutrition Today,* July/August, 1971, pp. 2–11.

Ringrose, Helen and Zimmet, P. "Nutrient Intakes in an Urbanized Micronesian Population with a High Diabetes Prevalence." *American Journal of Clinical Nutrition,* June, 1979, pp. 1334–1341.

# 4 GOOD DIGESTION: WHY WE CAN'T TAKE IT FOR GRANTED

In nutritional medicine, gastroenterology, and medicine in general, it appears we've only scratched the surface in investigating and uncovering problems of digestion and absorption. Although many details are known about a few nutrients, we really don't know much about the exact steps involved in the absorption process of most vitamins or minerals. Although medical textbooks list dozens of causes of "the malabsorption syndrome" (many of them rare), much more appears to be *unknown* about the subject than is known.

Certainly, I can't claim to know everything about digestion and nutrient absorption. What I can do, however, is underline their importance, hoping that if you're doing everything right with your diet, taking supplements, and still not feeling well, you'll consider faulty digestion and absorption as one possible explanation.

# Too Little Stomach Acid—A Common Problem

By far the most common digestive problem seen at our clinic is failure of the stomach to produce enough acid for digestion to procede normally. According to one medical textbook, *The Pharmacological Basis of Therapeutics,* from 10 to 15 percent of "the general population" has that problem. Among persons not in good health, the percentage is much higher. By actual measurement, we find many more individuals with too little stomach acid than with too much.

If you watch much television you might find that fact surprising. Thousands of advertisements every year recommend antacids for digestive difficulties. These products, which "absorb up to 47 times their weight in excess stomach acid," appear to be your only answer.

Yet when we actually measure stomach acid in people who've been taking antacids regularly, better than half have subnormally low levels of acidity. Taking antacids when not needed doesn't improve health; if anything, it makes it worse. I've found that switching to hydrochloric acid supplementation when laboratory testing indicates low or no stomach acid resolves not only the digestive symptoms but improves overall health. So why isn't television promoting sources of hydrochloric acid (and pepsin) as much as it does antacids?

The answer is simple: Hydrochloric acid is not an accepted part of medical practice. The commonly held medical opinion that it's not necessary or useful is best represented by a prominent introductory medical textbook, *A Digest of Digestion,* which states plainly: "Acid and pepsin are *not* essential for protein digestion." Pancreatic enzymes are said to be sufficient for the job. That view is taught at most medical schools. So students soon learn to ignore the importance of acid and pepsin in proper digestion, and to be concerned only with it when there may be an ulcer due to oversecretion of acid.

When physicians recommend antacids for digestive complaints, actual laboratory measurement of stomach acid is almost never recommended or performed. To make matters worse, on the rare occasion when measurement is performed, the usual and "approved" procedure includes the injection of histamine or pentagastrin, hormones which none of us injects regularly with lunch or dinner.

At my clinic we actually measure the stomach's secretion. What we find is that one-quarter to one-half of the people seen each day have low stomach acidity. Over the years I've found that while the stomach may not be a "vital organ" (we can survive for years without one), its function is essential to the best attainable health. I simply can't agree with those who feel that the stomach's secretion is of useless function—a vestige like our appendixes. If stomach acid isn't necessary, why then does nature give us the ability to concentrate acidity in our stomachs one million times stronger than in the surrounding bloodstream? It takes a large amount of metabolic energy to accomplish this. And under normal conditions, it goes on all our lives.

Abnormally low stomach acid is one of the most common reasons why good diet, vitamins, minerals, and other supplements may not produce much (if any) health improvement. So how will you know if your digestion isn't working at its best?

Look for telltale symptoms.

My patients with low stomach acidity (technically called hypochlorhydria) or no stomach acidity (achlorhydria) frequently report bloating, belching or burning immediately after meals; a feeling that food just sits in the stomach not digesting; and an inability to eat more than a small amount of food without feeling full. A large percentage are constipated, some have diarrhea, yet others have normal bowel function. Not everyone has all these symptoms. Many have just one or two. And some individuals with absolutely no stomach acid at all have absolutely no digestive symptoms at all.

Physical signs frequently found in association with low acidity include weak, easily broken, peeling fingernails as well as hair loss in women. Many people have "gassiness" in the upper abdomen, detectable on physical examination. Unusual dilation of the capillaries in the cheeks and on the nose (in a nonalcoholic) is often associated with the problem.

A long list of diseases frequently associated with low stomach acidity includes: diabetes mellitus, both underactive and overactive thyroid, childhood asthma, eczema, gallbladder disease, osteoporosis, rheumatoid arthritis, chronic hives, lupus erythematosus, weak adrenals, chronic hepatitis, vitiligo, and rosacea. Unfortunately, simply getting older is also associated with an increasing frequency of low stomach acidity. In fact, some investigations have found it in more than 50 percent of those over 60.

Whenever I'm working with anyone past 60, anyone with one of the diseases noted above, or anyone with symptoms or physical findings frequently associated with low or no stomach acid, I recommend direct measurement of gastric acidity by radiotelemetry using the Heidelberg capsule. At present, it's the best test available for functional determination of the stomach's ability to secrete acid normally.

I also use other laboratory clues to help my diagnosis. One is a mineral analysis of a hair specimen. If six or more minerals are low, excluding sodium and potassium, stomach acid should be checked. Even five low minerals are suspicious.

The other test we routinely do in our laboratory is on stool specimens, to check for completeness of digestion. It's not unusual to find an excess of undigested meat fiber in such an analysis. And measurement of the stomach acid in those cases usually discloses an insufficiency.

Once the problem is found, what can be done? Should anything be done? Will it make any real difference?

Present widespread medical opinion is negative to all three questions! One review published in the *New England Journal of Medicine* is typical, concluding that in cases of no stomach acid at all, "treatment with bland diet, sedation, and adequate attention to colonic evacuation appears to be more efficacious than substitution [hydrochloric acid] therapy." Many other journals and textbooks support the same sort of opinion.

Obviously, I disagree, despite having read the standard textbooks and medical journal reviews. My opinion is based in a small part on theory: Why do our stomachs bother to concentrate acid so highly if it isn't needed? But mostly it's based on direct experience, observing health improvement in individuals using appropriate hydrochloric acid therapy. I've also seen improvement from replacement of nutrients deficient as a result of defective stomach function and other digestive and absorptive problems.

I believe that the key to successful hydrochloric acid use is in recognition that low stomach acidity is hardly ever an isolated condition existing by itself with nothing else the matter. It's usually only part of an overall problem, but a key starting place if nutritional-biochemical treatment is going to have a chance to work.

That same *New England Journal of Medicine* review article noted that symptoms often returned after an initially successful period of hydrochloric acid treatment, even though the treatment was continued unchanged. This observation was used as part of the argument that replacing hydrochloric acid makes no difference.

Unfortunately, these authors didn't add pepsin along with the hydrochloric acid they recommended, usually a standard part of my treatment. They also didn't try supplemental vitamin $B_{12}$ by injection, even though all of their test subjects had achlorhydria (of the worst sort, histamine resistant) and could be assumed even in standard medical practice to have problems absorbing vitamin $B_{12}$. No calcium or iron was added, minerals known even at that time to be less well absorbed by individuals without stomach acid. And despite their stated observation of cases where symptoms were "provoked by specific food groups," they didn't recommend elimination of those foods for the duration of their test of hydrochloric acid. Food allergy and sensitivity is so frequently associated with low stomach acidity that the finding of one should automatically lead to a consideration of the other.

Such "tests" of hydrochloric acid treatment serve only to prove that a complete picture cannot be painted with only one color.

How do I know that hydrochloric acid treatment is actually doing anything? Well, besides reported symptomatic improvement, there are at least two other ways: The mineral analysis improves, and the undigested meat fiber usually present in the stool analysis disappears.

Before going over how I use hydrochloric acid supplementation, however, it's important to consider one obvious question: Isn't there a way to get the stomach to produce more acid and pepsin on its own, and return to normal function, so that supplementation would be unnecessary?

Unfortunately, there's no reliable method. One problem is that the cause or causes of failed stomach acid secretion aren't known. Solving a problem usually requires finding the cause. If, as it appears, there are many separate causes, there may be no standard solution.

Older medical writing reports the return of normal stomach function associated with a variety of treatments, including: raw liver, raw hog stomach, "lavage" (washing) of the stomach with hydrogen peroxide, injections of parathyroid extract, and prefrontal lobotomy (a type of brain surgery). None of these methods is either well proven or practical enough to be generally used.

## The Basics of Treatment

In my treatment with hydrochloric acid, I always emphasize that it can be dangerous. I only use it when testing indicates a need, and follow with careful supervision. Though problems occur rarely, they can be bad ones. Hydrochloric acid should *never* be used at the same time as aspirin, Butazolidin, Inodicin, Motrin, or any other anti-inflammatory medications. These medications themselves can cause stomach bleeding and ulcers, as can corticosteroid preparations, the most frequently prescribed of which is prednisone. Using hydrochloric acid with them increases the risk. Occasionally, when the potential benefits outweighs the risk, I'll recommend hydrochloric acid anyway, but *only* after an explanation of those possible risks, benefits, and precautions. And I carefully monitor the patient through the therapy.

I also rarely recommend hydrochloric acid supplements by themselves, but in combination with pepsin. Stomachs that don't produce adequate hydrochloric acid are presumed not to produce enough pepsin either. This assumption is not usually directly tested. In any event, I have found that hydrochloric acid usually gives better results with pepsin than without. And except in individuals sensitive to it, pepsin is usually recommended with hydrochloric acid.

Hydrochloric acid (except the prescription-only liquid form) doesn't come as just plain hydrochloric acid. It comes attached to "carriers"—betaine or glutamic acid. Carriers make it possible to provide the hydrochloric acid in a more convenient capsule or tablet form that is much more portable and safer for the teeth. The full names of the supplements usually recommended are either "betaine hydrochloride with pepsin" or "glutamic acid hydrochloride with pepsin."

Except on rare occasion, I don't recommend the tablet forms anymore. Follow-up analysis of stool specimens has shown that powdered preparations in capsules are much more effective in decreasing the amount of undigested meat fibers than solid tablet form. In some cases, a maximum dose of hydrochloric acid and pepsin in the solid tablet form has produced no change at all in undigested meat, but substituting the powdered form in a capsule has produced quick results. And, in addition to verifiably better digestion, there are fewer reported side effects.

What are the side effects to watch out for? Anything that feels bad: pain, burning, additional gas. Even when the gastric analysis is clear-cut, leaving no question about low stomach acid, some individuals have problems with hydrochloric acid in capsules. In such cases, I recommend very small doses of liquid hydrochloric acid dissolved in water and increased very slowly over intervals of several weeks. I also find that small, gradually increased quantities of lemon juice or vinegar will usually do the same job.

To minimize even minor side effects, I always start with just one capsule (5, 7½, or 10 grains) taken just before the meal. After two or three days, if there are no problems, I suggest adding two capsules before meals, then three another two to three days later.

The dose is gradually increased in this stepwise fashion until the recommended amount is reached. When numerous capsules are taken, I recommend half before eating and the other half during the meal.

The amount of hydrochloric acid that's usually effective for adults is at least 40 to 90 grains of betaine hydrochloride (or glutamic acid hydrochloride) with pepsin per meal. That is about 4 to 9 ten-grain (8 to 18 five-grain) capsules per meal. It makes sense to lessen the dose with smaller meals, but no firm guidelines can be given about how to do so.

One pharmacy textbook, *The Pharmacological Basis of Therapeutics*, states that the dose of powdered glutamic acid hydrochloride is to be considerably less than I recommend—5 to 15 grams. In my experience this amount is inadequate.

Presently, there also are no clear-cut guidelines for which form of hydrochloric acid—betaine or glutamic acid—is preferable. Generally, I find that if there's any side effect with one, it's worthwhile trying the other, since a few individuals are sensitive to one but not both.

In some cases, pepsin may cause adverse reactions such as loose stools, gas, diarrhea, or burning. In these instances, preparations of glutamic acid hydrochloride without pepsin are available.

When the powdered glutamic acid hydrochloride or betaine hydrochloride forms can't be used or are found to be ineffective, I recommend a 10 percent solution of liquid hydrochloric acid, one to two teaspoons, in four to eight ounces of water.

The liquid does, however, have several disadvantages, including inconvenience, poor portability, and the possibility of acid damage if the bottle breaks. More serious is its tendency to slowly dissolve away tooth enamel. For this reason, it's traditionally been recommended to sip it through a glass straw, and to rinse out the mouth with an alkaline solution such as bicarbonate of soda after meals.

Also, the 10 percent liquid hydrochloric acid solution doesn't have pepsin, so a separate pepsin supplement is recommended.

Unfortunately, pepsin tablets are hard to find. But one to two ten-grain (two to four five-grain) capsules per meal appear adequate.

To make sure that hydrochloric acid and pepsin in whatever form are working, I take repeated follow-up analyses of stool specimens until digestion appears improved. (Further details about this test are found in "ABCs of Nutritional Testing.") I also find follow-up hair mineral analysis to be helpful.

Even though the dosages of hydrochloric acid mentioned above may seem large (particularly when compared with the usual label recommendations), a normally functioning stomach is capable of manufacturing considerably more. You may be wondering why I recommend an amount of hydrochloric acid that is less than a normally functioning stomach is capable of making. Because, in practice, it usually works.

Individuals anemic for years despite taking iron (because of iron malabsorption associated with low stomach acidity) routinely achieve a normal blood count by adding this amount of supplemental hydrochloric acid. Others with progressive loss of bone from the jaw, documented on x-ray and not helped by calcium supplementation, have had reversal of the process, again documented on x-ray, by adding hydrochloric acid supplements along with the previously ineffective calcium. A wide variety of other health problems in hypochlorhydric individuals, previously resistant to treatment, have been improved with a "practical" dosage range of 4 to 9 ten-grain (8 to 18 five-grain) capsules.

In addition, the stool analysis usually normalizes, and the mineral analysis shows improvement. So, even though I suspect results might occasionally be better if it were practical to use the higher hydrochloric acid dosage ranges, I rarely recommend them.

## Nutrients Fail to Be Absorbed

Individuals with insufficient stomach acid also don't absorb many nutrients well, so they frequently have the greatest need for dietary supplementation. If I first recommended 25 to 30 capsules of glutamic acid hydrochloride (or betaine hydrochloride) with pepsin at each meal, and then find all the minerals and vitamins deficient or necessary, the overall number of pills and capsules required for them to take would be overwhelming. So I stay with the "practical" dosage range, as it usually works well enough.

The vitamin that offers the greatest benefit to people with insufficient stomach acid is $B_{12}$. I have individuals with laboratory-verified low stomach acidity try a series of $B_{12}$ injections (1,000 micrograms) once or twice weekly, along with folate (folic acid) (2.5 milligrams). To cut cost and to make it convenient, I teach these patients to administer their own injections. Most people find that the injections make them sleep sounder, think more clearly, and feel more energetic and calmer than before. Occasionally others report less joint pain. And a minority experience no change at all. They're usually advised to eliminate the injections unless the degree of low stomach acidity is severe. In severe cases of low or no stomach acidity, $B_{12}$ injections are preventive insurance against "pernicious" anemia, a type brought on by vitamin $B_{12}$ malabsorption. It seems that more men than women are unaffected by the injections.

The majority, however, report beneficial effects. After this length of time, I can't believe that it's a mass hallucination or placebo effect—an objection often made to $B_{12}$ injections.

There's good scientifically derived evidence indicating why vitamin $B_{12}$ might have a useful effect. The same evidence also tells us why injections are necessary, and why swallowing vitamin $B_{12}$ often won't do the same job.

The cells lining the stomach that produce hydrochloric acid also produce the "intrinsic factor," a special substance without which vitamin $B_{12}$ can't be absorbed by the small intestine. When the cells lining the stomach cease functioning normally, slowing or stopping hydrochloric acid secretion, the intrinsic-factor secretion also slows down. Under these circumstances, $B_{12}$ taken orally either in food or pill form isn't well absorbed. Presently, there is no economical, sufficient dose intrinsic-factor preparation for oral use, so $B_{12}$ is only effective when injected. Folate is a metabolic partner with $B_{12}$, so it's included in the injection, too.

To my knowledge, an overdose with vitamin $B_{12}$ or folate hasn't been reported. The maximum vitamin $B_{12}$ dose I've seen reported anywhere was 30,000 micrograms given intravenously daily for 20 days. No ill effects were observed and the condition under study improved.

There is concern expressed by a few British doctors that cyanocobalamin, one "natural" form of vitamin $B_{12}$, might (in theory) cause problems over a long period. They recommend the use of another naturally occurring form, hydroxycobalamin. Although the concern is so far purely theoretical, I recommend hydroxycobalamin for long-term use.

Whenever $B_{12}$ and folate injections are accompanied by beneficial results, I recommend that they be continued for self-determined periods of time. After several months of health improvement through upgraded diet, hydrochloric acid and pepsin improvement of digestion and absorption, nutrient supplementation, and in many cases allergy avoidance, most individuals report they don't need the injections as often.

Although vitamin $B_{12}$ injections are therapeutic for specific conditions written about elsewhere in this and my previous book, please note that they're not expected to improve digestion or stomach acid secretion. Routine vitamin $B_{12}$ injection trial is recommended when stomach acid is low, because the percentage of beneficial responses is high, but it doesn't normalize stomach acid or intrinsic-factor secretion.

At present there's no reliable way of returning stomach function to normal. Although I've certainly seen it happen in a few cases, especially in children and younger adults, most people with moderate to severe low stomach acidity (particularly those past 60) continue to need hydrochloric acid-pepsin supplementation indefinitely. Even though it's a nuisance, and not nearly as good as one's own normal stomach function, continued supplementation is preferable to poorer digestion, lessened nutrient assimilation, and the greater chance of ill health that follows on low or absent stomach acidity.

Hydrochloric acid supplements have other important functions aside from helping food digest better. In one study, Dr. Ralph Giannella and associates conclude: "We believe that the available data support the concept that hypochlorhydria [low stomach acidity] or achlorhydria [no stomach acidity] increases both susceptibility to and severity of bacterial and perhaps also of certain parasitic enteric infections." What that means is that normal stomach acid kills germs, decreasing the number and severity of gastrointestinal infections.

In another paper Dr. W. S. J. Ruddell and associates report a "highly significant increase in gastric juice nitrite in hypochlorhydric [low stomach acidic] subjects." In more alkaline stomachs, nitrites turn into nitrosamines, which are known cancer-causing substances. The authors point out the known association between low stomach acidity and gastric cancer, and speculate that persistently high levels of nitrites found in low acidic stomachs could be part of the cause. In a normally acid condition, nitrites are unstable, and mostly break down before they can cause trouble.

In our own laboratory, we find a much higher frequency of clinically signifciant intestinal yeast infections in individuals with low stomach acidity, as well as a greater percentage with high levels of indican in the urine. Elevated urinary indican is associated with bacterial overgrowth in the intestine, as well as with a variety of "malabsorptive" diseases. For more information on urinary indican as well as other tests, see "ABCs of Nutritional Testing."

# Other Causes of Poor Digestion and Absorption

An insufficiency of bile is another cause of digestion problems. Like hydrochloric acid, bile is secreted for a reason—to aid digestion—and should be present in an adequate quantity. It's particularly important for digestion of fats and oils, and of course, fat- and oil-soluble vitamins.

Once food is processed by the stomach, it arrives in the uppermost part of the small intestine, where it's acted on by pancreatic enzymes and bile. Even without any medical testing, overall insufficiency of bile isn't hard to detect, since bile imparts most of the color to the stool.

As a general rule, the lighter the stool color, the less the bile content. As we've all learned, a medium-dark brown color is usual. Though it's unusual, a persistently yellowish, grayish, or very light brown stool can happen, and isn't normal.

It isn't something to ignore or try self-treatment for, either, at least at first. A lack of insufficient bile over a period of time can be a symptom of serious health problems. Before trying to do anything about it yourself, a thorough medical checkup is indicated. Remember, I'm writing about a persistent problem, not just a one-time thing brought on by dietary indiscretion.

Once a medical check is completed, and nothing found, correcting the problem is a good idea. "Bile salt" preparations are available at health-food stores and some drugstores.

If you're thinking of trying them, try first to persuade your own liver to manufacture more bile on its own. Vitamins generally called lipotropic can help the process. Most lipotropic formulas contain choline, inositol, and methionine. Lecithin can also be of use.

If you do use bile salts, it's not hard to ascertain the right dose. A normal dark brown color of the stool will result. An overdose of bile salts is easily done, and produces an unpleasant, usually greenish-tinged diarrhea, so proceed cautiously. As bile salts are from animal sources, allergy is possible.

One group of individuals who have a malfunction of bile flow are those who've had their gallbladders removed. One of the functions of the gallbladder is to store bile so that a large quantity is available when a fatty or oily meal is eaten. Fat or oil in the upper small intestine triggers the release of a hormone which causes the gallbladder to contract, squeezing its contents through a duct into the intestine, onto the fatty or oily meal. If the gallbladder is gone, there's no place for the extra bile needed for fats and oils to be stored. Even though there's a steady bile flow from the liver, there's no reserve as when the gallbladder is intact. Although many persons without gallbladders experience no problems, others say digestion feels better and they feel better overall if they take bile salts with any oily or fatty meals.

All of this concerns only the quantity of bile, whether it's enough or not enough. Even now, there are no tests available for physicians in practice to check the quality of bile secreted.

Reasoning from natural function, both normal quantity and quality of bile are important to good digestion and thus good health. Strangely, comparatively little research meaningful or useful to practicing doctors has been done on this subject.

## Enzymes Are Important, Too

Not having enough pancreatic enzymes can be another cause of poor digestion.

Despite the observations of nutritionally oriented physicians, prevailing medical opinion has been that pancreatic enzyme supplements are hardly ever necessary except in cases of cystic fibrosis and chronic pancreatitis. Yet it's been my experience that sometimes nutrients which should work don't work in certain circumstances unless pancreatic enzyme supplements are added. Members of that group include: vitamin A; zinc; essential fatty acids; and vitamins E, D, and K. Many individuals report that digestion works better when supplemental enzymes are added after meals. As with hydrochloric acid, this observation is more common in older age groups.

A relatively reliable sign of inadequate fat digestion due to low levels of pancreatic enzyme secretion can be observed if stools float. Abdominal gas starting one to two hours after eating is also a clue.

Fortunately, the only hazard in trying enzyme supplements is allergy. Although the most effective (and the only pancreas-derived) enzyme preparations are from pig sources, there are usually adequate substitutes, bromelain and papain, derived from pineapple and papaya respectively. Until recently, the availability of dosage-strength bromelain or papain capsules or tablets has been poor, but much better capsule and tablet strengths have appeared in the 600 to 1,000 milligram range.

If a trial of two to four capsules or tablets of pancreatin, bromelain, or papain taken after meals produces better digestion, then it's usually advisable to continue taking them. If allergy occurs, the most frequent symptom is looser stool or diarrhea, although skin rash and other allergic symptoms are possible.

Low pancreatic enzyme secretion and low stomach acidity frequently occur together; the possibility should always be kept in mind.

## Food Allergy Causes Poor Digestion

Food allergy can be yet another cause of poor digestion and absorption. Some severe cases have been documented in medical journals, but less obvious cases often escape detection. I find them only in retrospect, when measures of nutrient status such as the hair mineral analysis improve after food allergies are removed. Quite often, discovery of allergy-related digestive malfunction requires the help of a nutritionally oriented, allergy-aware physician.

Lastly, many instances of poor digestion or absorption can only be labeled "cause unknown" at present. Poor absorption of nutrients for no apparent reason isn't unusual, especially in older individuals. When a nutrient which usually helps a certain condition isn't effective, and digestive aids don't help, I always find it's worth trying an injectable form if it's safe, practical, and available.

Many reports have demonstrated a relatively high frequency of vitamin deficiency in older individuals. In one study, Doctors Baker, Frank, and Jaslow checked blood vitamin levels in 228 individuals between 60 and 102 years of age. None had undergone major surgery, and their diet was said to be good. All had been taking a daily multivitamin tablet with content greater than the RDA. Despite this, 39 percent were found to have vitamin deficiency. Other studies noted by Dr. Baker have shown similar results.

After one injection of multivitamins, *all* deficiencies were corrected, even though oral supplements were discontinued. Since vitamin intake prior to the injections was known to be "more than adequate," the doctors had no explanation for the study results other than poor digestion and absorption in older persons, or interference with vitamin absorption caused by drugs taken more frequently by older individuals.

Considering the demonstrated frequency and diversity of malabsorption problems in older people, I frequently recommend injectable multiple vitamins (emphasizing the B complex) on a trial basis in cases where no specific illness can be found but the individual "just isn't feeling right." If results are favorable, the injections are continued indefinitely, as I don't expect the presumed digestive or absorptive defect to correct itself. Again, home injection is taught to minimize cost and the bother of travel.

Based on many studies among older persons there also appears to be a good case for periodic preventive multivitamin injections, again with emphasis on the B complex, especially since the cost is low, side effects are negligible, and the potential benefits are a healthier old age.

For those purists who critize this practice as useless shotgun therapy for no specific illness and not grounded by secure scientific knowledge of why it works, I can only hope that research establishes sufficient reasons for the frequent necessity and efficacy of such injections by the time these purists are old enough to need them.

I don't want to create the impression that injectable vitamins (or other nutrients) are only useful and necessary in older age groups. Sometimes they're very valuable for younger persons, even children, when the same nutrient or nutrients won't work by mouth.

I hope that in this chapter I've given you an idea of the importance of good digestion and absorption and offered you a new clue if you've already adapted what I call the "new traditional" diet, but still aren't feeling as well as you'd like. We're now ready to go on to the third important question in an evaluation of nutrition and health: "Are you sensitive or allergic to the food you eat?"

# REFERENCES

## Anemia

Howitz, Jette, and Schwartz, Michael. "Vitiligo, Achlorhydria, and Pernicious Anemia." *Lancet*, June 26, 1971, pp. 1331–1334.

Jacobs, A.; Rhodes, J.; and Eakins, J. D. "Gastric Factors Influencing Iron Absorption in Anaemic Patients." *Scandinavian Journal of Haematology*, vol. 4, 1967, pp. 105–110.

## Asthma

Caruselli, M. "Upon Therapy For Asthma Using Vitamin $B_{12}$." *Riforma Medica*, August 2, 1952, pp. 849–851.

Gillespie, Marjorie. "Hypochlorhydria in Asthma with Special Reference to the Age Incidence." *Quarterly Journal of Medicine*, vol. 4, 1935, pp. 397–405.

## Atrophic Gastritis

Schiff, Leon, and Goodman, Sander. "Desiccated Hog's Stomach Extract (Ventriculin) in the Treatment of Atrophic Gastritis." *American Journal of Digestive Diseases*, vol. 7, 1940, pp. 14–17.

Schindler, Rudolf; Kirsner, Joseph B.; and Palmer, Walter Lincoln. "Atrophic Gastritis: Gastroscopic Studies of the Effects of Liver and Iron Therapy." *Archives of Internal Medicine*, vol. 65, 1940, pp. 78–89.

## Carcinogens

Ruddell, W. S. J. et al. "Gastric-Juice Nitrite." *Lancet*, November 13, 1976, pp. 1037–1039.

## Diabetes

Hosking, D. J. et al. "Vagal Impairment of Gastric Secretion in Diabetic Autonomic Neuropathy." *British Medical Journal*, June 14, 1975, pp. 588–590.

Rabinowitch, I. M. "Achlorhydria and Its Clinical Significance in Diabetes Mellitus." *American Journal of Digestive Diseases*, September, 1949, pp. 322–332.

## Digestion

Davenport, Horace W. "Gastric Secretion." In *A Digest of Digestion*. Year Book Medical Publishers, 1975, pp. 41–55.

Gilman, Alfred, and Goodman, Louis. "Gastric Antacids and Digestants." In *The Pharmacological Basis of Therapeutics*. 4th ed. Macmillan Publishing, 1970, pp. 1002–1019.

Goldberg, David M., ed. "Disease of the Gastrointestinal Tract." In *Clinical Biochemistry Review, Volume 2*. John Wiley & Sons, 1981, pp. 94–97.

## Elderly

Baker, Herman; Oscar, Frank; and Jaslow, Seymour P. "Oral Versus Intramuscular Vitamin Supplementation of Hypovitaminosis in the Elderly." *Journal of the American Geriatrics Society*, January, 1980, pp. 42–45.

Davies, Daniel T., and James, T. G. Illtyd. "An Investigation Into the Gastric Secretion of a Hundred Normal Persons Over the Age of Sixty." *Quarterly Journal of Medicine*, vol. 24, 1930, pp. 1–14.

Montgomery, R. D. et al. "The Ageing Gut: A Study of Intestinal Absorption in Relation to Nutrition in the Elderly." *Quarterly Journal of Medicine*, April, 1978, pp. 197–211.

Rafsky, Henry A., and Weingarten, Michael. "A Study of Gastric Secretory Response in the Aged." *Gastroenterology*, vol. 8, 1947, pp. 348–352.

## Food Sensitivity

Kokkonen, J.; Simila, S.; and Herva, R. "Impaired Gastric Function in Children with Cow's Milk Intolerance." *European Journal of Pediatrics*, vol. 132, 1979, pp. 1–6.

Werner, M., and Wettwer, L. "Capacity for Gastric Acid Secretion in Adults with Milk Allergy." *Journal of the American Medical Association*, January 13, 1969, p. 395.

## Gallbladder Disease

Capper, W. M. et al. "Gallstones, Gastric Secretion and Flatulent Dyspepsia." *Lancet*, February 25, 1967, pp. 413–415.

Fravel, R. C. "The Occurrence of Hypochlorhydria in Gall-Bladder Disease." *American Journal of the Medical Sciences*, vol. 159, 1920, pp. 512–517.

**Hives**
Rawls, William B., and Ancona, V. Charles. "Chronic Urticaria Associated With Hypochlorhydria or Achlorhydria." *Review of Gastroenterology*, vol. 18, 1951, pp. 267–271.

**Hydrochloric Acid**
Alverez, W. C. "How Often Is There Value in the Giving of Hydrochloric Acid?" *Gastroenterology*, vol. 12, 1949, pp. 895–898.
Rappaport, Emanuel M. "Achlorhydria-Associated Symptoms of Response to Hydrochloric Acid." *New England Journal of Medicine*, May 12, 1955, pp. 802–805.

**Infections**
Giannella, Ralph A.; Broitman, Selwyn A.; and Zamcheck, Norman. "Influence of Gastric Acidity on Bacterial and Parasitic Enteric Infections." *Annals of Internal Medicine*, vol. 78, 1973, pp. 271–276.
Greenberger, Norton J.; Saegh, Samad; and Ruppert, Richard D. "Urine Indican Excretion in Malabsorptive Disorders." *Gastroenterology*, August, 1968, pp. 204–211.

**Mental Disorders**
Horstmann, Paul. "Investigations into Gastric Secretion in Patients with Manic-depressive Psychosis." *Acta Psychiatrica et Neurologica*, vol. 16, 1941, pp. 69–78.
Reed, John A. "A Study of Gastric Acids in Prefrontal Lobotomy." *Gastroenterology*, vol. 10, 1948, pp. 118–119.

**Mineral Absorption**
Hunt, J. N. and Johnson, C. "Relationship Between Gastric Secretion of Acid and Urinary Excretion of Calcium After Oral

Supplements of Calcium." *Digestive Diseases and Sciences,* vol. 28, 1983, p. 417.

Mahoney, Arthur, and Hendricks, Deloy G. "Role of Gastric Acid in the Utilization of Dietary Calcium by the Rat." *Nutrition and Metabolism,* vol. 16, 1974, pp. 375–382.

Mahoney, Arthur; Holbrook, Reid Scott; and Hendricks, Deloy G. "Effects of Calcium Solubility on Absorption by Rats with Induced Achlorhydria." *Nutrition and Metabolism,* vol. 18, 1975, pp. 310–317.

Personal Communication with Walter Mertz, M.D., director of the Human Nutrition Research Center, United States Department of Agriculture, 1983.

**Rheumatoid Arthritis**
DeWitte, T. J. et al. "Hypochlorhydria and Hypergastrinemia in Rheumatoid Arthritis." *Annals of the Rheumatic Diseases,* vol. 38, 1979, pp. 14–17.

**Skin Disorders**
Ayres, Samuel. "Gastric Secretion in Psoriasis, Eczema and Dermatitis Herpetiformis." *Archives of Dermatology,* vol. 20, 1929, pp. 854–857.

Ryel, J. A. et al. "Gastric Analysis in Acne Rosacea." *Lancet,* December 11, 1920, pp. 1195–1196.

**Stomach Acidity**
Hartfall, Stanley J. "Achlorhydria: A Review of 336 Cases." *Guy's Hospital Reports,* vol. 82, 1932, pp. 13–39.

Oliver, T. H., and Wilkinson, John F. "Critical Review Achlorhydria." *Quarterly Journal of Medicine,* vol. 2, 1933, pp. 431–455.

Schiff, Leon, and Tahl, Toba. "The Effects of Desiccated Hog's Stomach in Achlorhydria." *American Journal of Digestive Diseases,* vol. 1, 1934–35, pp. 543–548.

Williams, Robert H. "The Adrenals." In *Textbook of Endocrinology.* 5th ed. W. B. Saunders, 1974, p. 271.

**Thyroid Disorders**

Dotevall, Gerhard, and Walan, Anders. "Gastric Secretion of Acid and Intrinsic Factor in Patients with Hyper- and Hypothyroidism." *Acta Medica Scandinavica*, vol. 186, 1969, pp. 529–533.

**Vitamin B$_{12}$**

Matthews, D. M., and Linnell, J. C. "Vitamin B$_{12}$: An Area of Darkness." *British Medical Journal*, September 1, 1979, pp. 533–535.

# 5 FOOD SENSITIVITY: OFTEN THE HIDDEN REASON FOR PERSISTENT PROBLEMS

I haven't had to refer anyone for gallbladder surgery since 1979. That's a remarkable statement considering the fact that gallbladder disease isn't on the decline and that I still continue to see the same number of people with the problem that I did before.

Such an accomplishment certainly is not because I recommend any vitamins, minerals, or magic potions—or because I've devised some special treatment. In fact, I'm sorry to say that I can't claim any credit at all for such a dramatic success rate. All I did was read both a book and a paper authored by the same person— James C. Breneman, M.D., past chairman of the Food Allergy Committee of the American College of Allergists. Since that time, every gallbladder sufferer I've worked with is no longer having attacks, and still has been able to hold on to his or her own gallbladder.

Actually, what Dr. Breneman reported was that gallbladder attacks could be completely avoided by eliminating allergenic m the diet. And to date, I haven't found him to be

y, then, doesn't the number of people admitted to hospitals for gallbladder surgery continue to decline? And why hadn't I known about such treatment before 1979? After all, Dr. Breneman's original article was published in 1968. And other similar research had appeared in print nearly 30 years earlier. A 100 percent success rate certainly can't be swept under the rug, or shall we say hidden behind barricaded operating room doors . . . or can it?

It can and it does remain hidden, probably because prevalent medical opinion considers food sensitivity and allergy to be an insignificant cause of illness of any sort. For decades, medical journals have been replete with derogatory references to the "overdiagnosis" of food sensitivity and allergy.

Another reason is probably the economics of gallbladder surgery. The surgical removal of the gallbladder, called cholecystectomy, is a giant industry. According to a helpful information officer at the National Center for Health Statistics, approximately 482,000 gallbladders were removed in 1981, the latest year for figures.

So let's do a little arithmetic. If the average surgical fee is $1,000 and the approximate charges for the hospital, x-rays, and anesthesia are $2,500, then the cost for the 482,000 cholecystectomies in the United States in 1981 was more than $150 million.

Any "industry" of that size obviously would be resistant to the prospect of elimination.

# A 100 Percent Success Rate

Let's get down to Dr. Breneman's actual cases. What he did was to locate 69 individuals, 51 with proven gallstones and 18 who'd already had their gallbladders removed but still suffered from attacks of gallbladder pain. He put them on an elimination diet made up of foods he felt had minimum allergic potential—like beef, rye, soybean, rice, and spinach. According to Dr. Breneman, "All the patients [100 percent] were relieved of their symptoms at the end of one week's use of the basic elimination diet." It usually took three to five days for their symptoms to disappear.

He then had them add back foods they ordinarily ate, one at a time. When a food was found to provoke a gallbladder attack, it was eliminated, and not retested for several weeks. Each "guilty" food was retested several times to make sure it reproduced symptoms. Some individuals had sensitivities to medications as well. An average of four to five foods had to be finally excluded from each person's diet in order to put an end to the attacks of gallbladder pain. A few reacted to only one food, while others reacted to as many as nine and a medication. Interestingly, 64 of the 69 individuals (93 percent) reacted to eggs.

And contrary to standard gallbladder diet recommendations, Dr. Breneman didn't ask anyone to eliminate fats, oils, or "rich foods." Despite that, there were no further gallbladder attacks as long as proven allergenic foods were kept out of each person's diet.

That "allergy removal" system, however, doesn't dissolve or do anything else to gallstones if they're already formed. Dr. Breneman explains that allergy causes swelling of the bile ducts, slowing or stopping the flow of bile away from the gallbladder. That "backing up" of the bile is what causes the pain, which explains why allergy elimination works in the postcholecystectomy syndrome, too. What's really being stopped are episodes of swelling in the bile ducts, not a gallstone problem. It also suggests why some people have typical gallbladder attacks but x-rays show no gallstones.

Other research work has shown a difference in bile composition between gallstone formers and nonformers, but the discovery of how to prevent attacks of gallbladder pain, whether or not stones are present, casts doubt on the theory that gallstones themselves are the cause of most of the painful attacks. Given the "allergy explanation," it's quite possible that the only instances in which gallstones would be directly responsible for a gallbladder attack or other gallbladder pain would be if a stone slipped into the bile-drainage duct and got stuck, causing backing up of the

pain; or if stones were responsible for infection
: and bile ducts. Both of these circumstances
prise only a small proportion of the causes of
s.

h a successful explanation of gallbladder disease
that when there's a past history of the problem, even gallbladder
removal, I automatically suggest that allergy testing be done if the
person presently doesn't feel well.

# Allergies and Food Sensitivities: A Major Cause of Ill Health

Surprisingly enough, allergies or food sensitivities aren't only
associated with gallbladder problems. I believe, as does Dr.
Breneman and a host of other doctors and researchers, that they're
a major cause of ill health in general.

In fact, some 40 to 50 percent of the individuals I work with
have partial to complete relief of from one to all of their symptoms
when they uncover their allergies and/or sensitivities and avoid
the offending foods or chemicals.

"Food allergy can do anything to any part of the body," says
Dr. Breneman in his book, *Basics of Food Allergy.*

The list of some of the more common symptoms of food
allergy seems to go on indefinitely. It includes:

- asthma
- bedwetting
- bladder infections
- bronchitis
- bursitis
- canker sores
- celiac disease
- chronic low back pain
- depression
- diarrhea
- duodenal ulcer
- eczema
- edema (fluid retention)
- fainting
- fatigue
- gas
- gastritis
- headache
- hives
- hyperactivity

- hypoglycemia
- irritable colon
- itching
- joint pain and swelling
- learning disabilities
- malabsorption
- minimal brain dysfunction
- nephrosis

- personality changes
- protein in urine
- recurrent infections
- seizures
- sinusitis
- skin rash
- ulcerative colitis

Of course, not all of these problems are due to allergy, clarifies Dr. Breneman, but allergy is a *frequent* cause.

By ignoring—in fact denying—food sensitivities and allergies, present-day standard medical practice misses innumerable diagnoses. Food allergies and sensitivities can either cause or contribute to literally thousands of otherwise mysterious symptoms, and much serious illness.

One of the major reasons that many illnesses may be overlooked is because there's such a widespread disagreement on definitions of allergy and an unwillingness to accept food sensitivities as a cause of real problems. So before we go any further, I'd like to clarify just what the difference between allergy and food sensitivity is, as well as my opinion on the subject.

When the term allergy was introduced to medicine in 1906, it meant "altered reactivity." Unfortunately, over the years this meaning has been lost from medical practice. What allergy has come to mean is any reaction to molecules in the body called antigens, to which white blood cells make antibodies and become sensitized, so that each time the body is exposed to the same molecule it will again make antibodies, causing the familiar allergic symptoms.

If a reaction doesn't include one of these components, it's considered "not allergic," and frequently not "real" by many doctors. Unfortunately, as so aptly put by Dr. Breneman, we can become just as ill whether the reaction is an allergic one or not.

"Food sensitivity" (or food intolerance, as it's sometimes called) is a broader term which means any bad reaction attributable to food or food components, including artificial colors, flavors, and preservatives. Food sensitivities are entirely individual—what affects one person may have no effect on another. Many sensitivities occur through "nonallergic" means, thereby creating considerable confusion within the medical profession. Unfortunately, while doctors are being confused, many people remain sick because of food sensitivities, both allergic and nonallergic types. As Dr. Breneman says: "The patient suffers as much regardless of the basic mechanism involved." So why bother to make any distinction?

Because different means of diagnosis mean differences in treatment. And because most of us work with physicians unfamiliar with nutritional biochemistry, food sensitivity (including allergy), and the importance of these topics to health. When talking to them about the subject, it's necessary to be careful about terminology and definitions. Physicians are trained from their first days in medical school to be as precise as possible about diagnosis. Yet food sensitivities don't always wrap themselves up in neat scientific packages.

Despite the lack of scientific confirmation, working with food sensitivity every day as I do, I know Dr. Breneman's statement that "60 percent of illness involves food intolerance" is quite accurate.

That's why I pursue the question of food sensitivities during my nutritional-biochemical investigation.

## A Common Food Sensitivity

One of the most common nonallergenic food sensitivities is lactose intolerance. Except among those of Northern European descent, lactose intolerance is a condition suffered by almost 100 percent of the people in many areas of the world. In the United States, 95 percent of Orientals are lactose intolerant, 75 percent of blacks, 60 percent of native Americans, and from 2 to 24 percent of Caucasians, depending on the group studied.

Lactose is the naturally occurring sugar found in all milk (human, cow, goat, etc.). It's made up of two sugars coupled together—glucose and galactose. In the scientific community it's known as a "disaccharide." An enzyme in the intestine called lactase is necessary to split the glucose and galactose apart in order to digest lactose.

Since lactose is found in mother's milk, almost all infants of nursing age are able to digest it. But past weaning and with increasing age, progressively fewer children retain this ability. One study of black children found lactose intolerance in 11 percent of four- to five-year-olds, 50 percent of six- to seven-year-olds, and 72 percent of eight- to nine-year-olds. Other studies have found close to 85 percent lactose malabsorption among black teenagers. Mexican-American children studied were 18 percent intolerant to lactose among two- to five-year-olds and increased to 56 percent among teenagers. It's usually rare among North American white children under six years of age, but increases to 30 percent in adolescents.

Not all individuals with proven lactose intolerance have symptoms, particularly if only small quantities of milk are drunk. When symptoms do occur, however, they can include gas, abdominal distention, diarrhea, and recurrent abdominal pain (especially among children). Infrequently, though, severe cases of lactose intolerance in children have been shown to cause damage to the lining of the intestine, and severe diarrhea.

Lactose intolerance, as mentioned earlier, is a good example of a nonallergenic yet food-sensitive condition. But there can be an overlap of the two. People with a true milk allergy suffer both the intestinal and systemic symptoms and may have problems including nasal congestion, headache, urinary frequency, hives, and protein loss in the urine. They can also have a food sensitivity. Of 24 milk-allergic individuals studied, half were found to be lactose intolerant.

Such a reaction to milk illustrates the importance of distinguishing types of food sensitivity—in this case true allergy versus intolerance due to enzyme deficiency. Not using milk is the preferred treatment option in either case. Adding sufficient acidophilus bacteria or commercial preparations of the enzyme lactase to milk-containing meals will prevent symptoms and improve nutrient absorption for individuals with lactose intolerance, but not for those allergic to milk. Conversely, milk allergy can sometimes be treated by desensitization. This is a procedure that is still somewhat mysterious; it introduces a very small dose of an allergic substance into the body and blocks the body's response to the allergy. The process simply controls but doesn't cure the allergy. And it won't help lactose intolerance, either.

Another common problem heavily influenced and frequently caused by food sensitivities is arthritis. Although, and unfortunately for arthritics, that connection is vehemently denied by most "authorities" on arthritis.

There are various types of arthritis, the most commonly diagnosed being gout, rheumatoid arthritis, and osteoarthritis (frequently called degenerative arthritis).

Gouty arthritis has the least allergic involvement and appears to be caused by overactivity in the enzyme xanthine oxidase, which leads to the production of too much uric acid—the substance responsible for the gouty symptoms like joint pain, especially in the big toe.

## Sensitivities Aggravate Arthritis

Rheumatoid arthritis doesn't appear to be caused by food sensitivity, but in most cases food (and chemical) sensitivities definitely aggravate it. In his book *An Alternative Approach to Allergies* (must reading for anyone interested in successful nontoxic approaches to health care), Theron Randolph, M.D., precisely describes cases of rheumatoid arthritis greatly improved by removal of sensitizing foods as well as chemicals. Improvement of rheumatoid arthritis by diagnosis and removal of food allergy has been documented elsewhere in medical journals. Cure isn't claimed, but a distinct reduction of symptoms and medication can be achieved.

In my own practice, I've found that rheumatoid arthritis can almost always be improved, from a little to a lot, by strict adherence to a diet free of food allergens and synthetic chemicals of any type. Of course, vitamins, minerals, and amino acids are recommended, too, but people always tell me that certain allergens cause problems every time they're added back, accidentally or on purpose.

Many individuals who have been told they'll have to "live with" their joint pains are surprised to find that their symptoms can be alleviated or even completely eliminated by avoiding foods to which they are allergic. Although osteoarthritis frequently involves joint deterioration, that process appears to be aggravated and in a few cases even caused by allergy.

Recently a nonallergenic, food-sensitivity cause of many cases of osteoarthritis has been found. That food sensitivity is limited to one plant family—the nightshades—and though the exact cause isn't known it appears likely to be a natural food-chemical sensitivity.

Nearly all of us have been eating potatoes, tomatoes, and peppers—members of that family—since we were very small. Some of us eat eggplant, and quite a few smoke tobacco. These foods all belong to the plant family solanaceae, also called the nightshade. Some nightshade plants are very poisonous, but it wasn't until a horticulture professor, Norman Childers, Ph.D., found that tomatoes gave him joint pains that anyone suspected that this entire plant family might be a cause of osteoarthritis (as well as other health problems). Dr. Childers knew that potatoes, tomatoes, peppers, and eggplant all contain many of the same naturally occurring toxic chemicals found in much higher concentrations in belladonna ("deadly nightshade") and other poisonous members of the solanaceae family. He wondered if some individuals might be sensitive to those chemicals even though the chemical is in much smaller concentration in the edible members of the nightshade family.

Based on his own experience, and the cases of many he told his story to, Dr. Childers devised his own "no-nightshade" diet and detailed it in his book, *A Diet To Stop Arthritis*. When he persuaded many people with health problems to try it, he found that some discovered themselves acutely sensitive to nightshade-derived foods, others moderately so, and some not at all. Although many types of symptoms cleared in nightshade-sensitive individuals, the problem most often mentioned as vastly improved or entirely gone was that of osteoarthritis. Almost all who responded to the no-nightshade program proved Dr. Childers's theory, on purpose or by accident, by experiencing a rapid return of symptoms when a nightshade-derived food was entered back into the diet.

I've personally looked for biochemical signs of allergy in nightshade-sensitive individuals; sometimes they can be found, sometimes not. It's theorized that nightshade sensitivity may be due to inhibition of an enzyme, cholinesterase; whether this is true or not hasn't been proven. In any case, although we don't know the whys of such a sensitivity to the nightshade family, we do know that for some people, they are serious problems. As is so frequently the case in medicine, results based on practical observation seem to precede scientific understanding.

## Chemicals in Foods Cause Increasing Health Problems

Food sensitivities can also be triggered by food chemicals such as preservatives. Sensitivity to food chemicals is an area deserving of much more study than it's getting these days, especially since we're being bombarded with more and more unnecessary chemicals.

I simply don't believe artificial chemicals have any place in food at all. Human biochemical systems, functioning much as they have for at least two million years, have not had the time necessary to adapt to the synthetic food chemicals present in our diets for only the last 100 years. As food chemicals are increasingly studied, many more problems are being found.

A good example of a category of food chemicals that is an unnecessary cause of health problems is sulfites. They are used as preservatives to reduce food spoilage by microorganisms, and as antioxidants to retard the discoloration and browning of foods. They're widely found in beer, wine, many processed foods, juices, shrimp, and fresh fruits and vegetables. Restaurants use them heavily on salads, vegetables, and potatoes to give them that fresh, just-picked look.

Under normal conditions the body can usually break down sulfites by an enzyme called sulfite oxidase. However, in 1976 a case was reported of a man who had a severe reaction after eating a restaurant salad treated with sulfite. The reaction was later reproduced by a "challenge" test, in which a person is deliberately exposed to a substance suspected of causing the problem.

In 1977, some asthmatics were reported to become worse after drinking an orange beverage preserved with sulfur dioxide. And other asthmatics were found to react to the sulfite preservative found in an anti-asthmatic drug.

Evidence continues to accumulate in the case against sulfite use. Researchers at the Scripps Institute in La Jolla, California, have reported reactions such as flushing, faintness, weakness, wheezing, shortness of breath, cough, cyanosis (turning bluish), loss of consciousness, and death in sulfite-sensitive individuals. Episodes have often occurred after restaurant meals or after drinking wines. These symptoms can be reproduced with challenge tests with sulfite.

The Scripps researchers searched for evidence of sulfite-provoked abnormalities of the immune system that met the usual medical definition of allergy. None was found. Tentatively, it appears that sulfite sensitivity is caused by a relative deficiency of the enzyme, sulfite oxidase, which breaks down sulfites. Like lactase deficiency, this is a metabolic problem, not an allergic one—but a problem all the same.

It's been "guesstimated" by the Center for Science in the Public Interest that one in 11 asthmatics may be sulfite sensitive. Since there are natural, less-toxic alternatives to sulfites in most if not all of its uses, removing them entirely from the food supply would have a very favorable "benefit-to-cost" ratio. Until this is done, an awareness of the sources of sulfite contamination is important for any possibly sensitive asthmatic (or other individual) and an avoidance of such foods may be beneficial.

Many others, aside from myself, are looking into the question of food sensitivity. Pioneers like Theron Randolph, M.D., Marshall

Mandell, M.D., and William Philpott, M.D., have devoted decades of their careers to demonstrating chemical sensitivities to foods as well as nonfoods. Until recently, they were ignored or ridiculed. Even with interest in the topic increasing, food and other chemical sensitivity is only infrequently considered as an important part of a diagnostic evaluation in difficult health problems.

Times are changing, however, and the overall number of food-sensitive and allergic people appears to be increasing much more rapidly than the growth of the population. But not as fast as it would if there were a greater awareness on the part of the medical profession to identify the problem.

## Food Sensitivity More Frequently Diagnosed

There's an ancient medical school saying: "If you don't look, you won't find it." Food sensitivity as a major cause of illness was rarely looked for by past generations of physicians. Although the situation today is only slightly better, it is changing. Although the increase is small, the resultant successes with previously resistant cases has attracted considerable public and media attention. More frequent diagnosis adds to the impression that the problem of food sensitivity is increasing.

In addition to more frequent diagnosis, however, it appears to me that there has been a real increase in both the number and percentage of food- and chemical-sensitive individuals. There's probably no way this will ever be finally proven or disproven. Until investigators like Dr. Randolph came along in the 1950s and after, no one suspected the dimensions of the problem. Prior to Dr. Randolph, no one was asking the right questions in a systematic way, so comparative data is simply unavailable.

Two factors have, I think, increased the occurrence of food and chemical sensitivities: nutrient deficiencies due to several generations of soil depletion and food processing; and the enormous increase in both the number and quantity of chemicals to which we're all exposed. Again, there's no proof here, but the circumstantial evidence is considerable—and increasing.

In my practice, I've encountered two individuals who became intensely sensitive to foods as adults. Neither had any childhood history of allergy or sensitivity, nor any family history of these problems. The onset of food sensitivity in these two individuals was traced back to chronic exposure to chemicals emanating from photocopiers. Despite complete avoidance of photocopier chemicals for several years, the food sensitivities have persisted.

In another example of overexposure, millions of Michigan residents in 1974 became contaminated with polybrominated biphenyls (PBB) acquired from milk, meat, and other farm products. PBBs got into the food chain when they were accidentally mixed into livestock feed sold primarily to dairy farmers. A few years after the exposure, blood specimens from 45 Michigan dairy farmers were compared with 46 from Wisconsin dairy farmers, and 78 from New York City residents. All of the New York samples were normal, as were all but one from the Wisconsin dairy farmers. That one was from a person with cancer.

Eighteen of the 45 PBB-exposed Michigan dairy farmers showed seriously defective immune system function. The other 27 were described as "not entirely normal." Although the study wasn't concerned with food sensitivity or allergy, a normally functioning immune system is necessary for control of allergy and sensitivity, as well as resistance to infection and defense against cancer. And one of the effects of damage to the immune system can be an alteration in food and chemical sensitivity.

The PBB episode is a "worst-human-case" example. Very few of us have that much chemical exposure. It does forcefully demonstrate, however, the ability of a synthetic chemical to seriously disrupt immune system function. Many other chemicals to which we're frequently exposed have shown similar immune system disruption capability in animal experiments.

Nutrient deficiency is another well-known cause of immune system malfunction. There are many scientific studies proving this point. What's recently been demonstrated in an animal species is that nutrient deficiency in one generation can affect immune function in succeeding generations, even if they're not nutrient deficient. In that experiment pregnant mice were given a zinc-deficient diet. Their offspring had defective immune function, even though they and their mothers were fed a zinc-adequate diet as soon as they were born. Second and third generations of mice also had defective immune system function (although less severe), all while maintaining a zinc-adequate diet. "This study," the researchers said, "has important implications for public health and human welfare, as the consequences of fetal impoverishment may persist despite generations of nutritional supplementation. Dietary supplementation beyond the levels considered adequate might allow for more rapid or complete restoration of immunocompetence." Put another way, it's possible that immune system defects suffered by you or me (including overreactivity to foods) could be due to nutrient deficiencies suffered by our grandmothers in the months before they were born. It's also possible that diet supplemenatation (vitamins, minerals, and so on) above the usual levels might aid in more rapid recovery.

Food sensitivity is a major part of the large problem of environmental sensitivity, superbly covered in Dr. Randolph's book, *An Alternative Approach to Allergies.*

Until you've adopted a "new traditional" diet, made sure it's being digested and absorbed, and then made certain you're not sensitive to it, don't let anyone tell you your symptoms are "all in your head." And even if you're feeling well, checking into food sensitivities can be most rewarding. I'm frequently told that fatigue, aches, pains, and other minor problems accepted as "that's life" or "part of getting old" have actually disappeared when food sensitivities were finally identified.

## REFERENCES

**Arthritis**

Childers, Norman Franklin. *A Diet To Stop Arthritis.* Somerset Press, 1981.

Randolph, Theron G., and Moss, Ralph W. *An Alternative Approach to Allergies*. Lippincott & Crowell, 1979, pp. 129–137.

## Chemical Toxicity

Chen, Edwin. *PBB: An American Tragedy*. Prentice-Hall, 1979, p. 246.

Gunnison, A. F. "Sulphite Toxicity: A Critical Review of *In Vitro* and *In Vivo* Data." *Food and Cosmetic Toxicology*, October, 1981, pp. 667–682.

Gunnison, Albert F., and Farruggella, Thomas J. "Preferential S-Sulfonate Formation In Lung and Aorta." *Chemical-Biological Interactions*, vol. 25, 1979, pp. 271–277.

Stevenson, Donald D., and Simon, Ronald A. "Sensitivity to Ingested Metabisulfites in Asthmatic Subjects." *Journal of Allergy and Clinical Immunology*, July, 1981, pp. 26–32.

## Gallbladder Disease

Breneman, J. C. "Allergy Elimination Diet As the Most Effective Gallbladder Diet." *Annals of Allergy*, February, 1968, pp. 83–87.

———. *Basics of Food Allergy*. Charles C Thomas, 1978, pp. 67–69.

Necheles, H. et al. "Allergy of the Gall Bladder." *American Journal of Digestive Diseases*, vol. 7, no. 6, 1940, pp. 238–241.

Walzer, Matthew et al. "The Allergic Reaction in the Gall Bladder." *Gastroenterology*, vol. 1, 1943, pp. 565–572.

## Lactose Intolerance

American Academy of Pediatrics, Committee on Nutrition. "The Practical Significance of Lactose Intolerance in Children." *Pediatrics*, August, 1978, pp. 240–250.

Barr, Ronald G.; Levine, Melvin D.; and Watkins, John B. "Recurrent Abdominal Pain of Childhood Due to Lactose Intolerance." *New England Journal of Medicine*, June 28, 1979, pp. 1449–1452.

Flatz, Gebhard, and Rotthauwe, Hans Werner. "Lactose

Nutrition and Natural Selection." *Lancet*, July 14, 1973, pp. 76–77.

Kuitunen, P. et al. "Response of the Jejunal Mucosa to Cow's Milk in the Malabsorption Syndrome with Cow's Milk Intolerance." *Acta Pediatrica Scandinavica*, vol. 62, 1973, pp. 585–595.

Liebman, William M. "Recurrent Abdominal Pain in Children: Lactose and Sucrose Intolerance, A Prospective Study." *Pediatrics*, July, 1979, pp. 43–45.

McElroy, Ann, and Townsend, Patricia K. *Medical Anthropology In Ecological Perspective*. Duxbury Press, 1979, pp. 97–100.

Matsumura, T.; Kuroume, T.; and Amada, K. "Close Relationship between Lactose Intolerance and Allergy to Milk Protein." *Journal of Asthma Research*, September, 1971, pp. 13–29.

# 6 A GENETIC DEFECT WE ALL SHARE— HYPOASCORBEMIA

You have a genetic defect. I have it, too. It's in the family—yours and mine. We're not related? Of course we are, if only very distantly. That genetic defect is what we share in common with the entire human race. It's called hypoascorbemia and refers to the low levels of ascorbate we have in our blood.

Ascorbate? Isn't that a fancy word for vitamin C? Nothing new here! Lack of vitamin C has been known for years to lead to scurvy—a vitamin deficiency disease. There's vitamin C in our diets, and many of us take a little extra. So why all the fuss about a genetic defect?

Because that universal defect interferes with our production of vitamin C and appears to be responsible for a wide range of illnesses. Problems that *can* be prevented.

We all know that vitamins are substances essential to health, and that they can't be produced by our own bodies. Vitamin C fits this definition for humans, as do vitamins A, all the Bs except niacin (vitamin B₃), D, E, K, and so on. But vitamin C isn't a vitamin required by dogs, cats, horses, or the vast majority of living beings. They make their own.

The internal production of vitamin C is almost universal to animal life. An identical series of four enzymes transforms blood sugar, also known as glucose, into vitamin C in all animal species except guinea pigs, fruit bats, red-vented bulbul birds, other primates (gorillas, chimpanzees, monkeys)—and man. Aside from producing vitamin C, these enzymes serve no other purpose.

In the human liver, the first three enzymes required for vitamin C synthesis are present. Only the fourth enzyme is missing. In animals capable of vitamin C production internally (the vast majority), more can be made whenever it's needed. Humans have *lost* their automatic capability to adjust internal vitamin C production to demand, and must rely on whatever is found in the diet. Having the right amount of vitamin C available at just the right time can have a significant protective effect.

Most animals, for example, respond to drugs by producing much more vitamin C internally. Since vitamin C has been found experimentally to protect animals against a wide variety of toxic agents and physical stresses, increased internal synthesis is logically assumed to be one way animals protect themselves biochemically. In humans, on the other hand, taking drugs activates the three remaining enzymes of the ascorbate synthesis chain, producing more of the ascorbate precursors D-glucuronic acid, D-glucuronic acid lactone, and L-gulonolactone. Since the final step can't be completed without the missing enzyme, L-gulonolactone oxidase, more ascorbate can't be made.

As that is such a key point, let's look at it in another way. When an animal is given a drug (or other biochemical stress), four imaginary wheels start turning. The vitamin C assembly line churns out finished ascorbate as needed. In humans, the first three wheels spin, busily making previtamin C substances, but since the fourth wheel is missing, the first three spin in vain. The assembly line is broken. An no vitamin C is produced.

Compensation for that ascorbate synthesis defect could make an enormous difference to human health. Potent carcinogens, for example, have been shown to stimulate the synthesis of large quantities of vitamin C by those animals capable of producing it.

In humans, vitamin C has been shown to protect against some cancer-causing substances. If humans could produce *more* vitamin C when exposed to hazardous substances, as most animals do, it's very probable that some cancers could be prevented.

The potential health benefits from supplemental vitamin C aren't limited to cancer prevention or drug detoxification. Vitamin C could be a valuable defense against viral illness, which we all experience at one time or another. In a scientific study of winter illness, individuals were asked to take one gram of vitamin C daily, and to increase their intake to four grams at the first sign of any illness. In a very small way, that process would mimic the increased vitamin C production of stressed animals. Although the researchers claimed that one gram of vitamin C daily wasn't more effective than placebos (fake pills) in preventing winter illness, they pointed out that those who took four grams of vitamin C daily felt better more quickly than those who didn't. Millions of dollars could be saved each year in time lost from work, concluded the researchers, if everyone recovered more quickly with the help of ascorbate.

# Vitamin C Protects against Disease

The potential vitamin C has for disease prevention, treatment, and good health maintenance could fill an entire book—and has. Irwin Stone, M.D., a pioneer in vitamin C research, notes in his book *The Healing Factor* that experiment after experiment demonstrate vitamin C's protective effects against cancer-causing agents, viruses (including polio, hepatitis, herpes, encephalitis), bacteria, bacterial toxins (tetanus, staphylococcus, whooping cough), allergens, chemical poisons, toxic metals, extremes of heat or cold, radiation, and the physical stress of injury. Dr. Stone, who originated the concept of hypoascorbemia, and other vitamin C proponents have been severely criticized on the grounds that no one thing could be capable of so much. If we understand what almost all animals do biochemically in response to any of these stresses—increasing their internal vitamin C production—it becomes perfectly clear why added vitamin C might help humans.

Perhaps you take extra vitamin C already. And you add a little more when you're ill. Even if most physicians need to be convinced, you don't. Haven't you done all you can with vitamin C? Probably not, if you're still thinking of it as vitamin C, a vitamin like the rest, and not as the substance needed to fully correct your genetic disease.

Many biochemically oriented physicians, including myself, are convinced that lifelong full correction of hypoascorbemia is one major key to optimum health. Full correction means the amount needed to keep the system saturated with vitamin C, as it would be if our genetic deficit were truly corrected or hadn't happened. Although at present there's no way to know what an internally produced saturation level might be, there's an overwhelming likelihood that it would be higher than the Recommended Dietary Allowance (RDA) for vitamin C, which is 60 milligrams.

Dr. Stone notes that the 1962 National Research Council's committee on animal nutrition recommends 55 milligrams of vitamin C per kilogram (2.2 pounds) of body weight for monkeys. By contrast, the RDA for humans (also established by the National Research Council) is 60 milligrams—approximately *one* milligram per kilogram of body weight. Since neither monkey nor man can manufacture their own vitamin C, Dr. Stone suggests that one of those two figures must be wrong, and concludes that the amount recommended for monkeys (55 milligrams per kilogram) is closer to the true human daily requirement. When adjusted for human body weight, that calculates as nearly 4,000 milligrams (four grams) for the average adult human. Dr. Stone concludes that several grams of vitamin C daily may be necessary for full correction of our genetic defect.

# Vitamin C Needs Increase with Illness

Biochemically oriented physicians use the "body-tolerance" approach as a more individualized method of determining the quantity of vitamin C needed to fully correct hypoascorbemia. Body tolerance is the largest amount of vitamin C which can be taken without causing excess intestinal gas production, loose stools, or diarrhea. Starting with a small quantity, perhaps 500 to 1,000 milligrams with each meal, the amount is gradually increased every day until one of the foregoing symptoms is noted. Quantities are then decreased slightly to the largest amount tolerable, and continued (with adjustment as needed) indefinitely.

Individuals feeling well most often discover a body-tolerance quantity of 2 to 12 grams daily. Individuals who aren't feeling well frequently find their needs increase to 10 to 30 or more grams daily. Biochemically oriented physicians usually recommend that even these higher quantities be continued as long as tolerated, with appropriate precautions. Usually, as health improves, the amount tolerated gradually decreases.

Support for body-tolerance doses of vitamin C comes from the clinical work of two physicians, Frederick R. Klenner, M.D. and Robert Cathcart, M.D. Reviewing nine years of experience with over 9,000 individuals taking body-tolerance doses of vitamin C, Dr. Cathcart found that the more ill an individual was, the higher his or her body tolerance for vitamin C. Healthy persons could take 4 to 15 grams spread over 24 hours. Individuals with allergies had a body tolerance of 15 to 25 grams; those with mild colds 30 to 60 grams; severe colds 60 to 100 grams; burns, injury, or surgery 25 to 150 grams; mononucleosis 150 to 200 grams; and bacterial infections 100 to 200 grams daily.

Escalating ability to absorb with increasing stress of illness is exactly as predicted by the genetic disease concept of hypoascorbemia. Animals produce more vitamin C when stressed. Humans, on the other hand, unable to synthesize their own, should be able to absorb and use increasing quantities with increasing illness stress.

As long ago as 1949, Dr. Klenner, one of the pioneers in vitamin C therapeutics, reported in *Southern Medicine and Surgery* that up to 200 grams of vitamin C daily could successfully reverse a variety of severe viral illnesses, including polio and encephalitis. Since vitamin C was considered by nearly all physicians to be "only a vitamin," required in trace amounts, his work was ignored, even though the treatment was effective and non-toxic.

For routine use, Dr. Klenner recommends one gram of vitamin C daily for one-year-olds, two grams daily for two-year-olds, and so on until ten years of age, when ten grams daily becomes his recommended adult dose. In 1971, he reported in the *Journal of Applied Nutrition* on 104 infants born to mothers who took four grams of vitamin C daily for the first trimester, six grams daily during the second trimester, and ten grams daily thereafter. None of the infants had birth defects. Dr. Klenner reports they appeared healthier than infants of mothers who hadn't taken extra vitamin C.

In *The Healing Factor*, Dr. Stone details research concerning vitamin C and aging retardation, arthritis, atherosclerotic disease, diabetes, and other illnesses. Simply because any illness is stress, extra vitamin C is indicated, but the research cited does note specific beneficial effects of vitamin C on these and other disease processes.

Of all disease processes, aging and atherosclerosis deserve special mention. Research on aging has focused on free radicals and other molecules that cause oxidative damage to the body, and on gradual failure of the immune system as major factors in aging. Vitamin C is an effective antioxidant free-radical scavenger and immune system stimulant. In both those capacities, it can slow the aging process.

Vitamin C also normalizes elevated blood-fat levels. I've found high-dose vitamin C treatment effective in reversing moderately severe atherosclerosis (see "A Case of Poor Circulation"). And I believe that adequate vitamin C as well as other dietary habits are equally capable of actually *preventing* atherosclerotic changes.

Despite excellent results and apparent safety of high-dose oral vitamin C treatment, it's been rightly observed that any substance, including water, can cause some individual problems when used in much higher than usual amounts. Until considerably more experience with "full correction" of hypoascorbemia has been accumulated, it's advisable to work with a knowledgeable nutritionally oriented physician.

## Hazards of Large Doses of Vitamin C Are Few

What are the hazards of correcting hypoascorbemia with body-tolerance quantities of vitamin C? Few. They're preventable and, in my opinion, much less than the hazards of inadequate correction.

As the implications of hypoascorbemia as a genetic disease spread throughout the health professions, opposition to its full correction will probably fade, particularly since the emphasis in treatment of nearly all other genetic diseases is on complete correction whenever possible.

Present opposition to full-dose vitamin C is summarized by a textbook of pharmacology, *The Pharmacological Basis of Therapeutics:* "Any benefit that might be derived from such use of ascorbic acid seems small when weighed against the expense and risks of the megadose treatment. The latter include formation of kidney stones resulting from the excessive excretion of oxalate, rebound scurvy in the offspring of mothers taking high doses, and a similar phenomenon when subjects who are consuming large amounts of vitamin C suddenly stop. . . . Excessive doses of ascorbic acid can also enhance the absorption of iron and interfere with anticoagulant therapy. . . ."

Reference to "expense" reveals unfamiliarity with the cost of vitamin C. One major mail-order manufacturer/distributor offers a pound (454 grams) of ascorbic acid crystals for $7.95. If used at a rate of six to eight grams daily, an average adult body-tolerance quantity, a pound would last 57 to 76 days, or cost $3.20 to $4.20 per month. Other forms of vitamin C are more expensive, but still don't constitute a major financial burden.

Formation of calcium oxalate kidney stones is the only real "risk" on the list. It happens rarely—in ten years, I've observed it once. And I've worked with a few individuals who might have had a kidney stone if they hadn't checked their oxalate metabolism before taking relatively large quantities of vitamin C. So some caution is in order.

An occasional individual taking more than three to four grams of vitamin C daily may greatly increase his or her oxalate excretion. If excess oxalate excretion is sustained over months to years, it's possible that calcium oxalate stones could be formed. One investigator, Michael Briggs, tested 67 individuals for vitamin C-induced hyperoxaluria (excess urinary oxalate excretion). He found it occurred in three of those tested. Since two of the three individuals were related, he suggested that the response to vitamin C may also be genetically determined. "It would seem a reasonable precaution," concludes Briggs, "to recommend screening for ascorbate-induced hyperoxaluria in all people considering vitamin C supplementation." Given all the contradictory research on that point, Briggs's suggestion is quite reasonable, especially if there's a family history of kidney stones.

Those few persons who discover a problem can discontinue the amount of vitamin C causing it. Alternatively, vitamin $B_6$ and magnesium can greatly reduce oxalate stone formation from any cause.

Rebound scurvy in the offspring of mothers taking high doses isn't really a problem, if the newborn infant is nursed. Vitamin C transfers through the breast extremely well, so well that new mothers often need to cut back their own vitamin C intake because it gives the infant gas. Assuming that a mother is taking vitamin C to compensate for her own genetic defect, she'll want her children to stay healthy, too, and start them on their own vitamin C during weaning.

Rebound scurvy in the newborn is only a problem in the artificial circumstances of some hospitals, which keep infants separate from their mothers and off the breast too long, or worse, those advocating bottle feeding. Fortunately, the number of such hospitals is rapidly declining. Even under such circumstances, a small amount of supplemental vitamin C will eliminate that risk.

Likewise, rebound scurvy in "subjects who are consuming large amounts of vitamin C [and] suddenly stop" is possible, but whether it constitutes a risk depends on one's point of view. Presumably, an individual who's made the decision to fully correct his or her hypoascorbemia for health optimization is going to continue doing so for life. If for any reason a decision is made to stop, tapering down gradually will prevent rebound scurvy.

Vitamin C definitely enhances iron absorption. Why this should be viewed as a risk is a mystery, since iron deficiency occurs overwhelmingly more often than iron excess. Even in body-tolerance quantities, vitamin C will not lead to iron overdose in the vast majority of cases. For those rare individuals with hemochromatosis or otherwise at risk of iron overload, not taking large doses of vitamin C is wisest. If there's any question at all, a physician should be consulted.

Anticoagulants can only be obtained on prescription. Individuals taking full hypoascorbemia correction who are given a recommendation for anticoagulants should discuss the situation with their physicians. There are two options, and gradations in between: stopping all ascorbate and taking a smaller dose of anticoagulant; or maintaining ascorbate and taking a larger dose of anticoagulant to achieve the same blood-thinning effect.

In my opinion and that of Dr. Stone, individuals who use a lifelong adequate quantity of vitamin C considerably lessen the risk of stroke, heart attack, or other conditions for which anticoagulants might be prescribed.

Others have reported risks of high-dose vitamin C not mentioned in the pharmacology text. Vitamin C destruction of vitamin $B_{12}$ was found not to occur when more accurate means of measurement were employed. Similarly, improved techniques have shown that a previously reported vitamin C effect on uric acid may not exist.

Although it's never been reported as a risk of oral vitamin C, a possible risk (in some individuals) of high-dose intravenous vitamin C should be noted. In a single case, an extremely large quantity of ascorbic acid, 80 grams, was given intravenously on each of two consecutive days to an individual with second-degree burns of the hand. Four days later he was admitted to a hospital and subsequently died. It was found he had a red blood cell defect, deficiency of the enzyme glucose-6-phosphate dehydrogenase. The authors, G. Douglas Campbell and associates, who reported the case, suspected that individuals with this defect might be at risk for red cell hemolysis (breakdown) if given high doses of vitamin C intravenously.

Although only one case has been reported, and it can't be said for certain whether the 80 grams of intravenous vitamin C caused the problem, the possibility should be kept in mind. Glucose-6-phosphate dehydrogenase deficiency is the enzyme defect involved in fava bean and primaquine sensitivities. It occurs in 10 percent of North American black males, and in varying percentages among Sephardic Jews, persons of Mediterranean descent (particularly those from Sicily, Sardinia, Malta, and Tunisia), South American Indians, Chinese, Thai, and Melanesians. More than 100 variations of this defect have been described. The Mediterranean variety appears worst. Several drugs also cause hemolysis in individuals with this disorder, including high doses of the analgesics—aspirin and phenacetin; the anti-infectives—sulfisoxazole, primaquine, and chloroquine (antimalarials); nitrofuran antibacterials; and water-soluble vitamin K derivatives.

Glucose-6-phosphate dehydrogenase deficiency can be detected with a blood test, so any one at risk can be tested. Vitamin E has been found protective against hemolysis in glucose-6-phosphate dehydrogenase deficiency.

Considering the large quantities of vitamin C sold in the United States alone, it's probably safe to assume that any other serious hazards would have been found by now. Except for a small percentage of oxalate stone formers, the risks of taking 2 to 12 grams of vitamin C daily, the usual body-tolerance quantity (increased when ill), appears extremely small and the potential benefits enormous.

## Our Genetic Defect Is Correctable

For countless generations, the human race has suffered the effects of hypoascorbemia. Hundreds of thousands have died from scurvy, hypoascorbemia's terminal form. Dr. Stone's contribution has been to point out that hundreds of millions have suffered illness due to nonfatal but very inadequately corrected (through diet alone) hypoascorbemia. An unknown percentage of all cancer, heart disease, stroke, other atherosclerotic disease, asthma and allergy, diabetes, and bacterial and viral illness appears to be preventable or improvable with full correction of this genetic defect. Vitamin C enables more effective treatment of poisoning, injury, and a retardation of aging.

Until the 1930s, the identity of the substance needed to correct scurvy wasn't known. Until the 1950s, it wasn't understood that scurvy is simply the terminal form of an inborn error of metabolism, L-gulonolactone oxidase deficiency, a genetic disease usually manifested as hypoascorbemia. With this knowledge, each of us has an opportunity unprecedented in former generations. You and I can choose (or not choose) to fully correct our genetic disease. It's been estimated by Linus Pauling, Nobel Prize winner in biochemistry, that full correction of hypoascorbemia could increase the average life expectancy by five to six years. While living longer, we could be much healthier along the way.

Dr. Stone illuminated the path. Dr. Cathcart established the safety of large oral doses. The known risks of fully correcting hypoascorbemia appear small, and can be tested for in advance. Biochemically oriented physicians, knowledgeable about and capable of supervising hypoascorbemia correction, are located all around the United States. (Although their number is small, it's growing.) An inexpensive way to improve quality and length of life appears available to each of us.

You have a genetic defect. What you do about it is up to you.

## REFERENCES

### Cholesterol
Lee, Virginia. "Individual Trends in the Total Serum Cholesterol of Children and Adolescents Over a Ten-Year Period." *American Journal of Clinical Nutrition*, January, 1967, pp. 5–12.

**Colds and Flu**

Anderson, Terence et al. "Winter Illness and Vitamin C: The Effect of Relatively Low Doses." *Canadian Medical Association Journal*, April 5, 1975, pp. 823–826.

Pauling, Linus. *Vitamin C and the Common Cold*. W. H. Freeman, 1970, pp. ix–x.


**Enzyme Deficiency**

Beeson, Paul B.; McDermott, Walsh; and Wyngaarden, James B., eds. *Cecil Textbook of Medicine*. 15th ed. W. B. Saunders, 1979, pp. 1760–1761.

Campbell, G. Douglas; Steinberg, Martin H.; and Bower, John D. "Ascorbic Acid-Induced Hemolysis in G-6-PD Deficiency." *Annals of Internal Medicine*, June, 1975, p. 810.

Goth, Andres. *Medical Pharmacology—Principles and Concepts*. 7th ed. C. V. Mosby, 1974, pp. 549, 570, and 619.

Henry, John Bernard. *Clinical Diagnosis and Management*. 16th ed. W. B. Saunders, 1979, p. 1025.

Martin, Wayne. *Medical Heroes and Heretics*. Devin-Adair, 1977, pp. 72–77.

Schrier, Stanley L. "Anemia: Hemolysis." In Section 5: Hematology, *Scientific American Medicine*. Scientific American, pp. 8–11.

Wade, Ainley, and Reynolds, James E. F., eds. *Martindale—The Extra Pharmacopoeia*. Pharmaceutical Press, 1977.


**Genetic Defect**

Stone, Irwin. *The Healing Factor*. Grosset & Dunlap, 1972.


**Kidney Stones**

Briggs, Michael. "Vitamin-C-Induced Hyperoxaluria." *Lancet*, January 17, 1976, p. 154.

Gilman, Alfred Goodman; Goodman, Louis S.; and Gilman, Alfred, eds. *The Pharmacological Basis of Therapeutics*. 6th ed. Macmillan Publishing, 1980, pp. 1579–1580.

Hughes, Christine; Dutton, Stephen; and Truswell, A. Stewart. "High Intake of Ascorbic Acid and Urinary Oxalate." *Journal of Human Nutrition*, vol. 35, 1981, pp. 274–280.

Mitch, William E. et al. "Effect of Large Oral Doses of Ascorbic Acid on Uric Acid Excretion by Normal Subjects." *Clinical Pharmacology and Therapeutics*, vol. 29, no. 3, 1981, pp. 318–321.

Schmidt, Karl-Heinz et al. "Urinary Oxalate Excretion After Large Intakes of Ascorbic Acid in Man." *American Journal of Clinical Nutrition*, March, 1981, pp. 305–311.

**Niacin (Vitamin $B_3$)**

Marks, John. *A Guide to the Vitamins*. Medical Technical Press, p. 105.

Wilson, Eva D.; Fisher, Katherine H.; and Fuqua, Mary E. *Principles of Nutrition*. 3rd ed., John Wiley & Sons, 1975. pp. 265–266.

**Tolerance Levels**

Cathcart, Robert. "The Method of Determining Proper Doses of Vitamin C for the Treatment of Disease by Titrating to Bowel Tolerance." *Orthomolecular Psychiatry*, vol. 10, no. 2, 1981, pp. 125–132.

**Vitamin $B_{12}$**

Herbert, Victor, and Jacob, Elizabeth. "Destruction of Vitamin $B_{12}$ by Vitamin C." *Journal of the American Medical Association*, October 14, 1974, pp. 241–242.

Hogenkamp, H. P. C. "The Interaction Between Vitamin $B_{12}$ and Vitamin C." *American Journal of Clinical Nutrition*, January, 1980, pp. 1–3.

Marcus, M.; Prabhudesai, M.; and Wassef, S. "Stability of Vitamin $B_{12}$ in the Presence of Ascorbic Acid in Food and Serum: Restoration by Cyanide of Apparent Loss." *American Journal of Clinical Nutrition*, January, 1980, pp. 137–143.

Newmark, Harold L. et al. "Ascorbic Acid and Vitamin $B_{12}$." *Journal of the American Medical Association*, November 23, 1979, pp. 2319–2320.

## Vitamin C

Gilman, Alfred, and Goodman, Louis. *The Pharmacological Basis of Therapeutics*. 4th ed., Macmillan Publishing, 1970, pp. 1667–1668.

Klenner, Frederick R. "Observations on the Dose and Administration of Ascorbic Acid When Employed Beyond the Range of a Vitamin in Human Pathology." *Journal of Applied Nutrition*, vol. 23, 1971, pp. 61–88.

──────. "The Treatment of Poliomyelitis and Other Virus Diseases with Vitamin C." *Southern Medicine and Surgery*, vol. 111, 1949, pp. 209–214.

Kutsky, Roman J. *Handbook of Vitamins, Minerals and Hormones*. 2nd ed. Van Nostrand Reinhold, 1981, p. 254.

"Vitamin C Toxicity." *Nutrition Reviews*, August, 1976, pp. 236–237.

White, J. Douglas. "No Ill Effects from High-Dose Vitamin C." *New England Journal of Medicine*, June 11, 1981, p. 1491.

# 7 FOLATE: A WEAPON AGAINST BIRTH DEFECTS

Spina bifida. Myelomeningocele. Microcephaly. Anencephaly. These medical terms, designating split spine, deformity of the spinal cord and its coverings, abnormally small head, and a poorly developed head, are only some of the many birth defects of the nervous system generally grouped under the term *neural-tube defects*.

Defects of the neural tube (so named because of the appearance of the early embryonic brain and spinal cord) are a serious, relatively common birth defect. A comprehensive textbook on spina bifida and associated defects points out that about two of every thousand infants born live will have a neural-tube defect.

Children with neural-tube defects usually have lifelong handicaps. Many cannot walk. A large number have no bowel or bladder control. Many undergo a long series of surgical operations to compensate for those and other congenital deformities.

Yet it's very possible that such tragedies would be entirely preventable if mothers-to-be took small quantities of folate, a B vitamin (also called folic acid or folacin). Some observers would say not only possible, but probable. Let's review some evidence. Then you can make your own decision about folate, especially if your family has a history of neural-tube defects.

Evidence that lack of folate might be involved in neural-tube defects has been accumulating for years. As far back as 1952, it was observed that aminopterin, a powerful folate antagonist, caused several cases of anencephaly. However, the most positive evidence is recent.

In 1980, Dr. R. W. Smithells of the University of Leeds (England) reported a study involving women who had previously given birth to babies with neural-tube defects. For these women, the anticipated recurrence rate of neural-tube defects in subsequent pregnancies is 5 percent. One group of mothers took a multivitamin formulation providing 0.36 milligrams of folate daily. Another group took no vitamins, or started them too late. (The daily formula also provided 4,000 international units of vitamin A, 400 units of vitamin D, 1.5 milligrams of $B_1$, 1.5 milligrams of riboflavin [$B_2$], 1 milligram of $B_6$, 15 milligrams of niacinamide [an active form of niacin], 40 milligrams of vitamin C, 75.6 milligrams of iron, and 480 milligrams of calcium phosphate.)

## Start Supplements before Conception

Dr. Smithells emphasized that timing of the vitamin supplementation is critical. Normal neural-tube closure takes place during the fourth week after conception; most women have not missed the first menstrual period by then and frequently aren't aware of the pregnancy until this crucial time has passed. Supplementation should be started at least 28 days (approximately one menstrual cycle) before conception to insure adequate folate throughout the early days following conception.

In Dr. Smithells's study, only one baby with neural-tube defect was born to the 178 mothers who took the vitamins (0.6 percent). Thirteen babies or fetuses with neural-tube defects were delivered by the 260 women who took no vitamins (5 percent, the predicted recurrence rate). For scientists, the difference between 0.6 percent and 5 percent is significant.

Of course, one study is not considered conclusive, even if it shows a significant result. However, criticism of Dr. Smithells's study was principally on other grounds, a classic confrontation between scientific objectivity and ethical considerations.

Currently, many scientists do not consider a scientific point proven unless subjected to a "random double-blind, placebo-controlled" trial. In such a trial, roughly half the participants (randomly chosen) are given the substance to be tested, and half are given a nontherapeutic placebo (fake pill) identical to the test substance in every other respect. Neither the participants nor the investigators know who gets the placebo or the active substance until the trial is completed. In this way, all psychological, subjective influence is said to be eliminated, and the results are interpreted as objectively valid. A typical comment about Dr. Smithells's study from this point of view was made in a letter to the British medical journal *Lancet:* "Had a properly controlled, randomized trial been conducted, doctors would now have no doubt as to whether or not they could reassure a high-risk patient that she would decrease the risk of a neural-tube defect (NTD) by periconceptional vitamin supplementation."

On the other hand, many people, including some scientists, are troubled by the ethical implications of withholding possibly effective treatment to prove a scientific point. From this point of view, it would be unethical in the extreme to allow the birth of even one baby with a lifelong crippling disease if there is good reason to suspect the defect could be prevented. Dr. Smithells's study was originally designed with a placebo, but this aspect was disallowed by the three ethics committees that reviewed it.

## No Recurrence of Defects

An even more recent study used the double-blind, placebo-controlled, randomized model. Reported by Professor K. M.

Laurence and co-workers of the Welsh National School of Medicine, the study tested the effect of four milligrams of folate daily
(started well before potential conception) against a placebo, once
again with mothers who had previously borne a child with a
neural-tube defect. The trial started with 60 women in the vitamin
group, 51 in the placebo group, but finished with 44 women who
actually took their vitamins, and 67 who didn't. (Sixteen of the
women who were supposed to take their vitamins did not.)

The result: There were no recurrences of neural-tube defect
among the offspring of mothers who took folate. There were six
recurrences in the group who didn't take folate—four in the
placebo group and two in the group who were supposed to take
folate but didn't. Again the difference is meaningful: zero recurrences of neural-tube defect versus six.

Thus, both recent studies—the smaller double-blind, placebo-
controlled test and the much larger nonplacebo comparison
study—have reported a significant effect of folate in preventing
neural-tube defect recurrence.

In his second study published in 1981, Dr. Smithells reported
that of 200 folate-supplemented women, only one child was born
with a neural-tube defect. Yet, 13 children with the problem were
born to 300 women who didn't take folate. The difference, 0.5
percent versus 4.3 percent, was statistically significant to the
scientific community.

According to *Pulse*, a publication for British physicians, a
third investigator, Professor Norman Nevin of Queen's University,
Belfast, has found a sevenfold reduction in the occurrence of
neural-tube defects with folate (folic acid) supplementation.

The Medical Research Council of Great Britain considers
these studies to be promising enough to launch a governmentally
funded, larger study. However, the council doesn't consider
Dr. Smithells's results "scientifically valid" because no placebo
was used. Professor Laurence's investigation did use a placebo, but
the research coordinator for the council said it did not include
enough women to be considered conclusive. So the medical
research council intends to proceed with a much larger double-
blind, placebo-controlled investigation.

The ethics of this study have created a controversy in Great Britain. According to *Pulse*, newspaper headlines have accused the council researchers of using women as guinea pigs. The company that supplied the vitamins for Dr. Smithells's research declined to manufacture them with matching placebo for the Medical Research Council study. According to *Pulse*, a spokesman for the company said: "We declined to supply the latter [the placebo tablets]. The difference between today and when Dr. Smithells did his original study is that we now have considerable evidence that supplements administered in the right dosage and at the right time will reduce the incidence of NTDs [neural-tube defects]—that means there are ethical considerations to withholding them."

# Folate May Prevent
# Other Birth Defects

Folate appears to be important in the prevention of another type of birth defect, cleft lip and cleft palate. Following up in 1976 on previously suggestive studies reported in 1958, 1960, and 1964, Dr. M. Tolarova studied the recurrence of cleft lip with or without cleft palate in children born to women who had previously had a child with this problem.

Eighty-five women were asked to take 10 milligrams of folate (folic acid) along with multiple vitamins (containing 6,000 international units of vitamin A, 3 milligrams thiamine [vitamin $B_1$], 3 milligrams riboflavin [vitamin $B_2$], 3 milligrams vitamin $B_6$, 150 milligrams vitamin C, 300 units vitamin D, 9 international units vitamin E, 30 milligrams niacinamide, and 3 milligrams calcium pantothenate) starting three months before conception. In another group 212 women were advised not to take any supplements.

Of the 85 supplemented women, only one child was born with cleft lip, whereas 15 were born with this defect in the unsupplemented group of 212 women. This recurrence rate, 1.2 percent versus 7.4 percent, was highly significant.

Although cleft lip and cleft palate are not usually as disabling as neural-tube defects, anyone who's ever seen a child with these problems would agree it's another birth defect well worth preventing.

A study in the *South African Medical Journal* of mothers giving birth to low weight for gestational age infants found that 49 percent of the mothers had low red blood cell folic acid (folate) levels. A related study in *Acta Obstetricia et Gynecologia Scandinavia* reported the effects of five milligrams of folate started at the twenty-third week of pregnancy (versus no folate) on the birth weight of infants. Although the age at birth was full term (281 days) in both groups, the babies born to the folate-supplemented mothers were 12.7 percent heavier than the babies in the control group. There was a significant correlation between red blood cell folate and birth weight in this study also.

Some researchers have suggested that yet another type of birth defect, associated with an inherited chromosomal abnormality (the fragile-x chromosome) might be treatable with folate. Individuals with the fragile-x syndrome (all male) were relatively normal in physical appearance, but had I.Q.s from 20 to 80, considerably below the average of 100. Cells taken from individuals with fragile-x chromosomes only show the abnormality when grown in a culture medium low in folate. When more folate is present, cells cultured from the same individual appear normal. This suggests (although it doesn't prove) that if mothers carrying the fragile-x chromosome were given sufficient folate before conception and throughout pregnancy, and if the infants were immediately started and maintained on supplemental folate if necessary, the mental retardation characteristic of the syndrome might be prevented.

Prenatal prevention of disease is not unprecedented. It's already been done in another rare genetic condition, using the vitamin biotin.

The list of congenital conditions possible or probably preventable with folate is continuing to grow:

- cleft lip
- cleft palate
- mental retardation associated with fragile-x syndrome

- some cases of low birth weight for age
- delayed infant development in the first months and years.
- spina bifida
- microcephaly
- anencephaly

Anything we can do individually and collectively to encourage researchers to study the potential of folate for preventing these and other birth defects is very important. The prospective payoff in terms of whole, happy children capable of reaching their full potential as adults is enormous.

Even more important, prospective mothers can ensure for themselves and their own infants a sufficient supply of folate before, during, and after pregnancy with no known toxic potential. But folate alone isn't enough. Carefully planned whole-food "new traditional" diets, supplemented where safe and necessary, can go even further in minimizing the number of infants born with birth defects.

## Folate Supplementation: A Question of Safety?

If this evidence is reliable—and so far it appears to be—then it is reasonable to expect that folate supplementation starting well before conception will likewise prevent spina bifida and other neural-tube defects as well as the other birth defects mentioned.

Before deciding to take folate (or any other vitamin supplement), there are other aspects to consider. Is it safe? How great is the risk to your baby if you don't take it? Do you, personally, really need it?

According to a textbook of pharmacology, *The Pharmacological Basis of Therapeutics*, "orally taken folic acid [folate] is nontoxic in man." The same text reports that folate might counteract the effects of anticonvulsant medications but also says these reports have been contradicted. Since it's also known that anticonvulsant medication increases the risk of folate deficiency, it's possible that women taking these medications have an increased risk of bearing babies with neural-tube defects.

Even on prescription, the Food and Drug Administration limits the maximum dose of folate to one milligram. This is not because of considerations of safety, but because folate might interfere with the diagnosis of vitamin $B_{12}$ deficiency, which, if prolonged, could lead to degeneration of the spinal cord. Fortunately, the chances are remote of that happening in women in childbearing age. Besides, vitamin $B_{12}$ can also be taken safely.

Folate is generally considered safe to fetuses as well; in fact, many American-made prenatal vitamins contain one milligram of folate, more than the amount used in Smithells's study, for example.

Not every folate-deficient mother will give birth to a child with a neural-tube defect. The available evidence indicates that, as is often the case, it's an interaction between genetics and environment (in this case, diet). However, there are other risks of folate deficiency in pregnancy. In 1974, R. L. Gross, M.D., showed abnormal or delayed development in 57 percent of children born to mothers who received little folate during pregnancy.

How likely is it that anyone needs extra folate? It depends on the adequacy of the diet. Folate-rich foods include spinach, liver, kidney, wheat germ, asparagus, beet greens, kale, endive, turnips, broccoli, orange juice, Swiss chard, black-eyed peas, and lima beans.

# Folate Destroyed by Cooking

Unfortunately, folate is among the easiest-to-destroy vitamins. Both cooking and freezing have been reported to significantly lower the folate content of food. Food processing destroys much folate. And it has been widely reported that oral contraceptives, taken by millions of women, frequently cause folate deficiency.

So, if you might become pregnant, should you take extra folate? Perhaps one milligram? Although the risk of a neural-tube defect is small, it is significant (2 out of 1,000). It appears probable that even a small dose—one milligram or less—will lessen the risk. Taking vitamin $B_{12}$ with folate is wise. Both vitamins are generally considered safe. Remember it's very important that folate be started prior to conception.

What if, as forecast a letter to *Lancet*, "everyone" takes folate on the chance of preventing neural-tube defects, thus interfering with "final" objective proof that it really works? There are other ways of demonstrating whether or not folate works, including the accumulated weight of statistics, and observation. After all, digitalis, aspirin, penicillin, and many other agents known to work have not had randomized, double-blind, placebo-controlled trials, either.

As always, it's your baby, and your decision.

## REFERENCES
**Cleft Palate**

Peer, L. A.; Gordon, W. H.; and Bernhard, W. G. "Effect of Vitamins on Human Teratology." *Plastic Reconstructive Surgery,* October, 1964, pp. 358–362.

Tolarova, M. "Periconceptional Supplementation with Vitamins and Folic Acid to Prevent Recurrence of Cleft Lip." *Lancet,* July 24, 1982, p. 217.

**Folate**

Burton, Benjamin T. *Human Nutrition.* McGraw-Hill, 1976.

Goodman, Louis S., and Gilman, Alfred, eds. *The Pharmacological Basis of Therapeutics.* 5th ed. Macmillan Publishing, 1975, pp. 1342–1343.

*Handbook of Nonprescription Drugs.* 6th ed. American Pharmaceutical Association, 1979.

**Fragile-x Chromosome**

Lubs, Herbert A., and Lujan, Enrique. "The Mystifying Marker." In *1983 Science Year.* World Books, 1983.

**Neural-Tube Defects**

Kirke, Peadar N. "Vitamins, Neural Tube Defects, and Ethics Committees." Letter to *Lancet*, June 14, 1980, pp. 1300–1301.

Laurence, K. M. et al. "Double-blind Randomised Controlled Trial of Folate Treatment Before Conception to Prevent Recurrence of Neural-tube Defects." *British Medical Journal*, May 9, 1981, pp. 1509–1511.

Mason, Ian. "Neural Tube Defects." *Pulse*, December, 1982.

———. "Why We Will Go On with Neural Tube Defect Trials." *Pulse*, December, 1982.

Smithells, R. W. "Neural Tube Defects: Prevention by Vitamin Supplements." *Pediatrics*, April, 1982, pp. 498–499.

Smithells, R. W.; Sheppard, S.; and Schorah, C. J. "Vitamin Deficiencies and Neural Tube Defects." *Archives of Disease in Childhood*, December, 1976, pp. 944–950.

Smithells, R. W. et al. "Possible Prevention of Neural-Tube Defects by Periconceptional Vitamin Supplementation." *Lancet*, February 16, 1980, pp. 339–340.

———. "Apparent Prevention of Neural Tube Defects by Periconceptional Vitamin Supplementation." *Archives of Disease in Childhood*, vol. 56, 1981, pp. 911–918.

**Pregnancy and Infant Growth**

Gross, R. L.; Newberne, P. M.; and Reid, J. V. O. "Adverse Effects on Infant Development Associated With Maternal Folic Acid Deficiency." *Nutrition Reports International*, November, 1974, pp. 241–248.

Rolschau, J.; Date, J.; and Kristofferson, K. "Folic Acid Supplement and Intrauterine Growth." *Acta Obstetricia et Gynecologia Scandinavica*, vol. 58, no. 4, 1979, pp. 343–346.

Thiersch, John B. "Therapeutic Abortions With a Folic Acid Antagonist, 4-Aminopteroylglutamic Acid (4-Amino P.G.A.), Administered By the Oral Route." *American Journal of Obstetrics and Gynecology*, June, 1952, pp. 1298–1304.

**Spina Bifida**

    Brocklehurst, Gordon, ed. *Spina Bifida for the Clinician.* J. B. Lippincott, 1976.

# 8 ABCs OF NUTRITIONAL TESTING

Once a comprehensive health history has been recorded and a complete physical examination done, it's usually time to go to the laboratory for tests. Let's take an imaginary trip to our lab, and go over what we do here. As you'll see, some tests are used for general screening and might be done for nearly everyone. Others are more specialized.

We'll cover laboratory tests specifically useful or relevant to nutritional biochemistry. Although our laboratory does routine blood counts, urinalysis, and other standard tests, I won't go over them unless they're performed or interpreted in a different way. No implication is intended, however, that routine standard testing isn't important; it certainly is. We do it every day. But there's information on standard testing available elsewhere. So this visit to the laboratory will concentrate almost entirely on tests frequently or specifically used as a part of the nutritional-biochemical evaluation.

# Allergy

Investigation, reading, and observation have convinced me that the most accurate testing for food sensitivity is done in environmentally controlled inpatient hospital units by allergists specializing in clinical ecology. That type of testing is well described by Theron Randolph, M.D., and Marshall Mandell, M.D.

Unfortunately, controlled environment testing is expensive, time consuming, and (as yet) not widely available. There's no environmental unit in the Northwest where my practice is, so I've looked for a test that can be done on nonhospitalized individuals.

## RAST (RADIOALLERGOSORBENT TEST)

At present, the RAST test is the most useful in identifying food sensitivities. It's far from perfect, however. It only uncovers *allergy* to food, not the category of nonallergic *sensitivity*. And although it's not nearly as expensive as in-hospital testing, it isn't cheap either. Despite those drawbacks, it can be useful in clinical practice to ferret out food intolerances.

There are two methodologies for performing the RAST test. A comparative evaluation at our laboratory found one method far preferable to the other, which actually appeared of no use. Obviously it's important to use the specific method giving the most clinically useful results.

If an individual is allergic, antibodies against each specific allergen are produced by white blood cells. The worse the allergy, the higher the level of antibodies. The RAST test detects antibodies to specific allergens in the blood, and measures relative quantities.

A radioactively labeled specific food antigen is added to the serum in a test tube. If antibodies to that specific antigen are present, an antigen-antibody complex is formed. Antigen-antibody complexes weigh more than antigen alone, and so can be separated and measured by radiation detectors. The level of radioactivity in the separated fraction indicates the level of antigen-antibody complex. Thus the relative amount of antibodies measurable reflects the degree of allergy to that specific food.

Initially, it was thought that a single measurement of a category of antibodies called total IgE would indicate who should be tested further for specific food allergies. For nearly two years, with the cooperation of the RAST testing laboratory, total IgE was determined with every specific food allergy test done at our office. There was absolutely no correlation at all. After that lack of association was documented elsewhere, we dropped the total IgE test entirely.

Routine scratch tests for the detection of food allergies are well-known but, from my perspective, entirely unreliable. The RAST test has been favorably reviewed by authorities in traditional medicine. Despite that, many insurance companies refuse to cover such testing on the grounds that routine scratch testing is "usual and customary." It's a sad reflection on the goals of these insurance companies, who will pay for ineffective procedures because they're customary, but refuse to pay for effective procedures which aren't.

# Blood Sugar

## GLUCOSE-INSULIN TOLERANCE TEST

The glucose tolerance test is one standard means of determining abnormal blood sugar metabolism. A five- or six-hour test is used by nutritionally oriented practitioners to look for diabetes, hyperglycemia, and hypoglycemia (low blood sugar).

Hypoglycemia continues to be a controversial topic. Nutritionally oriented physicians universally recognize the enormous range of symptomatic relief that hypoglycemia recognition and treatment can bring, but most other physicians ignore the problem or deny its existence.

The criteria used to inspect six-hour glucose tolerance tests for evidence of hypoglycemia vary. Many nutritionally oriented physicians use the criteria published by H. L. Newbold, M.D., in his book *Mega-Nutrients for Your Nerves*. His criteria are as follows:

Hypoglycemia is indicated:

1. When the blood sugar, in the course of a six-hour glucose tolerance test, fails to rise more than 50 percent above the fasting level;
2. By a glucose curve which falls during a six-hour test to 20 milligrams percent [20 milligrams of glucose per 100 milliliters of blood] below the fasting level;
3. By a glucose tolerance test in which blood sugar falls 50 milligrams percent or more during any one hour of the test;
4. By a glucose tolerance test in which the absolute blood sugar level falls in the range of 50 milligrams percent or lower (anything below 65 milligrams percent is suspicious);
5. By clinical symptoms such as dizziness, headache, confusion, palpitations, depression, etc., appearing during the course of a glucose tolerance test—regardless of what the blood sugar readings may be.

The last criterion is important, because glucose levels may fluctuate quickly in the course of a tolerance test. The low point may occur *between* the blood sugar levels measured at one-hour intervals. You should, therefore, take into account any symptoms you exhibit during the test. Ideally, if any clinical symptoms make their appearance, extra blood should be drawn at once, to find out what the sugar level is at that point.

However, our laboratory no longer does simply glucose tolerance testing. Each time a blood specimen is drawn for glucose analysis, it's checked for insulin also, a procedure called glucose-insulin tolerance testing. In maturity-onset diabetes (which refers to noninsulin-dependent diabetes), the person usually develops insulin resistance, and the tissues don't respond to insulin. To try to keep blood sugar under control, the pancreas secretes more insulin than usual.

By measuring the insulin response to sugar (as well as the glucose response), potential maturity-onset diabetes can be identified before it becomes a real problem. That's because in the early stages of abnormality the insulin levels rise too high, even though the blood glucose is still normal. Early detection and correction of potential or latent maturity-onset diabetes is thus possible and certainly desirable.

In a series of 3,650 individuals referred for glucose-insulin tolerance testing, Joseph Kraft, M.D., of Chicago identified 1,713 as normal using glucose-curve interpretation alone. Looking beneath the glucose response at the insulin curve, he found potential or latent diabetes in 1,145 of the 1,713, or 67 percent. Although our percentages haven't been as high, I agree with Dr. Kraft, who wrote "identification of this phase of diabetes has far-reaching clinical implications."

## GLYCOHEMOGLOBIN (Hgb Alc)

Although the Hgb Alc test is relatively new, it's become available in nearly all commercial labs, and is widely used in traditional medical practice. The major advantage of using this test over the traditional urinary and blood sugar tests is that the latter measure circulating blood sugar (glucose) levels at one particular point in time, while Hgb Alc measures the average glucose levels over prolonged periods of time. It's extremely helpful in establishing whether a patient is being adequately controlled on a particular regime. It's also not influenced by daily changes due to meals, exercise, or medication.

Many laboratories report results of from 4 to 9 percent to fall within the expected range, with over 12 percent considered abnormal. Nine percent to 12 percent is said to be indeterminate. I consider anything above 9 percent abnormal, however, and in need of attention.

# Cholesterol

## HDL (HIGH-DENSITY LIPOPROTEIN)

HDL is the "good" cholesterol and is a measure of that fraction of cholesterol—high-density lipoproteins—that has been found protective against cardiovascular disease.

The more HDL cholesterol you have in proportion to your total cholesterol, the greater your protection against developing diseases of the heart and circulatory system.

To determine your own cholesterol ratio you need only to take your total cholesterol value and divide it by your HDL levels. If you get five, you would be considered to be at "average risk." An answer of under five means less than average risk, and over five means more than average.

A total cholesterol level of 300, for example, divided by an HDL of 100 is 3. The person with that value would have a less than average risk of developing cardiovascular disease.

It's possible through diet and supplementation to produce a more favorable HDL to total cholesterol ratio. For a further discussion, be sure to read "A Case of Irregular Heartbeat."

# Circulation

## PLETHYSMOGRAPHY (PRONOUNCED PLE-THIS-MA-GRA-FEE)

It's important to measure blood flow in the extremities (almost always the legs), particularly when pulses can't be found. Plethysmography is one way of doing that. Thermography (which measures tiny changes in skin surface temperatures) and Doppler testing (which uses ultrasound echoes in blood vessels) are two other methods in common use.

Individuals with symptoms of compromised circulation have abnormal plethysmograms to varying degrees. In these persons, testing is helpful to document just how bad the problem is, and to monitor treatment (see "A Case of Poor Circulation").

Plethysmography is particularly helpful for asymptomatic individuals with unfindable pulses. Since it measures a pulse wave present in the extremity without needing to precisely locate the artery or arteries, it can distinguish those individuals with truly compromised circulation (who need prompt treatment before becoming symptomatic) from those who have good circulation passing through areas where pulse waves aren't easily findable.

Cuffs much like blood pressures cuffs are placed around a toe, the calf, and the thigh of each leg. (If necessary, the cuffs can be moved to more precisely locate a problem.) Each cuff contains a transducer which translates pulsations into electrical signals. The cuff is connected by wires to an electrocardiograph machine, which prints out a pulse wave that can be analyzed and compared.

If circulatory compromise isn't severe enough to require surgery, various nutritional and supplemental treatments can be used and plethysmography can monitor the progress. The dramatic potential for change can be seen in the before and after treatments for Inez Cerillo, as shown in Figure 1.

# Clotting

## PLATELET AGGREGATION TIME

Research has shown that people with diabetes, high blood pressure, atherosclerotic disease, and transient ischemic attacks (a temporary, reversible block in the blood supply) are more likely than average to have abnormal platelet aggregation. If platelets aggregate (or clump together) too quickly, clots are likely to form in both small and large blood vessels, and cause heart attacks, strokes, or other vascular complications.

Working from a preventive perspective, I've found that individuals with a family history of these problems are more likely to have abnormally short platelet aggregation time also. The many natural measures that lengthen aggregation time and are likely to

# The Plethysmograms of Inez Cerillo

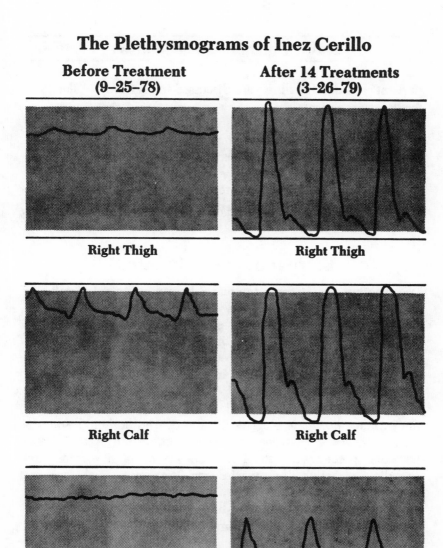

Figure 1: These are the plethysmograms of a woman in her late 40s, before and after treatment. Note the dramatic changes in the pulse wave heights and shapes in all measured areas, indicating significant improvement in her total circulation. Just 14 treatments in a short span of six months, using only nutritional therapy, made all the difference!

prevent considerable illness are discussed in "A Case of 'Blackout' Spells."

Individuals with autoimmune disease like arthritis, multiple sclerosis, severe allergies, and those past 70 years of age are also more likely to have shortened platelet aggregation times.

Abnormally short platelet aggregation time is a cardiovascular risk factor. The test is simple to perform, and if a lab does many of them, likely to be moderate in cost. Despite its usefulness, it isn't widely available at present.

## Estrogens (Fractionated)

Another almost-forgotten test of enormous potential value in disease prevention, particularly estrogen-related cancer, is the determination of fractionated estrogen levels. That test determines the levels of three types of estrogens called estrone, estradiol, and estriol. How much of each one a women has as well as their relative proportions appear to be of major importance in preventing cancer.

Women's bodies make all three types of estrogen. Estradiol is the primary hormone secreted by the ovaries, although some is made elsewhere. Estrone is made from estradiol and other hormone precursors. Estriol is made from both estrone and estradiol, although the ovaries may make a small amount directly.

Both estrone and estradiol have been implicated as carcinogenic (cancer causing) under some circumstances. And according to commentary by Alvin H. Follingstad, M.D., in the *Journal of the American Medical Association*, estrone is thought but not proven to be more cancer producing. According to the same commentary: "There has been a growing suspicion, if not a conviction, that estriol may not only be noncarcinogenic but indeed anticarcinogenic."

Animal experiments have shown that high levels of estriol protect against the tumor-causing effects of estrone and estradiol. Women in countries with a low incidence of breast cancer have higher levels of estriol excretion than women in countries with high breast cancer incidence. Henry Lemon, M.D., at the University of Nebraska, a longtime researcher into estrogens, asked women with breast cancer and metastases (cancer spread to other areas) to take estriol. Thirty-seven percent had arrest or remission of the metastatic lesions.

In 1966, Dr. Lemon published a research paper discussing the concept of the "estrogen quotient"—a calculation based on the fractionated estrogen test. To derive the estrogen quotient the quantity of estriol ($E_3$) is divided by the sum of the quantities of estradiol ($E_2$) and estrone ($E_1$). Mathematically, the formula appears like this:

$$Eq = \frac{E_3}{E_2 + E_1}$$

In his paper, Dr. Lemon reported that in 34 women without cancer, the median Eq was 1.3 before menopause, and 1.2 after. In 26 women with breast cancer and not receiving hormonal treatment, median Eq's were 0.5 to 0.8. (The higher Eq's reflect greater proportions of estriol.)

Dr. Lemon also measured the estrogen quotient before and after treatment in a group of women with breast cancer. No cancer remissions were observed in 12 women whose Eq decreased or remained unchanged; 10 objective remissions of cancer were observed in women whose Eq rose toward or exceeded 1.0.

What implications does Dr. Lemon's work and that of others have for nutritional-biochemical therapy? Like many others in this field, I don't work with individuals with cancer. (It's not that I don't want to, but political considerations make it inadvisable.) Aside from cancer treatment, estrogen quotient calculation from the fractionated estrogen measurement is an extremely useful tool in preventive medicine.

As noted by Dr. Lemon, "The low Eq of the few patients examined because of precancerous pathology of breast or uterus in this study suggests that a disproportionately large percent of the subnormal estriol excretors may develop precancerous or malignant tumors." Logically, then, if estriol excretion could be increased, the risk of cancer could be diminished. Not only Dr. Lemon's work but the work of other researchers strongly supports this possibility.

Through diet and specific nutrient supplementation, it's usually possible to induce an improvement in the estrogen quotient over 6 to 18 months' time, without the use of any drugs. There are many cases of such improvement on file at my clinic. The chances are excellent that women who substantially improve their estrogen quotients substantially reduce their cancer risk.

Who should have the fractionated estrogen test and estrogen quotient calculation? Women with fibrocystic breast disease (also called cystic mastitis), women who have a family history of breast, uterine, or ovarian cancer and those who (for whatever reason) must take estrogens. Estradiol and estrone are the estrogens associated with cancer, but ironically, estriol—the "safe" estrogen—is prohibited from use in the United States although it's available in Europe.

Breast cancer is the most common tumor among women— approximately 5 percent develop it—in the United States. If the fractionated estrogen test were sufficiently inexpensive, I'd recommend it for all women past the age of 25.

# Hair

A mineral analysis of a sample of hair taken from the nape of the neck can tell us what minerals are present. Information obtained from a hair analysis can be extremely useful, but only when properly correlated with other laboratory test results, health history, and a physical examination. Most frequently conclusions can't be based on it alone.

Toxic minerals including lead, cadmium, mercury, arsenic, and aluminum are probably exceptions to this general rule. Though debate in medical journals continues, the consensus of opinion appears to be that hair levels of toxic minerals are the best single indicator of exposure—considerably better than blood or urine determinations. I've found periodic hair mineral analysis the best indication that toxic mineral avoidance or bodily elimination techniques are successful. (See "A Case of Cadmium-Related High Blood Pressure.")

For other minerals, considerably more caution is required. Simultaneous hair, blood, and 24-hour urine tests are frequently very useful to unravel problems in mineral metabolism and distribution.

Clues to other problems are sometimes seen in mineral analysis patterns. Both the malabsorption pattern (a large majority of minerals lower than the reference range) and the early-bone-calcium-loss pattern (extremely high hair calcium and magnesium despite average or less than average calcium intake) are widely accepted by practitioners who work with hair mineral analysis all the time. However, causes still need to be found. For example, the early-bone-calcium-loss pattern is due with equal frequency to calcium malabsorption associated with hypochlorhydria, and an abnormal dietary calcium to phosphorus ratio. Sometimes it's both.

Despite the value and potential of hair mineral analysis, a principal problem has been variability of both testing procedures and results. The Hair Analysis Standardization Board in Annandale, Virginia, has reviewed most of the data in this field, and recommended that certain standards be adopted by the testing industry. The board has noted degrees of clinical significance for each mineral. Intense intra-industry rivalry and personality incompatibilities have so far led to nonindustry-wide adoption of these standards. Instead, a rival quality-control program has been instituted by an industry group, the American Society of Elemental Testing Laboratories in West Chicago, Illinois. This isn't as bad as it seems, however. Now everyone is paying more attention to test quality and reliability, so there's more chance of improvement than ever before.

If you're interested in hair mineral analysis, it can't hurt to inquire whether the laboratory you're considering conforms to the standards set by the Hair Analysis Standardization Board or the American Society of Elemental Testing Laboratories quality-control program. If the laboratory does neither, then more questions and serious reconsideration are in order. And if it's insurance coverage you want, you can forget it. Practically no insurance covers hair analysis—at least not at this writing.

# Minerals

Blood testing for minerals has many uses, but its limitations need to be understood more widely. It's often claimed to yield data beyond its capability. Much more attention to details of mineral regulation, distribution, and function in the bloodstream is needed before interpretations can be made.

## CALCIUM

Calcium measurement is the best example of that problem. I've heard over and over that "my doctor says my calcium is normal because my blood test is OK." A little thought shows the complete inaccuracy of such an interpretation.

You may have had an 85-year-old relative fall and break her hip (or break her hip and fall, as many suspect). When she's taken to the hospital and x-rayed, the radiologist almost always notes osteoporosis—a mild to severe calcium loss from the bones. Quite obviously, there's an overall deficiency in calcium, yet the routine blood test for calcium, the serum calcium, is normal (with rare exceptions).

Calcium in the bloodstream is regulated very closely. If it weren't, contraction of both the skeletal muscles and heart muscle would be immediately affected. Many other body functions would be adversely affected, too. So abnormalities of blood calcium are extremely rare, occurring almost exclusively in parathyroid abnormalities and some cancers.

Blood testing is often mistakenly relied on for measurement of toxic minerals. Lead, cadmium, and other toxic minerals don't belong in circulation, so the body tries to clear them from the blood. Some are excreted through the urine, but chronic overloads can't be handled entirely by the kidneys. Instead, they're stored away in other body tissues—lead in bone and teeth, cadmium in lung and kidney tissue. . . .

And hair! As noted in a *Lancet* article by Dr. Martin Laker, "Blood can be used only for immediate measurement of exposure to lead and cadmium, as it gives no indication of the cumulative levels of these elements." The *Lancet* reviewer cites several research reports which have shown blood to be less useful than hair to measure toxic metal exposure.

## IRON

Ferritin is the main storage form of iron in the liver, spleen, and bone marrow. It's been found that as iron-containing cells from these tissues deteriorate, small amounts of ferritin "leak" into the blood serum. Research has shown that under most circumstances, the serum ferritin is the most accurate reflection of total body iron storage. (Principal exceptions appear to be during some inflammatory diseases, and with some forms of cancer.)

Even with a normal blood count, serum ferritin levels are frequently low, especially in women. Since the test is relatively inexpensive, our laboratory does it routinely as part of an overall blood count.

Low serum ferritin levels in men are considerably less frequent, and suggest iron malabsorption investigation as well as a search for hidden gastrointestinal bleeding. After menopause, persistently low serum ferritin in women is equally suspicious.

Women with normal blood counts often note that "iron makes me feel better even when I'm not anemic." The serum ferritin—usually low in such individuals—explains why.

Although I've found no published research, it appears that serum ferritin is more accurate than hair iron as a reflection of total body iron storage.

## POTASSIUM

Only 0.4 percent of total body potassium is found in blood serum, while 89.6 percent is found inside body cells. The other 10 percent is found in lymph, cartilage, connective tissue, bone, and between cells. Despite this widely published information about potassium distribution, the almost universal potassium measurement is from blood serum. For emergency management especially, serum potassium is a critical measurement. If the levels go too low or too high, muscular contraction (especially that of the heart) and nerve conduction become abnormal. Serum potassium is the up-front inventory of potassium available for immediate use. Like calcium, the body regulates its level very closely.

Serum potassium, like serum calcium, is frequently used as a test of total body potassium deficiency. Since nearly 90 percent of potassium is found inside body cells, and serum is an extracellular (outside of cells) fluid, it's likely that this measurement, while important, isn't the most accurate overall potassium deficiency test.

Both red and white blood cells contain potassium. So theoretically, potassium within these cells should be a good reflection of total body potassium. Research has shown that theory to be accurate. As a measurement of total body potassium, whole blood containing red and white cells as well as serum is a more accurate test material. Testing of red cells only appears equally accurate.

Whole blood potassium is considerably more accurate than hair potassium or serum potassium for estimation of total body potassium.

Other minerals, notably magnesium and zinc, are predominantly intracellular. It's likely that whole blood or red cell measurements of predominantly intracellular elements will eventually be shown to more accurately reflect total body levels of each mineral.

# Oxalic Acid

## 24-HOUR URINE FOR OXALATE

An occasional individual will overproduce oxalic acid if he or she takes more than two to three grams of vitamin C daily.

Usually, normal urinary oxalate excretion is at or below 40 to 50 milligrams per 24 hours. The more it rises above that the greater the hazard. Since the most common form of kidney stone is calcium oxalate, kidney stone formation is a potential hazard of high-dose vitamin C.

In the past ten years, I've found only one individual who actually developed a kidney stone for that reason, but the hazard is totally avoidable by measurement of urinary oxalate excretion.

# Pancreatic Function

## TRYPSIN, AMYLASE, AND LIPASE

Trypsin, amylase, and lipase are three enzymes which digest proteins, carbohydrates, and fats. Trypsin is made exclusively by the pancreas; amylase is made by all salivary glands, although there is a pancreas-specific amylase function; and lipase is also produced by the pancreas and is used for the diagnosis of pancreatic disease. Although not the best measure, it's one of the few tests available.

According to a well-known textbook, *Clinical Biochemistry Reviews*, "A number of recent contributions suggest that trypsin immunoassays may be extremely useful in the detection and differentiation of pancreatic disease." The trypsin test is relatively new. In combination with measurement of amylase, lipase, and a digestive analysis, an overall picture of pancreatic function is possible, but there doesn't appear to be any single extremely reliable test yet available, short of research procedures involving passing a tube into the small intestine and collecting pancreatic secretions. We don't do that last test at our laboratory.

Sometimes estimation of pancreatic function is made on the basis of symptoms and physical signs alone. A trial of digestive enzymes can produce a clearer answer than a laboratory test. Fortunately, just trying enzymes is relatively safe. The only apparent hazard is allergy.

# Prostate

## MALE P.A.P.
## (PROSTATIC ACID PHOSPHATASE)

One promising method of prostate cancer detection, according to some experts, is the Male P.A.P., a blood test which measues the levels of an enzyme called prostatic acid phosphatase that appears to elevate in the presence of cancer. All scientists cannot agree, however, on the test's usefulness as a screening device.

In a major study sponsored by the National Cancer Institute (NCI) in 1978, the Male P.A.P. was put to the test to measure just how much cancer of the prostate it could detect. Reports from hospitals and clinics all across the U.S. revealed a 38 percent detection rate for localized prostate cancer and a 69 percent rate in prostate cancers that had spread to other parts of the body. Although these figures are far from the ideally desirable 100 percent detection rate, the test certainly appears to have an advantage over a low discovery rate during the physical examination.

Other scientists, however, don't agree. In a more recent study led by Lawrence A. Kaplan, Ph.D., and Evan A. Stein, M.D., of the University of Cincinnati, NCI's findings could not be confirmed. In some cases the test shows "positive" for cancer yet in a subsequent examination by a urologist no cancer was present, while in one person it shows "negative" for cancer when indeed cancer is present. In another study of 61 men who were symptom free, the test identified prostatic cancer in less than 50 percent of the cases. "You could get the same accuracy by flipping a coin," says Dr. Kaplan.

Until this controvery is settled or other methods of detection are developed, I'll continue to routinely use both the Male P.A.P. and the rectal examination to screen for prostatic cancer, especially in men who pass their fiftieth birthday.

# Stomach Acidity

Accurate measurement of stomach acid secretion is extremely important in nutritionally based health care. If stomach acid secretion is low, pepsin and intrinsic-factor secretion are usually low also. Research has shown that calcium and iron don't assimilate well in cases of hypochlorhydria (low stomach acidity). Vitamin $B_{12}$ doesn't fully detach from food if acid and pepsin are low. So if it remains bound to food protein, it can't attach to the intrinsic factor that helps it to be absorbed normally.

Observation at my office has made it clear that individuals with low stomach acidity have an excess of undigested meat fibers in their stool; lower than usual levels of nearly all minerals on hair analysis; abnormal bacterial, yeast, and fungus growth in the intestine more frequently; higher levels of indican in the urine; and several other minor biochemical abnormalities.

In the 1920s and 1930s, data from thousands of individual tests at major medical centers showed low stomach acidity to be a relatively common condition. Today, an analysis of levels of stomach acid by radiotelemetry confirms the same degree of frequency. Yet the older data is sometimes criticized as inaccurate because of obsolete testing methods, superseded by a more modern procedure. Before going over gastric analysis by radiotelemetry, let's briefly look at the most common stomach acid test in use today—gastric analysis by intubation.

After an overnight fast, a tube is passed into the stomach, and its contents are pumped out. Histamine, pentagastrin, or another stimulant to stomach acid secretion is injected. Stomach pumping goes on for a specified period of time. The stimulated acid production is measured and compared to normal standards. No food is eaten throughout the test.

By contrast, analyses performed in the 1920s and 1930s used various test meals, measured quantities of gruel or alcohol. The stomach's capacity to secrete acid after a test meal was measured, again by analysis of the pumped-out stomach contents. No stimulant injections were given.

I don't know anyone who takes injections of histamine with each meal. Histamine-stimulated stomach testing discloses how much acid can be secreted in response to histamine, but doesn't measure acid secreted in response to food or alkali in the stomach. For that reason, the thousands of tests done in the 1920s and 1930s actually were much closer to normal function testing than modern, histamine-stimulated testing.

When our laboratory started doing gastric analysis by radiotelemetry we tried to use foods—particularly milk—so that acidity could be measured under conditions as close to natural as possible. Two major problems became obvious with that test. It's practically impossible to standardize the alkalinity of food testing, and worse, food allergies for a particular individual can abnormally increase or decrease stomach acid production. Since food allergy and sensitivity is so common, especially in individuals not feeling well, the probability of an inaccurate test caused by allergy is high.

For these reasons, we've finally settled on a saturated solution of sodium bicarbonate as the test material. I'll admit that isn't a perfect state-of-nature test either, since few individuals eat sodium bicarbonate with meals. However, sodium bicarbonate doesn't appear to abnormally stimulate stomach acid secretion like an injection of histamine, pentagastrin, or a food allergen. Nor does it abnormally depress acid production as allergens can. So it appears at present to be the best compromise available.

The radiotelemetry capsule (called a Heidelberg capsule) is approximately $8/10$ inch long, $3/10$ inch wide—about the size of a large multivitamin capsule. It's mostly hard plastic, containing a miniature radio transmitter, a pH meter, and a battery. When wet it detects the exact pH (acidity-alkalinity) of its surroundings, and radios the information to an antenna attached to a receiver and recorder, which translates the radio signal. The receiver contains a display gauge which indicates pH changes as they occur, and a printer provides a permanent written record.

Following a fast, an individual is asked to swallow the "bugged" capsule. Once it's in the stomach, the pH is observed and automatically recorded. Only a tiny minority of people have an abnormally high fasting pH. A very large majority have a normal pH of 1.0 to 3.5. Abnormalities of stomach acid secretion are usually found after a challenge test, which introduces a small amount of saturated solution of sodium bicarbonate to the stomach.

If the fasting pH level is normal, the individual is asked to swallow about a teaspoon (5 ml's) of a saturated solution of sodium bicarbonate. The pH gauge rises to 6 to 8. If stomach function is normal and acid is secreted sufficiently in response to the alkali, the pH returns to normal in 20 minutes or less. That procedure is repeated three more times, occasionally four. Each time the teaspoon of sodium bicarbonate is swallowed, the pH should rise to 6 to 8, and return to 1.8 to 2.3 in 20 minutes or less. A normal gastric analysis, as printed by the recorder, should look like Figure 2, below.

If a person has no stomach acidity, then test results look like Figure 3. If that person is given an injection of histamine or other stimulant, acid will sometimes be produced, and pH will fall. Many physicians, however, will only use the description achlorhydria when even an injected stimulus doesn't cause acid secretion.

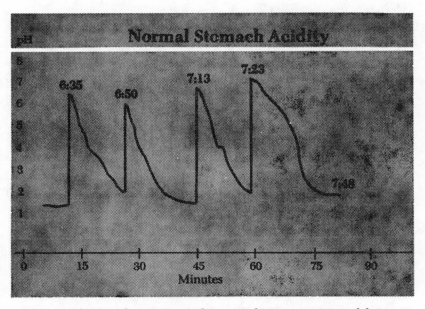

*Figure 2: This graph represents the type of reaction expected from a stomach producing a normal amount of acid. Each time the stomach is challenged, the level of acid returns to normal within 20 minutes.*

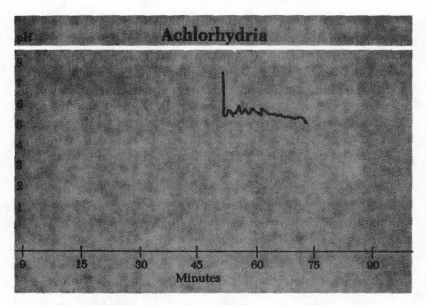

*Figure 3: When there's no stomach acid, the pH of the stomach is too high. A challenge test is, therefore, unnecessary.*

I disagree. Remembering that none of us inject histamine with lunch, I describe any test disclosing no fasting stomach acid as achlorhydric. (For the technical purpose of distinguishing between those whose stomachs respond to injected stimulus and those who don't, the terms stimulus-responsive and stimulus-resistant achlorhydria can be used.)

Hypochlorhydria is the term used to describe lower than normal degrees of stomach acid production, but still more than none. The degrees of hypochlorhydria (ranging from mild to severe) and hyperchlorhydria (overacidity) are shown in Figures 4, 5, 6, and 7, on the following pages.

Recommendations for hydrochloric acid and pepsin supplementation are made based on the degree of hypochlorhydria, as well as the digestive analysis. For more specific details, see "Good Digestion: Why We Can't Take It for Granted."

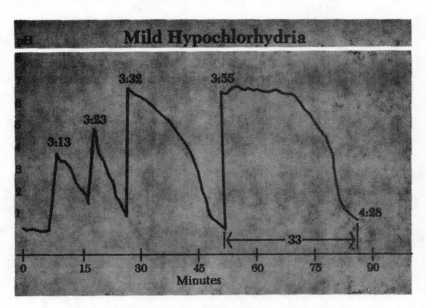

*Figure 4: Within the first two challenges with sodium bicarbonate, the levels of acid return to normal within 20 minutes, but by the third challenge the stomach tires and can't return to normal as quickly. After the third challenge it takes 23 minutes, and after the fourth it takes even longer—33 minutes.*

# Stomach Function

### SERUM GASTRIN

Gastrin is a hormone our bodies make which naturally stimulates stomach acid production. When acid production capability decreases, gastrin levels go higher, as if trying to keep stomach acid production normal by pushing harder. Since gastrin circulates in the bloodstream, blood levels can be used as part of an overall evaluation of stomach function. However, research has shown that serum gastrin can't be used by itself as an indicator of stomach function, since the relationship of high gastrin/low stomach acid isn't sufficiently reliable.

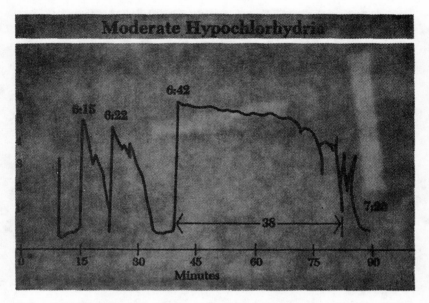

*Figure 5: This stomach is having increasingly more trouble reacidifying after being challenged with sodium bicarbonate. By the third challenge, it takes 38 minutes for the acid level to return to normal.*

## SERUM PEPSINOGEN I

Likewise, a precursor of pepsin called pepsinogen I can be measured in the bloodstream. There appears to be a rough correlation between serum levels of pepsinogen I and stomach pepsin production, which in turn correlates with stomach acid. Theoretically, a low pepsinogen I determination should predict hypochlorhydria. Unfortunately, our lab finds that to be the case only sometimes.

A research paper published in the *American Journal of Digestive Diseases* has shown that a combined finding of elevated serum gastrin and low serum pepsinogen I may be useful in uncovering severe stomach atrophy. Hopefully, as the costs of these tests decline and more research is done, that combination of tests, or others like them, may be able to reliably determine stomach function from blood tests alone.

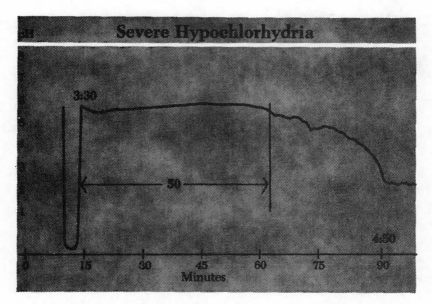

*Figure 6: When empty, the stomach is at normal acidity, but when the first challenge with sodium bicarbonate is given, the stomach has virtually no capability to respond with acid production. After 50 minutes, the pH begins to decrease, but normal acidity is never achieved.*

## Stool Analysis and Culture

A stool analysis is a test we use for general screening. It provides a relatively simple means of checking whether what's eaten is being digested properly, as well as other details of intestinal function.

Before describing the test in detail, proper credit should be given to Arthur Kaslow, M.D., a California GI specialist in nutritional-biochemical therapies, who collected many individual tests of intestinal function into one large group to be analyzed at one time. He has also taken his time at medical meetings to convince the rest of us in nutritional and preventive medicine of the importance of comprehensive stool testing.

The test I'll describe is my adaptation and isn't exactly the

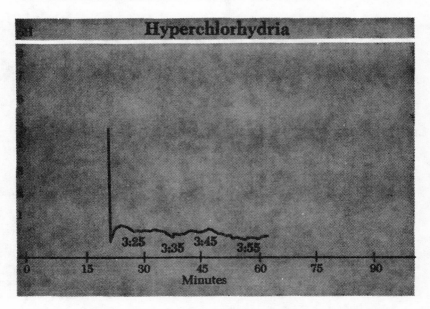

*Figure 7: There's so much acid in this stomach that even a challenge with sodium bicarbonate appears to make little difference in changing its acid levels.*

same as Dr. Kaslow's. (Doctors frequently don't do things exactly the same way.)

Individuals tested at our clinic are asked to eat an average (for them) amount of meat (beef, pork, chicken, fish, lamb), starch (bread, potato, rice, etc.), fibrous vegetable (celery, carrot, turnip, etc.), and fat or oil (butter, fat untrimmed from meat, salad dressing made with vegetable oil, avocado, etc.), all at one meal. Although selections of individual foods can vary, they're asked to eat meals of that general overall composition for breakfast, lunch, and dinner. Twelve to 15 hours after the last such meal, a stool specimen is collected for analysis. If none is available at precisely that time, the next available specimen is used.

The test diet instructions are modified for individual circumstances, such as vegetarianism or allergy to food. But three meals of protein/starch/fiber/fat composition are eaten in any case, and one stool specimen collected as close to a set interval later as possible.

Examination of the stool is done under a microscope for undigested meat fiber, vegetable fiber, oil or fat droplets or globules, and starch residue. Categories most frequently showing an undigested excess appear to be meat fiber and vegetable fiber. Follow-up testing to find the reasons for excess undigested materials is then done. Although there are many possible reasons, the most common is low stomach acidity. Once a reason or reasons are found, and corrected or compensated for with appropriate supplementation, follow-up digestive analysis tells us whether it's working or not.

Follow-up testing is what convinced me that in many circumstances supplementary hydrochloric acid in hard tablet form doesn't do the job, particularly in the more severe cases of low stomach acidity. Most of the time, the powdered, encapsulated form does a better job of aiding digestion.

Although a single stool sample is a convenient and simple analysis of digestive adequacy, it's not done to the same exacting standards called for in serious cases. In more severe cases, stool specimens are collected for intervals ranging from 24 hours to several days and analyzed for total fat content and total nitrogen. Those procedures are frequently done in hospitals, and are much too cumbersome for general screening. Dr. Kaslow's procedure is quick, more convenient, economical, and finds a surprisingly large number of individuals with faulty digestion.

In addition to checking digestion, other tests are performed on the same specimen. It's checked for hidden bleeding (a more routine test called occult blood testing). White blood cells are looked for. The pH (acidity-alkalinity) is tested; when pH is abnormal, it's usually too alkaline, which can alter the growth pattern of intestinal microorganisms and make it easier for yeast (technically, *candida* species) to proliferate in the intestine. In fact, an alkaline pH is often a tipoff to low stomach acidity.

A routine examination is also done for parasites (amoebae, pinworms, etc.). Bacterial stains separate the types of bacteria into general groups, and bacterial cultures determine if an excess of unfriendly bacteria are present. Considering what unfriendly bacteria may do, that can be a very important part of the test (see "A Case of Acne Rosacea"). Cultures are also done for mold and fungus. As noted, the most frequently cultured is the common yeast (*candida*), but others turn up occasionally. Especially in allergic individuals, minimization or elimination of intestinal yeast appears very important. After treatment, follow-up testing is done.

Other observations occasionally may include crystals of calcium oxalate, uric acid, tyrosine, and other substances which sometimes give more clues to individual metabolism.

# Urine

### URINARY INDICAN (OBERMEYER TEST)

Although there are exceptions, a positive urinary indican test usually indicates the presence of an excess number of unfriendly bacteria in the intestines. Those bacteria transform the dietary amino acid tryptophan into indican, which is largely reabsorbed into the circulation and excreted through the kidneys. It's a simple, inexpensive test to perform.

When the urinary indican test is positive, treatment with *Lactobacillus acidophilus* taken for several weeks to months will usually result in a negative follow-up test. Occasionally it's helpful to add garlic to the treatment.

Indican is only one of a group of intestinal bacterial metabolites suspected of symptom- and disease-producing capability. So far, it's the only test of these metabolites easily available, although it appears that more comprehensive testing could be very useful.

# Vitamins

Like tests for minerals, those for vitamins are of limited availability and usefulness. As we in medicine become more convinced of the importance of studying minerals, vitamins, and other substances natural to our bodies as part of routine disease treatment and health maintenance, more tests will probably become available. The rather limited group which follows are those I've found most useful in laboratory evaluations.

## EGOT, ETK, AND EGR

These tests are the forerunners of an entire series of functional vitamin tests greatly needed for comprehensive laboratory evaluation of biochemical status. Each set of letters stands for an individual enzyme dependent on a particular vitamin for optimum activity. Technically, each enzyme or substance that speeds up chemical reactions in the body isn't dependent on the vitamin as originally found in food, but on the activated form of the vitamin as transformed by our bodies. So there isn't a precise correlation between normal enzyme function and adequate supplies of its particular vitamin. There could be a metabolic problem in transformation of the vitamin in its original food-derived form to the activated form. Such a metabolic problem would result in an abnormal enzyme activity test, even if supplies of the original vitamin are adequate.

However, with that exception, the relationship between vitamin adequacy and normal enzyme activity is very close. The test can be used as an individualized measure of vitamin adequacy, thus avoiding the major shortcoming of absolute-level vitamin testing and reliance on statistical normals for interpretation. What's normal for most individuals may not be normal for others, but if levels of enzyme activity are adequate, individual adequacy is more likely.

EGOT refers to erythrocyte glutamic-oxaloacetic transaminase—a red cell enzyme dependent on an activated form of vitamin $B_6$ (pyridoxal phosphate) for its activity. ETK means erythrocyte transketolase, which depends on thiamine pyrophosphate—an activated form of vitamin $B_1$ (thiamine). EGR is erythrocyte glutathione reductase, which requires flavin adenine dinucleotide, an activated form of vitamin $B_2$ (riboflavin).

Unfortunately, these tests are not widely available. As medical awareness of the importance of proper nutrition grows, their use will probably spread, and other tests for individual nutrients and individual nutrient adequacy will be developed.

# Neutrophilic Segmentation Index

Despite his opposition to nutritionally oriented medical practice, Victor Herbert, M.D., of Bronx Veterans Hospital in New York City, was instrumental in the development of that very inexpensive, sensitive test for early folate (folic acid) deficiency. Although on occasion an abnormal segmentation index indicates uremia, kidney failure, or vitamin $B_{12}$ or iron deficiency, it usually signals a problem with folate. Since folate appears to be so important in the prevention of a variety of birth defects (see "Folate: A Weapon against Birth Defects"), it's my opinion that this extremely low-cost screening measure should be used for every prospective mother, particularly as folate is one of the most common vitamin deficiencies.

The segmentation index is another functional vitamin test, since it measures an effect of folate, rather than the absolute level of folate itself.

## PROTHROMBIN TIME

Prothrombin time is one of the first functional vitamin tests. It measures one of vitamin K's functions—producing adequate amounts of prothrombin, a key blood clotting factor. Although it doesn't measure absolute levels of vitamin K at all, it tells us whether there's adequate vitamin K in the body to perform that crucial job. It's often abnormal in children with no other cause of nosebleeds, and in persons of any age who don't eat their green vegetables.

Prothrombin time measurement is widely available at low cost. That isn't especially to help nutritionally oriented doctors in monitoring adequacy of bodily vitamin K, but (ironically) because the test is usually done to control drug therapy with anticoagulants, which inhibit vitamin K activity. Whatever the reason, however, the test is available and can be put to use as a functional test for vitamin K adequacy.

Some laboratories will report that protime measurements of less than 100 percent are normal, using a lesser percentage, in the 60 to 90 percent range, as a cutoff point. I don't subscribe to that theory, particularly since a little extra vitamin K in the diet or as a supplement will almost always return the protime to 100 percent of normal.

## PROTOZOAL VITAMIN ASSAYS

Drs. Baker and Frank, professors of medicine at the University of Medicine and Dentistry of New Jersey, devised an ingenious system to evaluate levels of a broad range of vitamins in the blood—vitamins A, $B_1$, $B_2$, $B_3$, $B_6$, $B_{12}$, beta-carotene, biotin, C, E, folate, and pantothenate. They actually use live single-celled organisms called protozoa that grow in direct proportion to the amount of vitamin in the blood. Considering the convenience of the testing procedure, a cost of $10 per vitamin is quite reasonable.

Although the protozoal assay appears to be an excellent test, I haven't made great use of it for two reasons. Many individuals with whom I work are already eating whole-food diets and taking vitamins. Vitamin insufficiency is not usually a problem in that group.

Secondly, that assay measures absolute levels of each vitamin, but says nothing about how it is functioning in each individual's body relative to that person's needs. Functional vitamin testing is more useful information, and is just starting to be explored. (See "A Case of Vitamin $B_6$ Dependency" for further discussion of functional vitamin testing.)

## XANTHURENIC ACID

Xanthurenic acid is a normal by-product of tryptophan metabolism, and is excreted in the urine. When the body's supplies of vitamin $B_6$ are adequate, only a small quantity of xanthurenic acid is excreted after a test dose of tryptophan. When $B_6$ is inadequate, excretion of xanthurenic acid becomes abnormally high. Increased excretion of xanthurenic acid following a test dose of tryptophan is one of the early signs of vitamin $B_6$ deficiency.

In some diseases, however, including rheumatoid arthritis, lupus erythematosis, dermatomyositis, psoriatic arthritis, and polymyalgia rheumatica, elevated levels of xanthurenic acid and kynurenic acid (another tryptophan by-product) are found with no apparent vitamin $B_6$ deficiency. It's thought that this indicates another abnormality of tryptophan metabolism in these diseases.

This latter possibility becomes more intriguing in view of a 1977 letter to the editor of the *British Medical Journal* by Dr. Alan D. Broadhurst, reporting "a dramatic lessening of rheumatoid symptoms associated with a fall in the erythrocyte sedimentation rate" in a few individuals with rheumatoid arthritis who were also being treated for depression with tryptophan. Discontinuation of tryptophan led to recurrence of symptoms.

The author of the letter correctly points out that no specific conclusions can be drawn from his limited number of observations, but using that test for individuals with rheumatoid arthritis and the above-noted diseases has occasionally been rewarding.

# Nutritional Tests Are an Investment in the Future

As I noted at the beginning of this chapter, our laboratory tour has only included tests of particular relevance to nutritional-biochemical therapy and preventive medicine. Physicians specializing in those areas also do the more standard tests—routine screening, blood counts, liver function tests, urinalysis, and so on.

No implication is intended that those reviewed are the only useful tests in nutritional biochemistry. Other practitioners have found laboratory evaluations not listed here to be very helpful in their practices. At our laboratory, we're evaluating other procedures, including immune cell testing and fractionated amino acid analyses, that appear to have great potential.

Finally, a few words about costs. One of the most frequent criticisms of nutritional-biochemical practice is "excessive laboratory costs." Insurance companies (who don't particularly like paying claims for preventive health care) complain of "overutilization."

There's no way I can determine body levels of many nutrients without laboratory evaluation. If your selenium is low, your risk of cancer is probably higher, but I can't tell by looking at you. Cholesterol levels don't disclose themselves to the eye. Folate deficiency isn't obvious. Estrogen quotients aren't visible on physical exam.

If laboratory testing discloses a hidden folate deficiency and aids in averting a possible birth defect, how much money has been saved? Care for a child with spina bifida can cost hundreds of thousands of dollars. If laboratory testing determines low estriol excretion in a group of women and only one case of cancer is prevented through diet and specific supplements, tens of thousands of dollars are saved. Coronary bypass surgery costs $20,000 to $30,000; prevention of coronary artery disease aided by laboratory monitoring is considerably cheaper.

More extensive laboratory evaluation for disease prevention saves much more in later disease treatment costs. To paraphrase an old adage: $500 of prevention is worth $50,000 of cure.

But more important, no amount of money will compensate for the lifelong handicap of a preventable birth defect. Early death or the pain and suffering from preventable cancer, heart disease, or other illnesses can't be measured in dollars.

## REFERENCES

**Allergy**

Gleich, Gerald J., and Yunginger, John W. "The Radioallergosorbent Test: Its Present Place and Likely Future in the Practice of Allergy." *Advances in Asthma and Allergy*, Spring, 1975, pp. 1–9.

Moore, R. E.; Wright, J. V.; and Williams, B. F. "The Radioallergosorbent Test: A Comparison of Two Methods." *Journal of John Bastyr College of Naturopathic Medicine*, in press.

Wide, L. "Clinical Significance of Measurement of Reagnic (IgE) Antibody by RAST." *Clinical Allergy*, vol. 3 (supplement), 1973, pp. 583–595.

**Blood Sugar**

Kraft, Joseph. "Detection of Diabetes Mellitus *In Situ* (Occult Diabetes)." *Laboratory Medicine*, February, 1975, pp. 10–22.

Leslie, R. D. G. et al. "Fast Glycosylation of Hemoglobin." *Lancet*, April 7, 1979, pp. 773–774.

Newbold, H. L. *Mega-Nutrients for Your Nerves*. Peter H. Wyden, 1975, p. 73.

**Cholesterol**

"High HDLs May Offset Risk of Elevated Total Cholesterol." *Medical World News*, December 8, 1980, p. 37.

**Circulation**

Pinckney, Cathey, and Pinckney, Edward R. *The Encyclopedia of Medical Tests*, Facts On File, 1982.

**Clotting**

Al-Mefty, Ossama et al. "Transient Ischemic Attacks Due To Increased Platelet Aggregation and Adhesiveness." *Journal of Neurosurgery*, April, 1979, pp. 449–453.

Davis, James W. et al. "Platelet Aggregation: Adult-Onset Diabetes and Coronary Artery Disease." *Journal of the American Medical Association*, February 20, 1978, pp. 732–734.

Mehta, Jawahar, and Mehta, Paulette. "Platelet Function in Hypertension and Effect of Therapy." *American Journal of Cardiology*, February, 1981, pp. 331–334.

Yudkin, John; Szanto, Stephan; and Kakkar, V. V. "Sugar Intake, Serum Insulin and Platelet Adhesiveness in Men Without Peripheral Vascular Disease." *Postgraduate Medical Journal*, vol. 45, no. 527, 1969, pp. 608–611.

**Estrogens**
Follingstad, Alvin H. "Estriol, the Forgotten Estrogen?" *Journal of the American Medical Association*, January 2, 1978, pp. 29–30.

Lemon, Henry M. et al. "Reduced Estriol Excretion in Patients with Breast Cancer Prior to Endocrine Therapy." *Journal of the American Medical Association*, June 27, 1966, pp. 112–120.

**Hair Analysis**
Cranton, Elmer M. et al. "Standardization and Interpretation of Human Hair for Elemental Concentrations." *Journal of Holistic Medicine*, Spring/Summer, 1982, pp. 1–16.

Hambridge, K. Michael. "Hair Analyses: Worthless for Vitamins, Limited for Minerals." *American Journal of Clinical Nutrition*, November, 1982, pp. 943–949.

Katz, Sydney A. "The Use of Hair as a Biopsy Material for Trace Elements in the Body." *American Laboratory*, February, 1979, pp. 44–52.

Passwater, Richard, and Cranton, Elmer. *Trace Elements, Hair Analysis and Nutrition*. Keats Publishing, 1983.

Strain, William H. et al. "Trace Element Nutriture and Metabolism Through Head Hair Analysis." In *Trace Substance in Environmental Health—V*. University of Missouri, 1972, pp. 383–397.

Wright, Jonathan V., and Severtson, R. Bradley. "Observations on the Interpretations of Hair Mineral Analysis in Human Medicine." *Journal of the International Academy of Preventive Medicine*, April, 1982, pp. 13–16.

**Indican (Obermeyer)**
Yokoyama, Melvin T., and Carlson, James R. "Microbial Metabolites of Tryptophan in the Intestinal Tract with Special Reference to Skatole." *American Journal of Clinical Nutrition*, January, 1979, pp. 173–179.

**Minerals**
Bahemuka, M., and Hodkinson, H. M. "Red-Blood-Cell

Potassium as a Practical Index of Potassium Status in Elderly Patients." *Age and Ageing*, vol. 5, 1976, pp. 24–29.

Beck, William S. *On the Clinical Usefulness of Simultaneous Measurements of Serum Ferritin in the Diagnosis of Iron Deficiency and Iron Overload*. RIA Products, 1979.

Cook, James D. et al. "Serum Ferritin as a Measure of Iron Stores in Normal Subjects." *American Journal of Clinical Nutrition*, July, 1974, pp. 681–687.

"The Correlation of Serum Ferritin and Body Iron Stores." *Nutrition Reviews*, January, 1975, pp. 11–14.

Dawson, K. P., and Whimster, J. "Serum Ferritin Levels in Iron Deficient Children." *New Zealand Medical Journal*, August 13, 1980, pp. 96–97.

Ganong, William F. *Review of Medical Physiology*. 10th ed. Lange Medical Publications, 1981.

Johny, K. V. et al. "Studies on Total Body, Serum and Erythrocyte Potassium in Patients on Maintenance Hemodialysis." *Nephron*, vol. 7, 1970, pp. 230–240.

Keen, Carl L. et al. "Whole-Blood Manganese as an Indicator of Body Manganese." *New England Journal of Medicine*, May 19, 1983, p. 1230.

Laker, Martin. "On Determining Trace Element Levels in Man: The Uses of Blood and Hair." *Lancet*, July 31, 1982, pp. 260–262.

Peter, Frank, and Wang, Stephen. "Serum Iron and Total Iron Binding Capacity Compared with Serum Ferritin in Assessment of Iron Deficiency." *Clinical Chemistry*, vol. 27, no. 2, 1981, pp. 276–279.

**Oxalic Acid**
Pinckney, Cathey, and Pinckney, Edward R. *The Encyclopedia of Medical Tests*, Facts On File, 1982.

**Pancreatic Function**
Lentner, C., ed. *Geigy Scientific Tables*. Vol. 1. 8th ed., CIBA-GEIGY, 1981.

**Prostate**

Bates, Harold M. "Is Your Laboratory Measuring Prostatic Acid Phosphatase By Immunoassay?" *Laboratory Management,* February, 1980, pp. 11–16.

Gittes, Ruben F. "Serum Acid Phosphatase and Screening for Carcinoma of the Prostate." *New England Journal of Medicine,* October 6, 1983, pp. 852–853.

Horwitz, O. "Public Health Aspects of Cancer Deaths." *Acta Dermato-Venereologica Supplementum,* vol. 5, no. 85, 1979, pp. 85–89.

Personal Communication with Lawrence A. Kaplan, Assistant Professor of Pathology at the University of Cincinnati Medical Center, 1983.

**Stomach Acidity**

Andres, M. R., and Bingham, J. R. "Tubeless Gastric Analysis with a Radio-telemetering Pill (Heidelberg Capsule)." *Canadian Medical Association Journal,* May 21, 1970, pp. 1087–1089.

Kurt, E. J., and Kong, Supa. "Radiotelemetry pH Determination for Gastroesophageal Reflux." *American Journal of Gastroenterology,* vol. 58, 1972, pp. 390–395.

Steinberg, W. H. et al. "Heidelberg Capsule I: *In Vitro* Evaluation of a New Instrument for Measuring Intragastric pH." *Journal of Pharmaceutical Sciences,* May, 1965, pp. 772–776.

Williamson, J. M.; Russell, R. I.; and Goldberg, A. "A Screening Technique for the Detection of Achlorhydria Using the Heidelberg Capsule." *Scandinavian Journal of Gastroenterology,* vol. 4, 1969, pp. 369–375.

**Stomach Function**

Ganguli, P. C.; Cullen, D. R.; and Irvine, W. J. "Radioimmunoassay of Plasma-gastrin in Pernicious Anemia, Hypochlorhydria, and in Controls." *Lancet,* January 23, 1971, pp. 155–156.

Goldberg, David M., ed. *Clinical Biochemistry Reviews.* Vol. 2. John Wiley & Sons, 1981.

Voris, K. "An Appraisal of Tests for Severe Atrophic Gastritis in Relatives of Patients with Pernicious Anemia." *American Journal of Digestive Diseases,* March, 1979, pp. 187–191.

**Stool Analysis and Culture**

Kaslow, Arthur L., and Miles, Richard B. *Freedom From Chronic Disease*. J. P. Tarcher, 1979.

**Vitamins**

Bills, Terence, and Spatz, Lawrence. "Neutrophilic Hypersegmentation as an Indicator of Incipient Folic Acid Deficiency." *American Journal of Clinical Pathology*, August, 1977, pp. 263–267.

Kishi, Hiroe, and Folkers, Karl. "Improved and Effective Assays of the Glutamic Oxaloacetic Transaminase by the Coenzyme-Apoenzyme System (CAS) Principle." *Journal of Nutritional Science and Vitaminology*, vol. 22, 1976, pp. 225–234.

Lonsdale, Derrick, and Shamberger, Raymond. "Red Cell Transketolase as an Indicator of Nutritional Deficiency." *American Journal of Clinical Nutrition*, February, 1980, pp. 205–211.

Tillotson, J. A., and Baker, E. M. "An Enzymatic Measurement of the Riboflavin Status in Man." *American Journal of Clinical Nutrition*, April, 1972, pp. 425–431.

**Xanthurenic Acid**

Bett, Isabel M. "Urinary Tryptophan Metabolites in Rheumatoid Arthritis and Some Other Diseases." *Annals of the Rheumatic Diseases*, vol. 25, 1966, pp. 556–562.

Broadhurst, Alan D. "Tryptophan and Rheumatic Diseases." *British Medical Journal*, August 13, 1977, p. 456.

Georgy, Paul, and Pearson, W. N. *The Vitamins: Chemistry, Physiology, Pathology, Methods*. Vol. VII, 2nd ed. Academic Press, 1967, pp. 198–203.

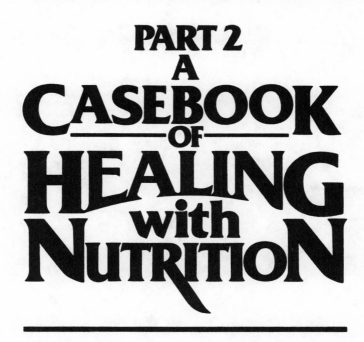

# PART 2
# A
# CASEBOOK
## OF
# HEALING
## with
# NUTRITION

The use of hydrochloric acid supplements clears up a long-standing case of acne rosacea in just two months—a simple solution for a complex problem.

# A CASE OF ACNE ROSACEA

# 9

Mrs. Cindy Krause came in cheerful and smiling. "I'm sure you can see what my problem is; everyone can. It's there all the time now. In fact, I seem to have worked up a particularly good demonstration for you today. My husband says I did it on purpose because I was coming in, but he's only teasing. It's been getting like this much more often in the last few years."

Her entire face was slightly reddened, like a mild sunburn or windburn. The redness was worse in the center of her forehead, over the bridge of her nose, onto the "blush" areas of her cheeks, and on her chin. She had two large pimples on her chin, three on her forehead, and one on her left eyelid. Her eyes appeared "bloodshot," and there were dilated capillaries in the worst of the reddened areas, particularly on her cheeks.

"You do have one of the most pronounced cases of rosacea I've seen in several months," I observed. "It's not always this bad?"

"No, but rapidly getting that way. My usual the last two or

three years has been redness mostly in the areas where it's bad today, with only a faint reddening anywhere else. My eyes are usually only a little red, and usually I don't have as many pimples. I've been taking an antibiotic, tetracycline, on and off, which does control the pimple part somewhat when I take it."

"What about the dilated capillaries?"

"Actually, I've had one of those on my right cheek and onto my nose since I was a teenager. But it was so faint that no one could see it except my boyfriends, and they mostly didn't get a chance because I covered it with makeup. The last three years the capillaries have gotten more numerous, and stay dilated all the time instead of just on and off. I've given up trying to use makeup. I'd have to use so much to cover all this that I'm thinking of going into the clown business. Why not take advantage of the situation?" She laughed.

"I suppose. Don't know if all that makeup would be good for your skin. Seriously though, have you noticed anything in particular that makes the capillaries dilate worse and your skin redder?"

"Alcohol will do it most of the time. I noticed that several years back when I first started getting rosacea, so I gave it up entirely. Haven't had a drink in over five years. Unfortunately it hasn't helped. It's really funny, too. One of my maiden aunts keeps telling everyone else in the family that I'm a secret alcoholic because my face keeps getting worse. But I don't drink, for sure—ask my husband. He tries to get me to have one with him every once in a while, but I won't."

"Anything else make it worse?"

"I don't go out in the sun much. That aggravates it a little. But what's odd is that just eating—it doesn't seem to matter what— will set my face off sometimes. It seems to go in spells. A few weeks, any meal will do it, then it stops for a while."

I made some notes. "Any other health problems?"

# Lifelong Constipation

"Nothing major, thank goodness. A little constipation from time to time, but that's nothing new. Even this rosacea, if that's the worst I get, I'm grateful. I could have cancer, or be disabled. No, I'm fairly healthy otherwise."

"Tell me about the constipation."

"It was worse when I was a little kid. My mother gave me enemas sometimes, otherwise I'd go a week or more. I got a lot better when I was a teenager. Now I sometimes go two or three days between bowel movements, sometimes every day. It varies."

"Were you an easy blusher as a child?"

"Wasn't I! I still am. Maybe this is just the natural consequence of all that blushing. You should have seen me when I was a teenager. I got embarrassed about being embarrassed, I was so bad. 'Stop Sign,' they used to call me, my face was always red." She smiled, then looked thoughtful.

"Do you think I got this just from overwork or wearing out of those blood vessels from too much blushing?"

"No. Although rosacea, acne rosacea technically, does seem to occur more often in the so-called easy blusher."

"That's good. Maybe there's some hope."

"Possibly. Besides constipation, do you have any other digestive troubles? Excess gas, belching, bloating?"

"Not that I've noticed."

We went through questions about her own and her family's health background. Except for tonsillectomy and a broken leg in a ski accident, she'd had no other problems. Her mother had developed high blood pressure at age 60, a cousin had hyperthyroidism, and her 16-year-old son had acne—"the regular kind, not this stuff," she observed.

## Split Fingernails

Her examination was also mostly normal. With the exception of the rosacea, the only other notable findings were two split, cracked fingernails. I asked about those.

"My fingernails have always been bad. I gave up trying to grow long ones in my early twenties; they'd break off. I didn't think to mention it because they're not really a problem. I keep them short. Now that you mention it, though, they have been breaking a lot more the last two or three years."

"You're how old now?"

"Same as Jack Benny, 39, although not as cute." She grinned. "At least, not today." Her expression changed to a more serious, wistful one. "Is there anything at all you think we can do? Anything new? Any vitamins or anything? My dermatologist said I was foolish coming over here, just wasting my time, but it is my time, and I was hoping. . . ."

"Why don't you get dressed again, and come back to my office. I want to get something from my files."

After she came in and sat down, I showed her two papers. "There's nothing new I know of for rosacea," I said. "But there is something old that works very well in the majority of cases. You have clues that indicate you may have the problem."

She looked at the dates on the papers. "1920? 1949? One of these is older than I am. Isn't this kind of obsolete?"

"If it's accurate, and the treatment based on it works, I don't care if it's from 1492 or 3003 B.C. In the case of rosacea, what have we got that's modern that works, anyway?"

"You have a point there. So what do I do"—she handed the papers back—"take charcoal and sulfur, or what?" She smiled.

"No, although it's odd you should mention those. What you should do, please, is have a gastric analysis done, as well as other nutritional screening tests."

"To see if my stomach's OK?"

"Specifically, to see if your stomach's making enough hydrochloric acid."

"I can see what that might have to do with my constipation or digestion, but what's it got to do with my face? You're implying there's some connection?"

"Yes, and with your fingernails, too. Poor fingernails like that frequently are associated with hypochlorhydria, or low stomach acidity. But about your face: The large majority of persons with rosacea, acne rosacea, have low stomach acidity and improve remarkably with hydrochloric acid supplements. I've seen it happen numerous times."

"What's hydrochloric acid in the stomach do for facial skin?"

"Frankly, I don't know. Perhaps it improves digestion and gives you more nutrients. Maybe it reduces intestinal putrefaction and cuts down on toxic substances absorbed into your system. There are many other theories, but the important point is that it works in most cases. Here, let me read you a line or two. From the 1920 report: 'The results obtained with this treatment [hydrochloric acid supplements] have been very satisfactory and frequently almost magical, even in the very worst cases.' And from the 1949 editorial: 'It is fairly common with dermatologists to find hypoacidity in association with acne rosacea and it is already known that the administration of acid supplements appears to assist control of this skin condition.' "

Mrs. Krause grimaced. "It hasn't been common with the dermatologists I've seen, and I'm more than ready for something almost magical. So why don't I just try taking hydrochloric acid capsules? I've seen them at my health food store."

"Because if you don't need them, and you take the dose required by people who do, you could give yourself gastritis or possibly even an ulcer. They should never be taken with aspirin, or certain other drugs. If you do have low stomach acidity, we recommend vitamin $B_{12}$ by injection. And a few other details. . . ."

"I get the picture. It's a little more involved than just taking hydrochloric acid capsules. There are possible complications, and I should find out if I really need them."

"Right. Remember, I said the large majority of people with rosacea are helped, but not absolutely everyone."

"Which way to the gastric analysis? I can live with rosacea if I have to, but if there's a way out. . . . By the way, do I have to have my stomach pumped?"

"No, we use gastric analysis by radiotelemetry. It's been proven just as accurate, and I find it more versatile."

## Results in Two Months

Mrs. Krause's gastric analysis was badly abnormal. She began taking 45 grains of betaine hydrochloride per full meal, an average adult dose, and had substantial clearing of her rosacea in just two months. Only the worst reddened areas remained, and they had subsided to a faint red. Her pimples were completely gone, none returned, and even the capillaries were less prominently dilated. She scarcely noted any "blushing" at all.

She also observed that her lifelong constipation was gone, and her fingernails weren't breaking as much and "even beginning to grow."

We then added vitamin $B_{12}$ and folate by injection, vitamin B complex, zinc, and numerous other nutrients she appeared to need, some of them probably due to poor assimilation related to low stomach acidity.

Two years later, her facial skin remains completely free of rosacea, except for traces of dilated capillaries near her nose.

## A Clue to Rosacea

Acne rosacea, sometimes called simply rosacea, is one of the many conditions commonly associated with low stomach acidity. The association is close, even in the mildest cases. In my experience, the use of hydrochloric acid supplements in adequate doses is extremely effective in reducing the severity of the problem, and in some cases nearly eliminating it. For reasons explained below, adding *Lactobacillus acidophilus* appears even more helpful than hydrochloric acid and pepsin supplements alone.

The usual present-day treatment for this skin condition is the antibiotic tetracycline. It's not known what tetracycline does for this condition, but it is partially effective.

According to the commentator in the 1949 reference below, "It is well known, however, that the administration of large amounts of dilute hydrochloric acid ... alters the putrefactive flora ordinarily dominant in the upper gut of achlorhydrics." Tetracycline kills bacteria. A reasonable explanation for the common effect of both of these substances on rosacea would be that it's a reaction of the facial skin to an as yet unidentified metabolite excreted by an "abnormal" intestinal bacteria. This would also explain why adding *Lactobacillus acidophilus* is helpful.

There's a small revival of research interest in the "intestinal toxemia" theory of the causation of some disease. Although I heard this theory ridiculed in medical school, it appears it may be true, after all, in problems other than rosacea.

Nicholas L. Petrakis, Ph.D., at the University of California, San Francisco, studied the cells in breast fluid taken from nonlactating women without cancer. Cells were classified as normal or showing "dysplasia." (As with dysplasia on a pap smear, this signifies "not normal but not cancerous, either." Dysplasia is sometimes considered precancerous; it's definitely an increased risk factor.) According to the researchers: "There was a significant positive association with dysplasia . . . in women reporting severe constipation, i.e., two or fewer bowel movements weekly, which was not seen in women reporting more than one bowel movement daily. Women who had one bowel movement daily or one every other day had [less chance of cell dysplasia]." Although the researchers made no mention of low stomach acidity, women and men with it are frequently constipated.

Whatever the cause of constipation, however, the researchers say: "Perhaps breast disease should be added to the list of conditions believed to be influenced by diet and bowel function."

British investigators, led by Dr. M. J. Hill, studied 44 individuals with colon cancer and 90 without. Eighty-two percent of the individuals with colon cancer had high levels of fecal bile acids, substances chemically similar to known carcinogens. Only 17 percent of those without colon cancer had similarly high levels. More important, 70 percent of those with colon cancer had both high levels of fecal bile acids and intestinal bacteria capable of tranforming bile acids into carcinogenic form. Only 9 percent of those without colon cancer had both high fecal bile acids and carcinogen-producing bacteria.

Returning briefly to low stomach acidity, two papers in the *Archives of Internal Medicine* and *American Journal of Clinical Nutrition* note that it's associated with bacterial contamination of the upper intestine, an area whose bacterial population is usually sparse. The full range of diseases associated with bacterial contamination is just beginning to be investigated.

Finally, in a series of publications, a French physician whose numerous works are reported in *The Biological Basis of Schizophrenia* has demonstrated that some causes of apparent mental disease have originated as reactions to toxic substances released by colon bacteria. He reports having cured some of them, relieving mental symptoms entirely, by treatment directed against the bacterial toxins. And he makes note of other European physicians who have published on the same topic.

# REFERENCES

**Acne Rosacea**

"Nutrition Notes and Abstracts on Nutrition: A Plug for Acid Therapy." *American Journal of Digestive Diseases*, vol. 16, no. 11, 1949, p. 418.

Ryle, J. A., and Barber, H. W. "Gastric Analysis in Acne Rosacea." *Lancet*, December 11, 1920, pp. 1195–1196.

**Intestinal Toxemia**

Barok, H. "Psychoses from Digestive Origins." In *The Biological Basis of Schizophrenia*. University Park Press, 1979, pp. 37–44.

Drude, Richard B., and Hines, C., Jr. "The Pathophysiology of Intestinal Bacterial Overgrowth Syndromes." *Archives of Internal Medicine*, October, 1980, pp. 1349–1352.

Gracey, Michael. "The Contaminated Small Bowel Syndrome: Pathogenesis, Diagnosis, and Treatment." *American Journal of Clinical Nutrition*, January, 1979, pp. 234–243.

Hill, M. J. et al. "Faecal Bile Acids and Clostridia in Patients with Cancer of the Large Bowel." *Lancet*, March 8, 1975, pp. 535–539.

Petrakis, Nicholas L., and King, Eileen B. "Cytological Abnormalities in Nipple Aspirates of Breast Fluid from Women with Severe Constipation." *Lancet*, November 28, 1981, pp. 1203–1205.

One of the principal causes of ill health, especially in small children, is allergies. Dark circles under the eyes, swollen lymph glands, enlarged tonsils, and fluid behind the ears are all telltale signs. This case shows you just how to track down the cause.

# A CASE OF "ALLERGIC SHINERS" 10

Aaron McKee was four years old, dark blond, blue-eyed. Beneath each eye, the skin was discolored dark blue. As he walked in with his mother, it appeared his abdomen was more protuberant than usual for his age. He was also a little thin. I thought I knew what his problem might be, but waited for his mother to tell me.

"He gets sick all the time," Mrs. McKee started. "I've tried to do everything right, but still he gets colds, flu, diarrhea, bronchitis, earaches, pneumonia . . . if it's going around, Aaron will catch it. It's really frustrating because he's never had any sugar, refined food, or artificial food chemicals. I nursed him entirely until he was eight months old. I read in *Prevention* about another little boy with recurrent infections and started Aaron on vitamin C, zinc, B complex, vitamins A and D, and thymus tablets when he was two. After I read about the right doses for two-year-olds, of course."

"Did it help?"

"If it had like the article said, we wouldn't be here! The

supplements seemed to help for two months or so, and then back to the same old thing."

"Have you continued them?"

"Well, yes. I figured he'd probably be worse without them. The next thing I tried was removing cow's milk, or anything with cow's milk in it. Thought he might be allergic."

"And?"

"No big change, except he did seem a little less stuffy in the nose when he got sick, after that. So I kept him off cow's milk, switched to goat milk. I still think he's food allergic, but I can't tell to what. I can't put him on a fast."

"Sounds like you're on the right track. You've not had allergy tests done?"

"No, I've read, and my pediatrician agrees, that skin tests for food allergy aren't all that accurate. He offered to have them done for inhalants, but Aaron's problems don't seem seasonal. Besides, I don't want him to have all those scratches."

"You're right. Standard skin tests for food allergy aren't helpful. There is a type of skin test done by clinical ecologists that seems much better, but particularly for a four-year-old, the blood tests for antibodies (RAST) is much better tolerated and accurate enough."

"You think he's allergic, then?"

## All the Right Clues

"That's always at the top of the list when you're 'doing everything right' . . . no refined sugar, no refined foods, no artificial food chemicals, only whole foods, the right supplements . . . and still there's chronic, recurrent illness. Besides, Aaron looks allergic."

"What do you mean?"

"It's not understood, but often observed that blond, blue-eyed children are more susceptible to allergy. Secondly, he has 'allergic shiners.'"

"You mean those bluish circles under his eyes?"

"Yes, one of the most frequent causes of those is allergy."

Aside from dark circles under his eyes, Aaron had larger-than-usual tonsils, slightly enlarged lymph glands in the neck, fluid behind his eardrums, and, as noted before, an abdomen a little more protuberant than most other children his age. I mentioned these things to Mrs. McKee.

## Signs of Excess Gas

"I've heard all of that before, except about his abdomen. I figured it was due to infection, allergy, or both. What does the part about his stomach mean?"

"Can't be sure yet. Does he have any problem with passing gas, or burping up a lot?"

"Sometimes, especially passing gas. I think I mentioned he gets diarrhea on and off. The rest of the time he's a little constipated."

"When he was smaller, did you ever see undigested food in his diapers? Besides, say, corn or seeds?"

"Yes, now that you mention it. Sometimes a bit of spinach or carrot. I remember watermelon, too. Thought it was a bit odd. Shouldn't those foods be digested?"

"Usually. Since he's been out of diapers, have you checked for undigested food?"

"No, I didn't think to."

"Does his abdomen ever get flat?"

"Sometimes, but now that I think of it, he does seem a little bulged out, usually. Especially after he eats. It's strange, since he's on the thin side. Maybe it's gas."

"Probably."

"Could gas be due to food allergies, too?"

"Excess gas is one of the most frequent symptoms. Since we have to draw a blood specimen for food allergy testing, though, we can also test it for digestive enzymes."

"What enzymes?"

"Pancreatic, amylase, lipase, trypsin."

"They show up in the bloodstream, don't they? I read that somewhere. You can tell whether he's digesting his food that way?"

"Indirectly."

"If he's not digesting his foods, he could develop more allergies, couldn't he?"

"That's one of the theories. It's also possible that allergies could lead to not digesting food properly. . . ."

"So it goes around in a circle."

"That's the way it seems. I'd also like to ask you to turn in a specimen of hair for mineral analysis."

"Sure, I expected that." She pulled an envelope out of her purse. "I thought checking to see what minerals he needed would be a good idea, too. Maybe he has too much of a toxic one, though I don't know where he'd get it."

## Hidden Allergy in Family

"I need to get your family health history, and your husband's, of course."

"That's what's so strange . . . that's why it took me a while to figure that Aaron might be allergic. No one on either side of the family has allergies, as far as we can tell, anyway." She pondered a moment. "I had all this memorized . . . my husband, Aaron's father, is well. No problems. His mother had gallbladder problems, finally had it out. His father and grandfather both died of heart attacks. One grandmother's still living. She has diabetes. The other two grandparents died in their nineties.

"On my side . . . my father's OK except for canker sores a lot. My mother has high blood pressure. One grandfather had pernicious anemia; one grandmother diabetes and gallbladder disease. That's all I know about."

"What about yourself?"

"Oh, yes. I'm fine except I get yeast infections a lot. Can't seem to get rid of them."

"You haven't mentioned any 'typical' allergy problems like asthma, hayfever, hives, or eczema, but you do have a strong history of possible hidden allergy in both families. Also, the history of pernicious anemia is intriguing."

Mrs. McKee looked puzzled. "Hidden allergy? Where?"

"Gallbladder problems, both sides of the family. Persistent canker sores, and you getting yeast infections a lot. Four probably food-allergic people."

I asked a few other background questions about Aaron. Then he and his mother left to have his tests done.

Most of his tests had to be mailed away, and weren't back for three weeks. Shortly after, Aaron and his mother were back.

"What's the news?" she asked.

"Not good, I'm afraid. Aaron's tests show high levels of antibodies to beef, Cheddar cheese, corn, egg, cow's milk, orange, peanut, pork, and soy. He's mildly allergic to apples and wheat."

"Good grief, no wonder he gets sick. What isn't he allergic to?"

"On this test, chicken, lamb, lettuce, potato, rice, tomato, tuna, brewer's yeast, and goat milk."

"Doesn't leave much."

"Believe it or not, it's better than some I've seen."

"I wonder how he got allergic?"

# Low Stomach Acidity

"I can't answer that, but his mineral analysis provides another clue. It appears quite possible he may not have enough acid secretion by his stomach. That would fit his symptoms of gas, undigested food, and protuberant abdomen."

"How can you tell lack of stomach acid from a mineral test?"

"Can't. We'd have to do a gastric analysis to know for sure. But the mineral test provides a strong piece of circumstantial evidence. Aaron's levels of calcium, magnesium, iron, manganese, zinc, chromium, selenium, nickel, and cobalt are all low."

Mrs. McKee counted. "That's eight. I've read that when that many minerals are low on an adult's test, it's a good clue for lack of stomach acid. I never heard of a child with stomach acid deficiency, though. How does it happen at such a young age?"

"I don't know. I've learned from experience that it's not at all rare in children with various illnesses, especially allergy. This isn't new information; around 1931, a Dr. Bray pumped the stomachs of 200 children with asthma, and found that 160 of them, 80 percent, were hypochlorhydric (not enough stomach acid production). Much lower but still significant percentages have been found in other allergic conditions."

Mrs. McKee looked dubious. "I don't think I want Aaron's stomach pumped. That's a bit much for a four-year-old. How about that radiotelemetry capsule thing?"

"You've read about the Heidelberg capsule test then. We've usually found that children can't swallow the capsule well until age six or after."

"So what do we do? Forget it?"

"No . . . remember, it's possible that if Aaron's food isn't digested properly, it might contribute to allergy formation. Experimentation suggests the possibility. Sufficient stomach acid is important to the activity of protein-digesting enzymes such as pepsin."

"What about his pancreatic enzyme test?"

"His level of amylase and trypsin were both low."

"So he should take digestive enzymes. Won't those do?"

"Not completely. Very little that nature provides is totally useless. There must be some good reason for stomach acid, or our bodies wouldn't go to all the work required to concentrate hydrochloric acid in the stomach. Remember, it belongs there naturally.

"Also, getting back to Aaron's mineral analysis, it's likely that many of his minerals are low because of insufficient stomach acid."

"Couldn't that be just from all those food allergies?"

"Possibly, but I've found it's not usually the case."

"So if he's too little to test, but probably needs hydrochloric acid supplements for mineral absorption, to digest food better and possibly cut down on allergies . . . what do we do?"

# A Cautious Plan

"Try having him take small quantities of hydrochloric acid supplements, in the form of glutamic acid hydrochloride or betaine hydrochloride, and watch out for adverse reactions."

"Adverse reactions? Could he get an ulcer?"

"Not likely. I haven't seen it happen . . . it probably would take prolonged unnecessary administration of hydrochloric acid supplements to produce an ulcer. No, I mean reactions like burning pain, stomachache, diarrhea, or other stomach symptoms. Another thing is to look for improvement of his gassiness, more normal bowel function, and watch to see if his stomach sticks out as far."

Mrs. McKee looked dubious. "You're sure it's safe?"

"If there are any adverse symptoms, give him a glass of goat milk or baking soda in water to buffer the acid immediately. Don't give him any more hydrochloric acid supplementation, either, and let me know what happened.

"Obviously, giving a small child a hydrochloric acid supplement should only be done when it really appears necessary, and under a doctor's supervision. There are other precautions to observe such as never giving aspirin and a hydrochloric acid supplement together. We'll give you all this, printed out, before you go."

"So . . . I don't feed him what he's allergic to, give him hydrochloric acid supplements, pancreatic digestive enzymes . . . and I suppose continue the supplements I've been giving him?"

"Anything you give him should be as nonallergenic as possible, at least at the outset. Pancreatin is usually made from pork or beef; he's allergic to those. Either pineapple or papaya enzymes are probably preferable, if he's not allergic to them.

"Similarly, any supplements containing allergenic substances, like soy in his case, should be avoided to start with."

Aaron's mother removed all his allergenic foods; his intermittent loose bowels and some of his gas cleared up. She then added, slowly and cautiously, glutamic acid hydrochloride supplementation, starting with 5 grains per meal, and working up to 15 grains per meal. His protuberant abdomen disappeared, becoming more flat, and he was no longer constipated. After just two or three weeks, she reported he'd gained some weight and "just seemed stronger." She added his supplements last, explaining that she wanted to do one thing at a time in case there were any difficulties.

Aaron and his mother continued to check in at intervals to make sure things were going well. Three years later, he was still doing fine with only a very occasional cold, and no other health difficulties.

# Recurrent Infection
## a Clue to Allergies

Unfortunately, Aaron's case is not unusual. Allergies are among the principal causes of ill health for children. "Allergic shiners," persistently swollen lymph glands, enlarged tonsils, and fluid behind the eardrums are the most common physical signs of allergy in small children.

However, a history of recurrent infections of any kind is also a key clue to allergy. Recurrent earache, sore throat, tonsillitis, or bronchitis are some of the most common, but any recurrent infection should raise the suspicion index for hidden allergy.

According to James C. Breneman, M.D., a well-known allergist, the majority of allergy in children is food allergy; only a minority is attributable to inhalants. The smaller the child, the greater the percentage of an allergy problem that's due to foods.

Until very recently, the overwhelming number of food allergy tests have been done by skin tests, sometimes called scratch tests. Since routine skin tests (as noted by Dr. Breneman) are inaccurate, generations of physicians have become discouraged about looking for food allergy in children, and frequently hold the opinion that it's of very minor importance in contributing to disease.

More accurate testing, including one type of RAST test; procedures followed by clinical ecologists; and properly supervised elimination diets make it very clear to physicians using them that food allergy is indeed a major cause of illness in children.

In my opinion, most of the tonsillectomies and "tubes in the ears" surgical procedures performed on children are preventable. Searching out and eliminating food allergies is a major part of what's needed to stop the recurrent infections that lead to such surgery.

For parents who may not have access to more accurate medical testing procedures for food allergy, the inexpensive self-help book, *Tracking Down Hidden Food Allergy,* by William Crook, M.D., a pediatrician, can be an invaluable aid. Written and illustrated especially for children, it enables many parents to eliminate their children's problems on their own, strictly through dietary means.

The problem of poor digestion due to hypochlorhydria or low stomach acidity and low pancreatic enzymes is also surprisingly frequent in allergic children. Exactly why it happens isn't certain, but there are clues.

George W. Bray, M.D., who demonstrated that 80 percent of asthmatic children in his tested group had low stomach acidity, noted that the problem appeared to occur after some viral infections, particularly more serious ones. Entirely by accident, this cause may have been rediscovered at two Texas hospitals.

Investigators were studying stomach acid secretion in 37 healthy volunteers. Between November, 1976, and June, 1977, 17 volunteers whose stomach secretion had previously been normal showed a sudden sharp drop in acid secretion. In 14 of the volunteers, stomach acid secretion returned to its original levels at intervals from 53 to 225 days. In three, low stomach acidity was persistent.

Nine of the 17 who developed sudden low stomach acidity reported experiencing a mild illness with stomach pain a few days before the problem developed. No fever occurred. Biopsies taken during the period of the problem showed only inflammation of the stomach lining.

The investigators could not identify the cause, but suspected a viral or toxic agent.

A medical newspaper report of this incident was headlined "A New Disease?" But to at least one observant clinician in the past, such an occurrence wasn't unusual. Writing to the *British Medical Journal* in 1949, Dr. Joseph Vine described two cases of low stomach acidity following gastroenteritis, and stated, "I have met with many such cases in the past."

In small children who have persistent low stomach acidity caused by (presumably) a virus, recovery sometimes doesn't occur for years. Many appear to recover at puberty.

However, children have one other factor working against them: Low stomach acidity has also been shown to be caused by cow's milk allergy. Particularly in the United States where cow's milk is often fed to human infants instead of their mother's milk, this may account for many children with low stomach acidity.

Researchers from the University of Oulu, Finland, studied eight children with cow's milk allergy and intolerance. Stomach acid production was markedly decreased; three children produced no acid at all. Biopsies of the small intestine disclosed atrophy of the absorptive surface in six of the eight, and slight changes in the other two.

After strict elimination of cow's milk, replaced with human milk or soy milk, stomach acid secretion returned to normal within an average of six months.

Although this study reported only on cow's milk allergy, it certainly raises the question, as yet unanswered, of whether other allergy can also lead to low stomach acidity and consequent nutrient malabsorption.

Low stomach acidity caused by milk allergy doesn't always go away at the end of childhood. In a study of adults with and without milk allergy, milk ingestion was found to significantly reduce acid secretion to those allergic to it.

Once low stomach acidity is caused—whether by virus, allergy, or other things unknown—digestion is poor, sometimes over a period of time. Food, particularly protein, may not be broken down. Other research has shown that it's quite possible for relatively large food particles to be absorbed intact through the intestinal wall, a process called "macromolecular absorption." In theory, these large molecules are capable of causing an allergic response. Thus it's quite probable that in some individuals (especially those with allergy-prone genetics) poor digestion could lead to the development of allergy.

Here we have a classic "chicken and egg" problem. Allergy can lead to low stomach acidity and poor digestion. However, something other than allergy—a virus, for example—can cause low stomach acidity and poor digestion, which could then cause allergy. Trying to determine what caused what in a child or adult with the common overlapping of both allergies and low stomach acidity is usually impossible.

At present, all that can be said is that allergy and low stomach acidity are frequently associated in children (as well as adults). In children like Aaron McKee, who have both problems, allergy removal will only deal with part of the causes of their ill health. Poor digestion also needs correction. Otherwise even the best diet and needed supplementation won't be as helpful as they should be, and the child with poor digestion will inadvertently be suboptimally nourished.

# REFERENCES

**Allergy**

Breneman, J. C. *Basics of Food Allergy*. Charles C Thomas, 1978.

Crook, William G. *Tracking Down Hidden Food Allergy*. Professional Books, 1978.

Randall, H. et al. "Milk Hypersensitivity: RAST Studies Using New Antigens Generated by Pepsin Hydrolysis of Betalactoglobulin." *Annals of Allergy*, October, 1980, pp. 242–245.

**Low Stomach Acidity**

Bray, George W. "The Hypochlorhydria of Asthma in Childhood." *Quarterly Journal of Medicine*, January, 1931, pp. 181–197.

Kokkonen, J.; Simila, S.; and Herva, R. "Impaired Gastric

Function in Children with Cow's Milk Intolerance." *European Journal of Pediatrics,* June, 1979, pp. 1–6.

Vine, Joseph. "Achlorhydria Following Gastro-enteritis." *British Medical Journal,* January 29, 1949, p. 196.

Werner, M., and Wettwer, L. "Capacity for Gastric Acid Secretion in Adults with Milk Allergy." *Journal of the American Medical Association,* January 13, 1969, p. 395.

A search for the cause of an anemic condition (present since childhood) in a young woman reveals low stomach acidity. Hydrochloric acid and iron supplements, as well as vitamin $B_{12}$ shots, finally relieve her problem.

# 11    A CASE OF CHRONIC ANEMIA

Jane Houghton looked tired and pale. Her skin color didn't quite match her dark brown eyes and hair. Her lips were more pale pink than red. Probably anemic, I guessed; she let me know right away that that was not an original thought.

"I'm anemic again, I'm sure," she started. "Hemoglobin probably around 10.5. I'm more than usually tired, and especially tired of being tired. I know I shouldn't have stopped taking my iron, but I'm tired of that every day of my life. No one else I know has to take iron pills all the time just to stay normal. Besides, they're constipating and that gives me hemorrhoids."

Since it sounded like a long-time problem, I thought perhaps it would be best to start at the beginning. "How long have you been anemic?"

"On and off since 1945, when I was eight years old. Actually, it must have been since before than, because I'd been unusually tired for a while before my parents decided to take me to the doctor. They gave me iron pills, made me eat liver and blackstrap molasses. Ugh!" She made a face.

"Did it work?"

"I guess so. I wasn't as tired anymore . . . or maybe I just didn't want to eat another bite of liver. So I stopped all that stuff for a while."

"Then what?"

"Well, after my periods started, I had two or three fainting spells. I just didn't feel good. My mother figured out what it was right away, but took me to the doctor just to make sure. That time my hemoglobin was 10. They put me back on the iron pills."

"And?"

"It helped again. It usually does, but I had to take three pills a day to get my blood count barely normal. I got very constipated. The doctor said it was either that or stay anemic. So I took them most of the time. But after I left home, I quit."

"With no problem?"

"I don't know for sure. Sometimes I felt fine, other times tired. Maybe I adjusted."

"But you've been anemic since?"

"Oh, yes. Every time I go to the doctor for anything, they always tell me my hemoglobin's borderline, right at 12, or a little bit low."

## Injections during Pregnancy

"Have you ever been in the hospital or had tests done to find out what is the matter?"

"Not actually in the hospital, although they were going to put me there the first time I was pregnant. I'd been away from home a few years, not taking my iron pills. I'd felt well, just a little tired as usual. Anyway, the first time I went in to see the doctor about the baby, he just about came off his chair. He wanted to put me in the hospital right away, saying something about a transfusion if I didn't improve. My hemoglobin was 9. I told him not to worry so much, it was usually between 10 and 12 unless I took lots of iron. So he put me back on iron pills, but they didn't work as quickly as he wanted. I got iron shots. They hurt a lot."

"Have you taken shots any other time?"

"Only with my other babies, when it was really important. It worked every time. The only advantage was I didn't get constipated or annoy my hemorrhoids."

"What about tests?"

"Oh, yes. About nine or ten years ago, I decided I'd had enough of being anemic. I told my doctor I wanted some tests done, and a referral to a blood specialist. About that time, I'd started having stomach symptoms on and off, so he ordered stomach and intestinal x-rays to make sure I didn't have an ulcer or slow intestinal bleeding. I didn't; it was all normal. The laboratory checked my bowel movements for any hidden blood, too. There wasn't any."

"How about the hematologist, the blood specialist?"

"He was very nice. He checked me for hereditary kinds of anemia . . . thala-something-or-other was one of them."

"Thalassemia?"

"That's it. He said it wasn't that, or any other hereditary kind. It's not pernicious anemia, either. My spleen wasn't destroying too many blood cells. I even had a bone marrow biopsy."

"What did that show?"

Mrs. Houghton looked discouraged. "Marginally low iron storage. The same story, after all those tests."

"Were you checked for copper deficiency? Sometimes iron doesn't work so well if copper is low."

"Oh, yes, the hematologist told me about that, too. It wasn't a problem."

"So you've been on iron since?"

"On and off, and anemic on and off."

"Had you tried taking your iron with vitamin C?"

"I heard about that two or three years back. What does it do?"

"Studies show that vitamin C increases iron absorption, sometimes as much as double."

"It helps a little, I think."

"Also, iron is absorbed better with animal protein."

"Really? That's why lots of iron pills have liver in them, then. I thought it was just because liver was high in iron."

"You're right, it is, but as animal protein it helps iron absorption, too. You know which foods are high in iron?"

"I've looked those up long ago. Liver, organ meats, brewer's yeast, deep green vegetables, wheat germ, fish . . . I make sure to eat lots of those."

"Good." I made a few notes.

"So, is that all I can do? Take iron, make sure it's with vitamin C and animal protein, stay constipated, and hope for the best?" She looked disappointed.

"No, I didn't say that. There are a number of other things I need to ask you though."

We discussed the rest of her health background. She'd had her tonsils out, but no other surgery. As far as she knew, she had no allergies. She didn't use tobacco or caffeine ("it makes me nervous") and drank alcohol only occasionally. Her father had hypertension; her mother "borderline" diabetes; two relatives had had cancer. A great-aunt had developed pernicious anemia in her eighties.

## On-and-Off Indigestion

"You mentioned you had stomach x-rays. Why was that?"

"Oh, I'd started to get a sort of indigestion. No real bad pains, just gas and heartburn occasionally. It's on and off; sometimes I go weeks with no problems. Then I'll have it for a few months. After the x-ray was negative, the doctor said it must be just acid indigestion, and to use antacids when I need to."

"Do they help?"

"Mostly."

"Did you have your stomach acid measured?"

"I don't think so. The x-ray doesn't do that, does it?"

"No. I think that's probably a test you should have done, along with checking your anemia, a hair mineral test, and other routine tests."

"Why? My stomach really isn't a big problem. Do you think I'm not absorbing my iron from my food? Does too much stomach acid interfere?"

"Not too much acid, too *little*. But that's not completely consistent: Some people whose stomachs make too little acid don't get anemic, while others do. Even textbooks aren't completely clear on the importance of stomach acid to iron absorption.

"Acid is apparently only one of several factors involved in iron absorption. For many people with chronic anemia, though, it appears to be a key."

"What makes you think I don't have enough stomach acid?"

"I don't know for sure, but your symptoms—indigestion, gas, heartburn—indicate you might."

"Even though antacids help?"

"Yes. Lots of people who take antacids for indigestion should actually be taking hydrochloric acid supplements instead. But it's not a completely safe thing to do without a test. Those who take hydrochloric acid supplements and don't need them run the risk of developing an ulcer. That's why I want you to have your stomach tested."

"I heard about that from my neighbor. You checked her last year. You use some little radio gadget, don't you?"

"Yes, it's called gastric analysis by radiotelemetry. We use challenge testing to see how your stomach does at making acid."

## Some Acid, But Not Enough

Nearly a month later, Mrs. Houghton was back for the results of her tests.

"What was my hemoglobin?" she asked.

"10.4."

"What about my stomach acid test?"

"Definitely low. Your stomach does produce acid, but less than usual and more slowly than usual. Since there is some acid, it's called hypochlorhydria—for too little acid—rather than achlorhydria, for none."

"What causes that?"

"I wish I knew. Then maybe I'd know how to help you get it better, rather than just compensate for it."

"What do you mean?"

"Ideally, the solution would be to get your stomach acid production up to normal on its own. But at present I don't know how that can be done. So, second best is to have you use hydrochloric acid capsules, betaine hydrochloride or glutamic acid hydrochloride, with meals."

"I've already started, after the medical technologist told me my test was low when I had it done. I'm taking three of the five-grain capsules. My digestion definitely feels better."

"That's a good start, but probably not enough. Please try to increase the dose, a little at a time, to at least 50 grains, taken with full meals. Use the ten-grain capsules if it's more convenient."

"Fifty grains? Isn't that an awful lot? Won't I get an ulcer?"

"Of course you should always stop if a higher dose of acid hurts your stomach; that might indicate you don't need that much, although not always. Actually, 40 to 50 grains is an average dose for good digestion."

"What about iron?"

"Try using 100 milligrams of chelated iron twice daily, with the hydrochloric acid capsules, some vitamin C, and, of course, food. Don't take vitamins E, A, D, K, lecithin, or any oily or fatty vitamins at the same time. Chelated iron is likely to interfere with these vitamins less than inorganic iron, but separate them by at least two to four hours if possible."

## Minerals Low

She got up to go. "Oh, what about my mineral analysis?"

"Most of the minerals were low. That's typical for low stomach acid problems."

"Shouldn't I take those, too?"

"Yes, but let's start later. I'd like you to work on getting the anemia better first. I think the hydrochloric acid capsules with meals and iron will do the job, but we can't be sure until you try it. Another thing I'll want you to try later are vitamin $B_{12}$ injections. I always try those in case of low or no stomach acidity."

"Vitamin $B_{12}$ injections? Aren't those for pernicious anemia like my great-aunt had? The hematologist said I don't have that, just iron deficiency."

"Pernicious anemia is an endstage of vitamin $B_{12}$ deficiency. It's always associated with no stomach acidity, though. Actually, your great-aunt's problem was one of the clues in your case. Who can say if your low stomach acidity might not slowly develop into no stomach acidity by the time you're 80, along with pernicious anemia? Since vitamin $B_{12}$ is generally considered safe, I'd rather prevent trouble than wait for disease and then try to cure it."

She nodded. "That makes sense. I'll take my iron with the hydrochloric acid capsules and see what happens this time."

Her hemoglobin subsequently rose to 14, an entirely normal level. She found that with the hydrochloric acid capsules and chelated iron she had only occasional constipation. Once her anemia was gone, it didn't return as long as she ate iron-rich foods. She no longer needs iron pills.

Most persons with low stomach acidity, especially if it's been present in childhood, have either obvious or hidden allergies. Mrs. Houghton's case is unusual in that so far none has been found.

## Low Stomach Acidity Causes Anemia

In my experience, unexplained persistent anemia or chronic intermittent anemia is more frequently caused by hypochlorhydria or low stomach acidity than anything else. Caused isn't exactly the right word, since something else in turn causes the low acidity which then leads to anemia, and is thus the probable true cause of both problems. However, at present the cause (if it is just one) of low stomach acidity isn't known, and it isn't easily correctable.

I always search for other conditions leading to chronic anemia. Heavy menstrual bleeding, bleeding from the bowel, and a variety of nutrient deficiencies are among the more frequent. Another diagnosis, "anemia of chronic illness" is often associated with low stomach acidity (although certainly not always), since individuals with other chronic illnesses are quite likely to have it, too.

The relationship of iron absorption to sufficient stomach acidity isn't a clear one. Although many iron-deficient individuals have low acidity, I've worked with several individuals with no stomach acid at all (actual measurement) who had adequate iron levels. Conversely, there are many iron-deficient people (women especially) who have perfectly normal stomach acidity. Despite the lack of a perfect correlation between adequate stomach acidity and iron absorption, the association is sufficiently frequent that whenever a serum ferritin (currently regarded as the best test for body iron storage) turns up low, I make sure to check for low stomach acidity as the cause. More often than not, it's present.

In my experience, low stomach acidity is the number one cause of iron deficiency anemia in men. That isn't sexist; men simply don't have monthly iron loss. I always check for gastrointestinal bleeding, and frequently other causes, too, but failure of iron assimilation associated with low acidity is far and away the most frequent cause of iron deficiency in men (at least at our lab).

There's entirely enough discussion of low stomach acidity in the chapter "Good Digestion: Why We Can't Take it for Granted," so I'll end here by saying that if your anemia won't get better and stay that way with a good diet, perhaps you should have your stomach checked.

## REFERENCE

**Therapeutics**
Goodman, Louis S., and Gilman, Alfred, eds. *The Pharmacological Basis of Therapeutics.* 5th ed. Macmillan Publishing, 1975, pp. 970–971.

A family history of angina and heart attacks, plus an increasing problem of angina in his own life, bring this 50-year-old man in for a checkup. A new supplement is recommended and six months later all evidence of his angina is gone. Drugs and exercise may not always be the answer.

# 12 A CASE OF ANGINA AND HEART ATTACK PREVENTION

"I think I'm making progress at preventing my heart attack," Mr. Sanders said. "At least I haven't had it yet. My angina's a lot less than three years ago. Maybe if I just keep doing what I'm doing it'll finally go, but there's a stubborn remnant that hasn't changed for nearly a year, so I thought I'd come in to see if there's anything else to do."

"What have you done so far?"

"Lots of things: exercise, diet, lecithin, vitamins. . . . But maybe I should start at the beginning. Do you mind? It's a long story."

"Go ahead. Let's get as many details as possible."

"Angina and heart attacks run in my family. My father's father started having chest pain at 67, died of a heart attack at 71. He never saw a doctor, didn't believe in them.

"My father had angina first at age 57. He remembered Grandpa, so he went to several doctors, took all the treatment recommended. He died of a heart attack at 61.

"I started having mild chest pain with exercise at 47." He

paused. "You know, it's been ten years younger each generation. If this keeps up, in two more generations angina should start at age 27."

"Wouldn't be surprised, considering what I see in some supermarket shopping carts," I mumbled. "But seriously, heart disease has been declining for about the last 10 to 15 years. It appears at least some of us are learning to prevent it."

"I'm hoping I have. Let's see, where was I . . . oh yes . . . when I first started having chest pain, I wasn't much of an exerciser, just chopped wood on weekends. When I started having chest pain with that, I tried to blame it on muscle strain. But it kept getting worse, so I checked in with the best cardiologist I could find. He ran some blood tests, and a treadmill electrocardiogram. My cholesterol and triglycerides were both high, and there were what he called 'disturbing changes' with exercise on the treadmill test."

"What did you do?"

"He told me to enroll in a medically supervised exercise program, and prescribed nitroglycerin tablets to be used under the tongue if I had more than just a mild pain." He reached into his jacket pocket, pulled out a small brown bottle. "See, I still have them. Haven't used one in a long time, though. I'd like to get rid of them entirely."

"So you exercised?"

"Yes, and still do. I think it's a good idea, but it hasn't been the whole answer in my case."

"What do you mean?"

## Better . . . Then Worse

"For the first two or three months, my chest pains seemed to get better. Then I started getting worse again. After a year I actually could do less exercise than I could at three months. I was getting more frequent episodes of angina, and they were more intense. So I was given a 'long-acting' form of nitroglycerin to take, and something called a 'beta-blocker.' Propranolol, it was called."

"That's fairly standard drug therapy."

"So I heard. Half the men at my exercise class were taking them. Well, the added medication seemed to help for about six months. Then I started getting worse again."

"Must have been discouraging."

"You're not kidding. I redid my will, and was making plans for my funeral at age 51. Figured that would follow the family pattern, too. My doctor put me on aspirin and another medication that's supposed to prevent heart attacks by blocking platelets, if I understand it correctly."

"You do. Too bad it's not more widely known that at least six nutrients do the same thing, and more safely."

"I know that now. I'm taking garlic oil. I hear that's the best."

"It's one of the best documented. When did you start?"

"I'm getting out of sequence here. . . . Well, there I was, age 49, able to do less and less exercise without pain, taking four drugs including aspirin, and generally feeling lousy. Starting to have a little impotence, too . . . my doctor said the propranolol could do that. He was talking about x-rays of my coronary arteries with dye, angiograms he said, and maybe bypass surgery in a year or two if I kept getting worse. Of course, I asked what was to keep the whole thing from happening all over again even if I had surgery. It wouldn't change whatever caused the artery problem in the first place."

"True."

"My doctor agreed, but pointed out it was better than dying from a heart attack like my father and grandfather. If surgery became necessary, it would buy time."

"Also true. But you say you're much better now, and you've not had surgery?"

# A Visit from Charlie

Mr. Sanders smiled. "Sure am. The week after I saw my lawyer about my will, one of the neighbors dropped by. I was out mowing the lawn . . . actually I was resting, waiting for the nitroglycerin I'd just swallowed to take away another spell of angina. It was almost like it was planned. He pulled out a little brown bottle of nitroglycerin tablets just like mine. I was surprised—I didn't know him that well—so I said, 'Small world. You have angina, too.'

"He laughed, asked me to look at the date of the bottle. It was four years old. He said he hadn't taken one nitroglycerin since then, but was keeping the bottle around just to remind him, in case he slacked off his program. I thought he meant exercise, and asked him when he had surgery. He laughed again and said he hadn't, that's why he wanted to talk to me. Seems his wife had talked to her best friend who's friends with my wife's best friend . . . you know how that goes. I guess I'd been doing a lot of complaining that week, giving my wife a hard time.

"He was really polite, said he hoped he wasn't intruding, but he wanted to tell me what he'd done about his angina. He caught me at a good time . . . a year before I wouldn't have listened. We talked for three hours."

Mr. Sanders looked at his watch. "Speaking of that, sorry to go on for so long. Don't want to make anyone else wait. To make it short, I changed my diet entirely. Much less animal protein; what there is, is mostly fish and chicken. Cut out the sugar and refined carbohydrates completely. Stopped all the caffeine and all but a little alcohol. I'm taking three grams of vitamin C a day, 800 international units of vitamin E, two tablespoons of lecithin, three dolomite tablets, and 100 micrograms of selenium. Not to mention a good strong multiple-everything vitamin, just in case."

"Sounds like you've been doing your reading."

"Mostly it's Charlie's help. At first I wasn't sure, but thought, he's better, and what's there to lose? I checked enough to make sure it was safe . . . I didn't have high blood pressure, so I didn't worry about the rare case of vitamin E aggravating that problem. I stayed skeptical for the first few months. After all, I'd seen initial improvement with drugs before. But not only did my angina improve, I felt better all over. The improvement felt solid.

"So, with my doctor's approval, I slowly dropped off the

drugs. Of course, I didn't tell him everything I was doing, just the diet part, because he'd told me that everything I needed was in food, and vitamins were just a ripoff. But as my exercise tolerance has gotten better and better, and my cholesterol, triglycerides, and even EKG have improved, he's gone along with less medication."

"But you still take some?"

"Only the nitroglycerin when needed, which isn't often. No aspirin, beta-blocker, or platelet blocker. I feel I'm about 80 percent better on chest pain. The trouble is, I got to that level about a year ago. My cholesterol and triglyceride readings haven't changed much since then."

"What are they, by the way?"

Mr. Sanders pulled out a slip of paper. "My last reading before 'H-Day'—that's Health Day, the first day I talked to Charlie—was cholesterol 388, triglyceride 417. A year ago it was cholesterol 255, triglyceride 165 . . . and a month ago, cholesterol 260, triglyceride 163. After a steady improvement for two years, it's stuck."

"Actually, that's quite a bit better. You and Charlie have done quite well. . . ."

"By the way, Charlie says hello. After a year, when he figured it was safe and I was better enough, he told me he'd been a patient here.

"Anyway, I know I'm doing a lot better than before, but there's still some change on my EKG with exercise . . . S–T segment, I think it's called. And even though the triglyceride and cholesterol are much better, they're still high-normal, and the HDL cholesterol isn't good."

"I was going to ask you about that."

"The HDL (or good cholesterol) was 38 a month ago."

"That's a cholesterol to HDL ratio of . . . about 6.8. Not the worst I've seen, but not so good, either."

"I've read it should be five or less?"

"In that area. The lower the number, the less the risk is supposed to be."

"So what else can I do?"

I went back over my notes. "You really have done just about everything commonly recommended. You did say garlic oil?"

"Six capsules daily."

"What about other vegetable oils? They help with both triglyceride and cholesterol."

"Did I forget to mention oil? I'm using about a tablespoon daily, sunflower or safflower, on my salads." He looked at his notes. "Let me see if I forgot anything else...oh yes, two tablespoons of brewer's yeast daily, for chromium and B vitamins, and 30 milligrams of zinc.

I reviewed the list again. "All of this for the last three years?"

"Actually, two. Charlie said he didn't want to scare me with all of it until I'd seen some results."

## A New Treatment

I thought for a moment. "You...and Charlie...do seem to have most everything covered. Could be it'll just take longer, or this is as good as you can get. However, there's something relatively new you could try. It's natural, actually manufactured by our bodies, and appears safe. It's been reported to improve exercise tolerance, triglycerides, cholesterol, and even HDL cholesterol. Appears worth a try, anyway, as it fits your circumstances."

"If it's manufactured by the body, why should I need more?"

"I don't even know for sure that you do. But remember there are other natural biochemicals synthesized in the body that are useful as supplements. Niacin is probably the best known example ... the body can synthesize it from tryptophan, if enough tryptophan's available and the enzyme systems are working well."

"What is it?"

"Oh yes ... sorry. It's carnitine. The active form is L-carnitine, but often the only type available is DL-carnitine. Please take 1,500 milligrams of DL-carnitine or 750 milligrams of DL-carnitine twice daily.

"What does it do?"

"Improves the burning of fats, particularly in heart muscle and liver cells. It appears to improve heart muscle exercise tolerance by increasing the heart's ability to oxidize—burn—fatty acids."

"So the heart muscle has more energy available to it?"

"Exactly."

I completed Mr. Sanders's checkup, but there was nothing to add, so he left to have a few screening tests done and then try the carnitine.

Six months later, his angina was gone, even with maximum exertion. He reported that changes on his exercise electrocardiogram were nearly gone. His triglycerides were 114, his cholesterol 195, and HDL cholesterol 46, giving him a cholesterol to HDL ratio of 4.2. We agreed that although we couldn't be absolutely sure, the carnitine had probably been responsible for the change.

As noted above, L-carnitine is a molecule natural to the body. Reference works say it's safe to use. Even though carnitine research is new for angina and lipid problems, at least part of the "biochemical mechanics" is known. Most of the work on heart problems involves intravenously given carnitine, but the work on lipids reports oral administration showing that carnitine is active by the "oral route." Like anything else, it won't help every time, but as shown by Mr. Sanders's case it can sometimes be very helpful.

## Carnitine Burns Up Fat

Although carnitine is synthesized within the body, research is finding an increasing number of uses for supplemental quantities. So far, relief of angina, lowering total cholesterol and triglyceride levels, increased exercise tolerance with visible electrocardiographic improvement, and prevention of some irregular heartbeat (arrhythmia) have all been documented.

The author of a comprehensive 1978 review of knowledge about carnitine wrote: "We know little about the content of carnitine in foods or diets." In general, there's much more carnitine in foods of animal origin, and less in foods of plant origin.

L-carnitine appears to be safe in its naturally occurring form. DL-carnitine (often found in carnitine supplements) is presently the most available form of carnitine. It's made of 50 percent D-carnitine and 50 percent L-carnitine. The D-carnitine half appears to be a problem only for those with kidney problems. Otherwise, it appears to be safe according to present research.

Carnitine hasn't been available for very long, so I haven't had time for extensive observation of its effects. So far, however, it's been extremely reliable as a "lipid-improvement" supplement.

## REFERENCES

**D-Carnitine**

Bazzato, G. et al. "Myasthenia-like Syndrome After DL—but Not L—Carnitine." *Lancet,* May 30, 1981, p. 1209.

McCarty, Mark F. "A Note on 'Orthomolecular Aids for Dieting'—Myasthenic Syndrome Due to DL-Carnitine." *Medical Hypotheses,* December, 1982, pp. 661–662.

**Exercise**

Kosolcharoen, Peter et al. "Improved Exercise Tolerance After Administration of Carnitine." *Current Therapeutic Research,* November, 1981, pp. 753–764.

**Fatty Acids**

Maebashi, M. et al. "Lipid-Lowering Effect of Carnitine in Patients with Type-IV Hyperlipoproteinaemia." *Lancet,* October 14, 1978, pp. 805–807.

Opie, Lionel H. "Role of Carnitine in Fatty Acid Metabolism of Normal and Ischemic Myocardium." *American Heart Journal,* March, 1979, pp. 375–388.

Pola, P. et al. "Carnitine in the Therapy of Dyslipidemic Patients." *Current Therapeutic Research*, February, 1980, pp. 208–216.

"The Regulation of Fatty Acid Synthesis and Oxidation by Malonyl-CoA and Carnitine." *Nutrition Reviews*, January, 1980, pp. 25–27.

Wittels, Benjamin, and Spann, James F., Jr. "Defective Lipid Metabolism in the Failing Heart." *Journal of Clinical Investigation*, vol. 47, 1968, pp. 1787–1794.

## General

Bach, A. C. "Carnitine in Human Nutrition." *Zeitschrift für Ernahrungswissenschaft*, vol. 21, no. 4, 1982, pp. 257–265.

Mitchell, Madeleine E. "Carnitine Metabolism in Human Subjects I. Normal Metabolism." *American Journal of Clinical Nutrition*, February, 1978, pp. 293–306.

## Heart

DiPalma, J. R.; Ritchie, D. M.; and McMichael, R. F. "Cardiovascular and Antiarrhythmic Effects of Carnitine." *Archives Internationales de Pharmacdynamie*, vol. 217, 1975, pp. 246–250.

Folts, John D. et al. "Protection of the Ischemic Dog Myocardium with Carnitine." *American Journal of Cardiology*, June, 1978, pp. 1209–1214.

Suzuki, Yoshikazu; Kamikawa, Tadashi; and Yamazaki, Noboru. "Effect of L-Carnitine on Cardiac Hemodynamics." *Japanese Heart Journal*, March, 1981, pp. 219–225.

Thomsen, James H. et al. "Improved Pacing Tolerance of the Ischemic Human Myocardium After Administration of Carnitine." *American Journal of Cardiology*, February, 1979, pp. 300–306.

A 37-year-old carpenter complains of deep aching muscles in his back, shoulders, and arms—the cause of which eludes many doctors. Tests show his early childhood allergies (manifested as persistent ear problems) now appear as muscle aches. Although controversial, allergies can and do cause muscle aches, which in this case are eliminated once milk products and other allergenic foods are avoided.

# 13 A CASE OF ALLERGY-RELATED BACKACHE

"I'm beginning to think this is more than backache from hard work. In fact, I know it is because it's spread to the rest of my muscles in the last three years. I've been through everything I can think of to get it better, and it isn't, so I thought I'd give this a shot."

Harley Dykstra was 37 years old, a carpenter like his father. "My back problems are just like his, too. I remember he used to come home from work complaining about his aching back, and sore shoulders and arms, now that I think of it. He took an aspirin bottle with him wherever he went his last few years, he got so bad."

"His last few years?"

"He died of a heart attack. Only 49."

"Do you use aspirin?"

"Have to. Can't get through a day without it anymore. I take it with milk, though, so I won't get an ulcer like Dad did."

"Have you taken any other treatment?"

"Cortisone for a few weeks last year. It really worked. I felt better than I had in years, but the pain came right back after I stopped. The specialist at [he named a large local referral center] told me about the possible long-run side effects of cortisone, so we decided I'd best go back to aspirin."

"How many do you take?"

"Twelve to 16 a day."

"When did your backaches start?"

Mr. Dykstra looked up and sighed. "It's a long story, but I've got it memorized talking to doctors, so here goes.

"Looking back, I remember muscle aches when I was a kid. I had mostly leg aches, occasionally a backache, when I was six or seven."

"Cramps?"

"Rarely. Mostly deep aching, like I have now. I'd tell my folks about it. They told me it was growing pains—everyone had them, don't worry. At that time, the aches lasted only a few hours, or at most two or three days, so I didn't say any more."

## "I Was Almost Proud."

"When did the aching get steady?"

"Not until I was 22 or 23. That's when I started having steady backaches, all the time. It got better after overnight rest, and worse after a long day's work. You know it's almost funny now, but at first I was almost proud of having steady backaches. I'd just gotten on full-time as a carpenter, like Dad, and now my back hurt like his. Almost a sign I was a grown man, finally." He smiled to himself.

"Are you still worse after a hard day, better in the morning?"

"Yeah, but it isn't the work that's doing it; that's just an aggravation. I get backaches when I'm off work doing nothing, too.

"Now . . . where was I? Oh, yeah . . . after two or three years of steady backaches, I started asking around at work. Sure enough, everyone had backaches now and again, but not every day, seven days a week. When they got one, they could usually trace it back to something specific. I couldn't. They stayed home a few days, or went to a chiropractor or osteopath, and got better. Not me."

"Did you go to an osteopath?"

Mr. Dykstra laughed. "I've been to . . . let's see . . . seven chiropractors and four osteopaths. For a while there, in my late twenties, I'd go to a new one every time someone told me they'd gotten some help. But I stopped, because it didn't help much."

"Too bad. Manipulation frequently helps back pain."

"That's what I hear."

"So, what next?"

"Nothing, until I met my wife. After we got married, she got tired of listening to me complaining about my backaches. So I went to see an orthopedic surgeon."

"What happened?"

"Nothing but a lot of tests and more doctors. I had stacks of x-rays, blood tests, even a muscle biopsy. I was in the hospital for a few days. They even wanted to send me to a psychiatrist, but I told them if I was crazy, so was my old man."

"You didn't go?"

Mr. Dykstra looked disgusted. "When they want to send you to a shrink, it means they can't find anything, so it's my fault. I talked it over with my wife. We decided I shouldn't go."

"Then what?"

"Well they told me I had 'idiopathic myalgia and low back pain,' nothing serious or life-threatening. I should take aspirin unless it made my ears ring. So, I went home and took my aspirin, with milk."

"And you've gotten worse?"

"Yeah, like I said, the last three years it's started to spread. First my shoulders, then my arms, upper legs. Only a little at first, and not all the time. I tried to ignore it, because I was still going to work every day, and playing ball all summer."

"Baseball?"

"Yeah. Still pretty good for an old man." His smile changed to a frown. "But I'm going to have to quit if I can't get rid of this aching. It's all the time in my shoulders, upper arms, and legs now. Aspirin isn't cutting it, anymore. That's why I went to see the neurologist a few months back, who had me try the cortisone."

"What else did he do?"

"She. Nothing much. She had a few tests repeated, but after looking over my records, said I'd been through everything already. She did suggest a referral to a pain clinic."

"Did you go?"

"Not yet. That might be next, but my wife has been doing some reading on vitamins and minerals, and suggested I come over here."

"Describe the pain a little more, please."

## "A Deep-In Aching"

"Well, it isn't a sharp pain, really, except when I've worked hard. It's more like a deep-in aching and incredible tiredness all at once. It hardly lessens anymore—it's steady."

"In all your muscles at once?"

"It always centers in my back, but the only places that don't ache anymore are my hands, feet, and forearms. Even my calf muscles have started lately."

We went over the rest of Mr. Dykstra's medical history, which was remarkably negative except for recurrent earaches between ages one and three. His father and grandfather had both had heart attacks, but his other grandparents had lived into their eighties and nineties. His six-year-old had had earaches "like me, and is starting to get muscle pains, too."

Mr. Dykstra's diet still contained some sugar and refined food. However, his wife had made considerable change towards a more whole-food diet in the past year. He was taking no vitamins or minerals except calcium, which didn't seem to help much.

His checkup was negative. Even deep pressure on his aching muscles produced only a slight increase in pain. There was no sign of muscle swelling or inflammation.

I requested that he have a mineral analysis done, as well as routine screening tests. Also, I recommended he have tests done for allergies to food.

"While we're waiting for your tests, please eliminate all milk and dairy products," I urged.

"Stop drinking milk? Allergy tests? What's this all about? I thought maybe I was missing some minerals or vitamins, but allergic? I've never been allergic!"

## Earaches Are a Symptom

"You've already said you probably were when you were two and three years old. Remember all those earaches you told me about? The vast majority of children with recurrent earaches are allergic to food."

"But that was over 30 years ago. I don't have earaches anymore."

"That's true. Most allergic children with earaches quit having them after age four or so; the allergies simply switch symptoms or go 'underground.' I think yours switched to muscle aching. Remember, you've had that since you were six or seven."

"Why haven't I heard this before?"

"Allergy, particularly food allergy, is still a very controversial area. What I just told you isn't 'generally accepted' by physicians. However, Dr. James C. Breneman, author of a basic textbook on food allergy, lists back pain as one of the common manifestations of food allergy."

"Why pick on milk? What will I take my aspirin with?"

"Take your aspirin with food, any other food. And about the milk: Doctors frequently learn things from people they work with. A few years back, another person with muscle aching like yours came in about it. He was taking 12 aspirin a day, too. After we spent nearly six months trying nearly everything else, he came back one day to tell me he'd solved his problem by going on a week-long fast. After four days, his aching was gone completely. No more aspirin. When he started eating again, he found that several foods caused problems, but that milk caused the vast majority. Really, I'm just guessing, but I'm fairly sure you're allergic. So while we're waiting for your tests, why not try it? Also, you've been through most everything else, including that muscle biopsy, and it was all negative."

"But I really like milk. . . ."

"I thought so, from what you said. Some allergists note that foods we crave are the ones likely to be causing problems."

"And I was taking it with my aspirin every time. . . ."

"Hold on, we don't know for sure milk's the problem. It's just a suspicion until tried."

Mr. Dykstra eliminated milk and dairy products; most of his muscle aching cleared within a week. When he stopped the other foods subsequently found to be allergenic by his tests, his aching stopped completely.

## More Than Just a Backache

Since my background is family practice, the vast majority of individuals with back pain with whom I work don't require surgery. They also don't require the large quantities of painkillers and antispasmodics dispensed on a routine basis. Maybe a little, in acute cases, but not much.

Allergy isn't the usual problem either, although, as Mr. Dykstra's case shows, it does cause back pain sometimes. In the large majority, however, what's needed is skilled manipulation by either a chiropractor or an osteopath.

There's no reason a medical doctor couldn't perform manipulation, too. Except that almost none, including myself, are trained in it. Most still believe the myth fostered in medical schools that manipulation of the spine is a fraud, or at best a fringe practice. Fortunately, a few medical doctors have observed the facts for themselves. There's now a professional society for M.D.s interested in spinal manipulation—the North American Academy of Manipulative Medicine.

Mr. Dykstra's case demonstrates the importance of a complete personal health history in a difficult problem. Many individuals who "outgrew" childhood allergies find that years later their allergies are still present, causing an entirely different set of symptoms. Unfortunately, as noted elsewhere, many recurrent childhood problems aren't recognized as allergy or sensitivity caused.

Except in cases of hypoglycemia (low blood sugar), serious underweight, or debilitating disease, a five-day fast (distilled water only) is often the quickest way to determine whether or not symptoms are caused by food sensitivity, including allergy. Younger children often can't fast, either, but for most adults, such a fast will settle the question. For individuals with sufficient time, persistence, and record-keeping ability, fasting with controlled reintroduction of foods is another way to diagnose sensitivities to foods. *Dr. Mandell's 5-Day Allergy Relief System* contains an excellent guide to fasting and self-testing, which you'll find most useful.

## REFERENCES

**Allergy**

Breneman, J. C. *Basics of Food Allergy*. Charles C Thomas, 1978.

Mandell, Marshall, and Scanlon, Lynne Waller. *Dr. Mandell's 5-Day Allergy Relief System*. Thomas Y. Crowell, 1979.

The changeable personality of this four-year-old from active and talkative to whiny and listless causes much worry and concern for her parents. Removing refined sugar and artificial chemicals as well as foods to which she is allergic leads to a more even emotional tone, with only the usual ups and downs of childhood.

# A CASE OF PRESCHOOL BEHAVIOR PROBLEMS 14

"We can't figure out what's the matter with Lisa. She's gotten so changeable. Some days she's running all over the house, getting into everything, talking a streak. I can't keep up with her. But other times she's whiny, listless, clinging to me. I can't get her interested in anything. She has temper fits, and gets into fights in preschool."

"That's 'cause Billy wouldn't give me his crayon, Mommy."

"We'll talk about it later, Lisa," Mrs. Armbruster replied. "Now stop pulling on the plant, come over here, and sit down. Remember what your father said."

Mr. Armbruster sat Lisa on his lap, where she began to wiggle. "Today's one of her 'active' days," he said. "We're used to those; she's been that way all her life. We didn't really think it was a problem, just put it down to childhood energy and exuberance. Besides, we didn't have any other children to compare her to.

"Now we're wondering, because her preschool teacher says her 'active' days are much more active than the usual four-year-old's."

"But that's not the main thing, Charles," Mrs. Armbruster put in. She turned to me. "It's her 'worn-out' days that really have us worried. She used to have them occasionally, which seemed normal, considering her energy output other days. She started having more of them when preschool started last fall. At first we thought it was just a reaction to the school."

"Over the winter, her 'worn-out' days got more frequent, and worse. Now she's having more 'worn-out' than 'active' days," Mr. Armbruster said, settling Lisa down in his lap again. "At least on active days, like this, we can take her to the zoo, the park, run her all around, have some fun. Sure, we have to watch her closely so she doesn't get into things, but lots of parents have to do that."

"Are we going to the park, Daddy?"

"Only if you behave yourself," Mrs. Armbruster answered. Lisa subsided with obvious effort.

"Now, on her 'worn-out' days we can't get her to do anything," Mr. Armbruster continued. "If we go out, she clings to Jane or me, whines, fusses. Nothing pleases her. If we stay home, she lies around, won't play with her toys, throws her dolls in the corner. She does sleep more those days, which is a relief, but there's got to be something the matter."

## Pasty Complexion

"Also, she just doesn't look well," Mrs. Armbruster said. "More pale than she used to be. Her complexion gets positively pasty. She's always had those circles under her eyes, but on 'worn-out' days they're worse. I took her to our family doctor. He checked her out, did a blood count, said everything was OK.

"My mother read in the newspaper about lead poisoning, and told me we ought to bring Lisa here, because she heard you do hair tests for that. I really don't think that's the problem. Lisa doesn't eat paint or anything abnormal, but we thought we'd come anyway, just in case. Besides, there's got to be something the matter. Her preschool teacher says Lisa won't do well in kindergarten next year if this keeps up."

"You've given me a good description of the problem," I said. "I should ask you a few questions, though, before we decide what to try first.

"Did you have a normal pregnancy, labor, and delivery with Lisa?"

"Well, I was a little nauseated the first few weeks, but otherwise no trouble. She was born two days from her due date, and went home with me."

"Did you nurse her, or bottle-feed?"

"Nursed for a few weeks, but switched to bottle-feeding at two months. I had to get back to work."

"When did Lisa start to crawl, walk, and talk?"

"Our doctor said she was really early. She was crawling all around at six months, walking before she was a year old, and saying whole sentences before she was two."

"Has she had ear infections, tonsillitis, bronchitis, bladder infections?"

"No, just a cold or two. We've only had to take her to the doctor once for anything but well-child checks."

"What was that for?"

"She got really colicky for several weeks after she was weaned. The doctor said that was common, and gave us some medicine. The colic disappeared gradually."

"I remember having a lot of earaches when I was that age, and older," Mr. Armbruster said. "I'm glad Lisa hasn't had to go through that."

"Let's get a family medical history now," I said. "Besides earaches as a child, what other health problems have you had?"

"Not much. Acne pretty bad . . . I still get a spot or two. Other than that, I've been really well."

"Remember your canker sores, Charles."

"Yes, but those aren't really an illness. I get them in spells, lots for a few months, then none for a while. I figure it's just when I'm run down."

I made some notes, then turned to Mrs. Armbruster. "What about you?"

"I get migraine headaches, but fortunately less often this last year. Otherwise I'm fine."

"Grandparents, other relatives?"

"My mother's had her gallbladder removed; so has her sister. My father has a little high blood pressure, but his medicine controls it. Charles's parents both died in an auto accident six years ago."

"What does Lisa eat?"

"I like hot dogs," Lisa said. "I'm going to have one at the park."

"What do you have for breakfast?"

"Cereal."

"She has a variety of cereals with milk, and orange juice sometimes."

"Sugar on the cereal?"

"Half a teaspoon of brown sugar."

"Lunches?"

"Peanut butter and jelly sandwich sometimes. Sometimes a hot dog with ketchup. I make sure she gets carrot or celery sticks. And milk."

"Dinner?"

"Meat . . . beef, chicken, sometimes fish, but Lisa doesn't like it. Potatoes, lettuce salad . . ."

"I really like the cucumbers," Lisa said.

"She'd eat cucumbers all day if I let her. But I figure they're good for her. . . . Let's see, rice, corn, peas. Then Jell-O or ice cream, sometimes some pie."

"What does she have for snacks?"

"Cookies, apples, oranges, Jell-O, mostly."

"Any soft drinks?"

"Only when we go out. We're trying to hold down the dental bills."

"Any vitamins?"

"Just a one-a-day chewable multivitamin that we get at the supermarket."

"I think I've got enough information now. Please bring Lisa in the exam room so I can check her over."

# Swollen Lymph Glands

Like her mother, Lisa was light skinned, blue-eyed, and blonde. She had notably dark circles under her eyes, and creases in each lower eyelid. The lymph glands in her neck were slightly swollen.

"Her lymph glands are usually a little swollen," Mrs. Armbruster said. "The doctor says it's nothing to worry about as long as her white blood count's OK. Lots of children have swollen lymph glands."

"That's true, many children do. But it isn't really normal. Persistently swollen glands, even if slight, are usually a sign of other problems, even if they're not a problem themselves."

"What sort of problems?"

"Most frequently, and definitely in Lisa's case, allergies."

"Allergies?" Mr. Armbruster declared. "We've never had any allergies in the family on my side, or on Jane's side either. Are you sure? You haven't run any tests at all!"

"There's no hay fever, sinus, asthma, or eczema anywhere in our families," Mrs. Armbruster said. "How could Lisa get allergies?"

"Just a minute. I'd like to show you a textbook . . . I think that would be the quickest way to answer your question. Actually, you've been telling me about allergies since you got here, both Lisa's and the rest of the family's." I went back to my office, and brought the book back.

"First, please look at the title page."

"*Basics of Food Allergy,* by James C. Breneman, M.D.," Mr. Armbruster read. "Let's see, he's chairman of the Food Allergy Committee, American College of Allergists. Seems authoritative enough."

"Now, let's turn to pages 225 and 226. This lists the common manifestations of food allergy. Remember, common ones, not even unusual ones."

"Good grief!" Mr. Armbruster said. "All that? Canker sores, cholecystitis . . . that's gallbladder disease, isn't it? . . . Migraine headaches? That's all possibly allergic? I guess we have been telling you about allergies, haven't we, if that's true."

"Now let's look at page 47 ... let's see ... here."

" 'The allergic fatigue syndrome is typified by the child who is constantly tired, is irritable, pepless, and lacks enthusiasm. He seems dull, even though his IQ might be high.' Sounds like a description of Lisa on her 'worn-out' days," Mr. Armbruster said. "But what about her 'active' days? They're almost the opposite."

"Early stages of allergic exposure frequently show up as abnormal excitation. Sometimes the 'excitation phase' lasts for years. In Lisa's case, it appears she's going into the 'depressive phase' of allergy response, as some textbooks call it.

"Also, I don't think Lisa's entire problem is caused by food allergy. Refined sugar and food chemicals aren't good for anyone, but they seem to cause some of the worst problems in allergic individuals, especially children. We could do a glucose tolerance test for Lisa, to see exactly how sugar sensitive she is, but it'd be a little hard for her at age four. It would be just as well to completely eliminate all refined sugar and artificial chemicals from her diet, and observe what happens."

"She really doesn't get much," Mrs. Armbruster said.

"I think if you start reading labels you'll find she's getting more than you think. However, the best amount for anyone's health is zero."

"We can work on that," Mr. Armbruster said. "But how do we find out what she's allergic to? Aren't scratch tests a lot of trouble for a four-year-old?"

"Not only a lot of trouble, but very unreliable for foods, according to Dr. Breneman. Actually, there are several ways, but we use a type of blood test called radioallergosorbent or RAST for short. We're careful about where it's done, too, for best accuracy."

Mr. Armbruster turned to his wife. "Sounds like the thing to do."

"We won't have the results for about two weeks," I said. "You could get started on eliminating the sugar and food chemicals in the meantime." I marked a laboratory form, and the Armbrusters left for the lab.

Lisa turned out to be allergic to milk, peanuts, soy, rice, eggs, wheat, oranges, beef, tomatoes, lettuce, and her favorite vegetable, cucumbers. With help from allergy cookbooks, several information sources, and a lot of hard work, Lisa's mother put together a diet program for her.

Once sugar was entirely removed from Lisa's diet, her parents discovered that "even just a little" would get her "high" for two days. Food chemicals made her irritable.

Lisa's a second-grader now, not a behavior problem, and, according to her mother, "usually a delight to be with." Her "active" and "worn-out" days are gone, replaced by a relatively even emotional tone, with only the usual ups and downs of childhood.

# Food Sensitivity
# Widespread among Children

Food sensitivity, including allergy, is the most widely under-diagnosed cause of ill health among children. At my office, recurrent ear infections, tonsillitis, bronchitis, bed-wetting, urinary tract infections, hyperactivity, eczema, asthma, headaches, and stomachaches are routinely eliminated in the vast majority of cases by proper diagnosis, eliminating foods and food chemicals causing the sensitivity, and adding certain nutrients.

I claim no credit for this record of success; I'm only applying what I've learned from observant, caring physicians both present and past, including (but not limited to) Drs. Randolph, Breneman, Philpott, Mandell, Crook, Miller, Rapp, Rinkel, Rowe, and Alvarez. Most of these physicians I've never met, but learned from them through their writings.

I've already gone over the crucial difference between the various procedures for the RAST test (see "ABCs of Nutritional Testing"), but it's important to emphasize again that doing the wrong type of test, the "scratch" test for food allergy, is a large part of the reason for discounting the importance of food allergy by so many physicians. Even though a properly performed RAST test is very useful, it's not perfect, either. Probably the most accurate testing for sensitivities (not just allergies) is that done by clinical ecologists which involves hospitalization, fasting, and repeated challenges. However, since those techniques are sometimes very difficult to use in small children, and even more expensive than RAST testing, I usually refer only the most difficult sensitivity cases.

If you have a child who has been ill often, food sensitivity might well be the problem. Why not check into it before much more time goes by?

## REFERENCES

**Allergy**

Breneman, J. C. *Basics of Food Allergy*. Charles C Thomas, 1978.

Crook, William G. *Tracking Down Hidden Food Allergy*. Professional Books, 1978.

———. *Your Allergic Child*. Medcom, 1973.

Mandell, Marshall, and Scanlon, Lynne Waller. *Dr. Mandell's 5-Day Allergy Relief System*. Thomas Y. Crowell, 1979.

Philpott, William H., and Kalita, Dwight K. *Brain Allergies*. Keats Publishing, 1980.

Randolph, Theron G., and Moss, Ralph W. *Allergies: Your Hidden Enemy*. Turnstone Press, 1980.

———. *An Alternative Approach to Allergies*. Lippincott & Crowell, 1980.

Rapp, Doris J. *Allergies and the Hyperactive Child*. Simon and Schuster, 1981.

———. *Allergies and Your Family*. Sterling Publishing, 1981.

Rinkel, Herbert J.; Randolph, Theron G.; and Zeller, Michael. *Food Allergy*, Charles C Thomas, 1951.

Rowe, Albert H., and Rowe, Albert, Jr. *Food Allergy*. Charles C Thomas, 1972.

**General**

Alvarez, Walter C. *Help Your Doctor Help You*. Celestial Arts, 1976.

Miller, Benjamin F. *The Complete Medical Guide*. Simon and Schuster, 1967.

Miller, Benjamin F., and Galton, Lawrence. *The Family Book of Preventive Medicine*. Simon and Schuster, 1971.

> A newly retired man suffers periods of "blackouts" and numbness in his limbs. A platelet aggregation test reveals his platelets clot much more quickly than normal. Rather than taking drugs, he takes garlic oil. In two weeks his symptoms are gone, and in three weeks his platelet aggregation time reaches normal levels. Drugs are rarely necessary when nutrients can do the same job just as effectively.

# 15 A CASE OF "BLACKOUT" SPELLS

George and Anna James came in together. They both looked worried—Anna more than George. "As soon as I found out what was going on, I made sure we got right back here," she said. "George has been having these *spells* for months and didn't tell me! I think he might have a stroke, if he hasn't already. I can't understand why he didn't tell me."

"Didn't want to worry her," Mr. James said. "Besides, they're not so bad, and I figured they'd just go away. They always pass in a minute or two."

"Just long enough to end up at the bottom of a cliff. To think I let him drive! I drove back all the way—wouldn't let him near the wheel. Cut our trip short, too."

Mr. and Mrs. James had been in to the office at intervals for several years. Neither had any serious illness. Mrs. James had become interested in diet, exercise, and lifestyle changes for health maintenance, and Mr. James went along with varying degrees of enthusiasm.

He'd recently retired. They'd planned for years to travel after retirement, but apparently had cut their most recent trip short when Mrs. James discovered her husband's difficulty.

"What sort of spells?" I asked.

"They're different. Lots of times I feel like I've blacked out for a few seconds. Sometimes I get a numb feeling in my arms or legs. I try to shake it out, but it doesn't go. The feeling passes in a few minutes."

"It's a lot worse than that, George," Mrs. James declared. "You're not telling the doctor everything you told me." She turned to me. "I think George is so scared he's going to have a stroke and be paralyzed that he won't even admit to himself that those spells are serious."

"I didn't spend 57 years working to end up in a wheelchair as soon as I retired. Too much I want to do. You're too worried."

## "Sitting Like a Zombie"

"Too worried! Tell the doctor. I found out about this in a motel halfway to Phoenix. I'd been out a few minutes, came back, and asked George a question. He was sitting on the bed like a zombie, like he didn't hear me at all. I'm used to him not answering, but usually he grunts or something. This time nothing—he just stared straight ahead. He looked peculiar. I went over and shook him. He acted like he was asleep, shook his head after a few seconds. I insisted he answer me, and he talked like he was drunk. George isn't much of a drinker, but I smelled his breath. Nothing. His speech was thick, not clear, some of the words came out wrong. I really got frightened, but he improved in four or five minutes. Then he was himself again. That's when I decided we weren't going anywhere but right here."

"Have you had this kind of speech difficulty before?"

"Never tried talking when I had a spell before."

"I think that really shook George up," Anna put in. "He didn't give me any argument about coming back."

"Was he having any motions, any jerkiness, anything like a convulsion?"

"Not that I could see."

I turned to Mr. James again. "Have you ever noticed any jerking or trembling in an arm or leg?"

"No. I've had some times when one leg or the other was kind of weak or clumsy, just didn't want to go right. Almost fell once or twice. Longest spell of that lasted three or four hours, but usually it's a few minutes."

"How about your arms?"

"Get kind of clumsy there, too. Sometimes funny tingly feelings, especially my fingers."

"Do you have tingly feelings in the same places, or is the clumsiness usually in the same arm or leg?"

"Sometimes, but more often it moves around."

"And those feelings last how long?"

"Usually a few minutes, sometimes longer. Never a whole day."

"What about the blackout spells? Do they go with any of the other symptoms?"

"Every once in a while I'll get a tingling, then wake up a minute or two later. But they don't overlap much."

"Does it affect your eyesight?"

"Sometimes both eyes get blurry for a while. Once or twice it's been as if my right eye wasn't working right."

## "It's Like I'm Just Not There"

"When you say blackout spell, do you mean you faint or fall over?"

"No, it's not like that. I mean I get confused or can't think straight or do anything. Or like I'm just not there for a few seconds. But I don't pass out."

"Have you been having any other symptoms besides the blackouts, numbness, tingling, muscle weakness, occasional clumsiness?"

"Isn't that enough?"

"Sure, but can you think of anything else?"

"Well, my insides haven't felt good. My digestion can't behave itself—sometimes good, sometimes not."

"A lot of gas?"

"Not really, just feels funny."

"Constipation, diarrhea?"

"No."

"Do you get any of those spells when you exercise, turn your head in a certain direction, or raise your arms above your head?"

"Not especially."

"Have you ever had high blood pressure?"

"No."

"Any high blood pressure, heart attack, or stroke in your family?"

"No stroke. My uncle had a heart attack. No high blood pressure I know of."

"Have you been having headaches?"

"Not a one. That means I don't have a brain tumor, doesn't it?"

"Your symptoms don't sound like brain tumor. But having no headache doesn't mean that for certain. How long has all this been going on?"

"Started six, seven months ago, just before I retired. I thought it was the stress, or maybe like the car breaking just after the warranty expires."

"How often do you have symptoms?"

"Varies. Sometimes not for two or three weeks, then several times a week."

"More frequent recently?"

He looked uncomfortable. "Yeah, I guess so."

"George, you should have told me!"

"I'd like you to come to the examining room," I said.

## All Signs Are Normal

Mr. James seemed quite normal, I told him and Mrs. James. His blood pressure was average; his heart sounded fine and quite regular. His neck pulses were normal; there were no noises that might indicate blood vessel obstruction.

"What do you think it is, doctor? George can't be imagining all that. I saw it myself!"

"I'm sure it's all real enough, but frequently nothing can be found on examination between spells of symptoms. There are some blood tests I'd recommend you have done, but I think we're going to need some additional help."

"What do you mean?"

"I think you need to see a heart and blood vessel specialist, and, just to be sure, a neurologist."

"Why?"

"The symptoms you're having sound like episodes of lack of blood flow to one area of the brain or another, which luckily have been passing. Technically, those are called transient ischemic attacks, or TIAs."

"What causes them?"

"All the answers aren't known, but it's thought that much of the cause is small clots of platelets, blood cells, or debris from obstructions in blood vessels that travel to the brain."

"That sounds serious," Mrs. James said. "Could it cause a stroke?"

"In some cases. One estimate is one-third strokes, one-third spontaneous remission, one-third continuing to have TIAs. But that's just an estimate.

"Now, this could be something else, too. That's why I think we need some help from a neurologist and a cardiovascular specialist." I wrote a few names. "Please see one doctor on each of these lists."

"We will—right away," Mrs. James said. "Oh . . . what tests should George have done here?"

"Cholesterol, high-density cholesterol, triglycerides, glucose tolerance test, blood count, platelet count, platelet aggregation time. . . ."

"That all has to do with heart and blood vessel stuff, doesn't it?"

"Yes. There are things you need the specialists for, though. X-rays of blood vessels, EKG monitoring, making *sure* there's no brain tumor, although I don't think there is one."

# "I've Been through the Works"

Two weeks later, Mr. and Mrs. James were back. In the meantime, I'd talked to the cardiovascular specialist and received a report from the neurologist.

"I've been through the works," Mr. James announced. "Head x-rayed, brain scan, arteriogram, 24-hour heart monitoring, pictures taken of the blood vessels in my eye. That was one specialist you didn't tell me about. All negative. Did I really have to go through all that?"

"I think too much testing is sometimes done when simpler measures should be taken first. But in your case, it could have been something serious. I'm happy nothing was found, but you could have needed blood vessel surgery, for example."

"I guess so. They finally decided it was that TIA you mentioned, but they couldn't find a reason for it. One doctor wants me to take aspirin all the time. The other wants me to take these." He handed me a prescription bottle of a drug used to help stop platelets from clumping. "But I didn't want to take any of that, yet. Besides, why aspirin?"

"Aspirin's like this drug. It inhibits platelet aggregation, too. It might be the thing to do if there were no alternative, but there is. Actually, there are several."

"Do I really have anything wrong with my platelets?"

"Looks like you do. Your test for platelet aggregation shows they stick together much too quickly. In this test system, the range of normal is supposed to be two to five minutes. Your time was 19 seconds."

"Nineteen seconds? If they stick together that quickly, why aren't I a giant clot?"

"That's 19 seconds in the test system, where they're stimulated to aggregate on purpose. There's nothing to stop or dissolve them, as there is in you and me. Your little clots are obviously dissolving again. What the test shows is that your platelets are unusually sensitive to stimulus to clotting."

"And that goes with my symptoms?"

"Usually."

"So what do I do about it? You said there were alternatives to those drugs?"

## Start with Garlic Oil

"The best-studied one is garlic oil. There are several papers reporting that garlic oil inhibits platelet aggregation. Linoleic acid works, too. That's found in most vegetable oils. Then there's pineapple enzymes, onions, vitamins C, E, and $B_6$. And mackerel."

"Mackerel?"

"Actually an oil found in mackerel. The researchers had people eat the whole fish, though."

Mr. James looked thoughtful. "Any of those things should stop my platelets from clumping and stop those TIAs?"

"Probably."

"How do I find out?"

"Your symptoms should go away. And we'll measure your platelet aggregation time to make sure it normalizes."

He turned to Mrs. James. "You've been trying to get me to take vitamins for years now," he said. "Looks like I'll try a few. No drugs?" he asked.

"Probably not."

"Where should I start?"

"Garlic oil."

Mr. James made a face. "I hate garlic. I suppose I'll smell like a pizza."

"Have you had symptoms lately?"

"Yes. Just yesterday. Got Anna all worried again."

"Then since garlic oil is the best studied, start there. Later on you can try to switch to something else. And keep close track of how quickly the platelets in your blood clump together to make sure it's working."

"By the way, how were George's other tests?"

"Glucose tolerance test OK. Sometimes hypoglycemia can be a source of weird symptoms. Cholesterol a little high, high-density cholesterol a little low, triglycerides OK, platelet count OK."

"What do we do about the cholesterol?"

"Frequently, the oils that help platelet aggregation help cholesterol levels, too. Let's wait and see."

Mr. James took a dozen garlic capsules daily. In ten days his platelet aggregation time was 1 minute, 30 seconds; three weeks later it was 3 minutes, 43 seconds—well within normal.

His symptoms went away the second week. However, he disliked the garlic, so he experimented with the other nutrients and was pleased to find that 2,500 milligrams (½ teaspoon) of flaxseed oil, 400 international units of vitamin E (which should always be used with unsaturated oils), three grams (3,000 milligrams) of vitamin C, along with two 250-milligram bromelain tablets with each meal also kept his platelet aggregation time normal. His cholesterol tests improved, and he's had no symptoms since.

Not all transient ischemic attacks can be helped that way. Some require surgery or other measures. But aspirin and other platelet-inhibiting drugs are hardly ever necessary with the wide variety of nutrients effective for the same job.

## There's a More Natural Way to Prevent Clogged Arteries

Platelets are blood components smaller than red cells. They're part of our clotting system. If platelets don't stick to each other and blood vessel walls after an injury, bleeding is prolonged. If they stick together (aggregate) too quickly, clots may form abnormally with little or no injury.

Platelet research is presently very "hot." Most research involves aspirin and other drugs which inhibit platelet aggregation. Research indicates that platelet-inhibiting drugs may prevent some heart attacks and strokes by preventing abnormal clotting in the arteries of the heart or brain. It's suspected that normalizing platelet function may be helpful in treatment of diabetes, especially diabetic eye problems.

Platelet aggregation testing is simple and relatively inexpensive. Despite this, platelet-inhibiting drugs are usually recommended without laboratory testing to determine whether the platelets really need inhibiting or not. Follow-up measurements of platelet aggregation to monitor treatment usually aren't done either. Considering the potential hazards of abnormal platelet aggregation, including death from heart attack, the almost complete neglect of platelet aggregation testing at present is a genuine mystery.

If platelet aggregation time (the time required for platelets to clump or aggregate) is abnormally short, effective vitamin (and mineral) agents will lengthen the aggregation time to normal or slightly longer than normal, but will not produce so much lengthening that abnormal bleeding may follow. I've not observed abnormal bruising or bleeding caused by the use of vitamins E, $B_6$, or any of the other supplements discussed here. It is possible, however, to "go too far" with drugs affecting platelet function. Even aspirin has been associated with abnormal bruising and bleeding when taken in large doses. Despite the relative safety of most natural platelet-effective agents, it's most wise to check with a doctor familiar with their use and with proper laboratory measurement of platelet aggregation times. For more information on this testing method, see "ABCs of Nutritional Testing."

There are so many supplements capable of normalizing abnormally short platelet aggregation that discussion of each one would take entirely too much space. Instead, I've made a list, taken from medical journals, of supplements and daily doses found effective. They may be taken alone or in combination.

| Supplements | Dosages |
| --- | --- |
| Bromelain enzymes | 2 tablets |
| Cod-liver oil | 20 milliliters (approximately ⅔ tablespoon) |
| Eicosapentaenoic acid (EPA) | 2,000 to 3,000 milligrams |
| Garlic oil | 25 milligrams |

| Supplements | Dosages |
|---|---|
| Primrose oil | 2,400 milligrams |
| Salmon oil | 60 to 80 milliliters (approximately 2 to 3 tablespoons) |
| Vitamin B$_6$ | 40 milligrams |
| Vitamin C | 2 grams (or more) |
| Vitamin E | 1,800 international units |

Other supplemental items found capable of affecting platelet function include magnesium, manganese, onion, salmon steak and mackerel.

Who should be particularly concerned about platelet function? Studies have shown that platelets are particularly likely to be "hyperaggregable" (clumping too quickly) in individuals with coronary artery disease, hypertension, diabetes, transient ischemic attacks, and those who have had strokes. Even if you don't have any of these problems, you should be particularly concerned if anyone in your family has had them. Preventing a problem is always better than waiting until later, when it may or may not be correctable.

Last of all, another word regarding that familiar enemy to good health—refined sugar. Research done by Stephen Szanto, Ph.D., and John Yudkin, M.D., Ph.D., has demonstrated that sugar's effect on platelets can be detrimental in some individuals, leading towards abnormally short platelet aggregation. This effect is seen particularly in persons with known atherosclerotic disease. Since body chemistry is similar within families, it's probable, although not absolutely proven, that the same effect would be seen in relatives of individuals with atherosclerosis.

The same research demonstrated that for other persons of the same age as those with atherosclerosis, but free of the disease, refined sugar didn't have the same adverse effect. Although present evidence doesn't totally exclude the possibility that atherosclerosis might cause "sugar sensitivity," the overwhelming likelihood is that sensitivity to sugar is one of the contributory causes to atherosclerosis (see "A Case of Sugar Susceptibility" for further material on sugar sensitivity and platelets, and atherosclerosis).

Before taking any platelet-inhibiting drugs, consider the variety of natural alternatives. One or a combination of them will probably work for you. "Proof" of their effectiveness can be obtained by laboratory measurement. Although finding a doctor or laboratory to do the test may be a little difficult, as a preventive measure it's quite worthwhile.

# REFERENCES

### Aspirin

Persantine-Aspirin Reinfarction Study Research Group. "Persantine and Aspirin in Coronary Heart Disease." *Circulation*, September, 1980, pp. 449–461.

### Beneficial Vegetables

Makheja, A. N.; Vanderhoek, J. Y.; and Bailey, J. M. "Effects of Onion (*Allium Cepa*) Extract on Platelet Aggregation and Thromboxane Synthesis." *Prostaglandins and Medicine 2*, 1979, pp. 413–424.

### Bromelain

Heinicke, R. M.; van der Wal, L.; and Yokoyama, M. "Effect of Bromelain (Ananase) on Human Platelet Aggregation." *Experientia*, July, 1972, pp. 844–845.

### Cod-Liver Oil

Sanders, T. A. B. et al. "Cod-Liver Oil, Platelet Fatty Acids, and Bleeding Time." *Lancet*, May 31, 1980, p. 1189.

### Diabetes Mellitus

Davis, James W. et al. "Platelet Aggregation: Adult-Onset Diabetes Mellitus and Coronary Artery Disease." *Journal of the American Medical Association*, February 20, 1978, pp. 732–734.

Kwaan, H. C. et al. "Increased Platelet Aggregation in Diabetes Mellitus." *Journal of Laboratory and Clinical Medicine*, August, 1972, pp. 236–246.

Mustard, J. F., and Packham, M. A. "Platelets and Diabetes Mellitus." *New England Journal of Medicine,* December 15, 1977, pp. 1345–1347.

**Drugs**
Anturane Reinfarction Trial Research Group. "Sulfinpyrazone in the Prevention of Cardiac Death after Myocardial Infarction." *New England Journal of Medicine,* February 9, 1978, pp. 289–295.

**EPA (Eicosapentaenoic Acid)**
Thorngren, M., and Gustafson, A. "Effects of 11-Week Increase in Dietary Eicosapentaenoic Acid on Bleeding Time, Lipids, and Platelet Aggregation." *Lancet,* November 28, 1981, pp. 1190–1193.

**Fatty Acids**
Goodnight, S. H., Jr.; Harris, W. S.; and Connor, W. E. "The Effects of Dietary Omega-3 Fatty Acids on Platelet Composition and Function in Man: A Prospective, Controlled Study." *Blood,* November, 1981, pp. 880–885.

**Fish**
Siess, W. et al. "Platelet-Membrane Fatty Acids, Platelet Aggregation, and Thromboxane Formation During a Mackerel Diet." *Lancet,* March 1, 1980, pp. 441–444.

**Garlic**
Bordia, Arun. "Effect of Garlic on Human Platelet Aggregation *In Vitro.*" *Atherosclerosis,* vol. 30, 1978, pp. 355–360.
Makheja, A. N.; Vanderhoek, J. Y.; and Bailey, J. M. "Inhibition of Platelet Aggregation and Thromboxane Synthesis by Onion and Garlic." *Lancet,* April 7, 1979, p. 781.

**General**
Beeson, Paul B., ed. *Textbook of Medicine.* W. B. Saunders, 1975, pp. 653–654.

Farber, Eugene M., and Abel, Elizabeth A. "Miscellaneous Dermatoses." In Section 2: Dermatology, *Scientific American Medicine*. Scientific American, pp. 2–6.

### Hypertension

Mehta, Jawahar, and Mehta, Paulette. "Platelet Function in Hypertension and Effect of Therapy." *American Journal of Cardiology*, February, 1981, pp. 331–334.

Vlachakis, N. D., and Aledort, L. "Platelet Aggregation in Relationship to Plasma Catecholamines in Patients with Hypertension." *Atherosclerosis*, vol. 32, 1979, pp. 451–460.

### Linoleic Acid

Fleischman, A. I. et al. "Beneficial Effect of Increased Dietary Linoleate upon *In Vivo* Platelet Function in Man." *Journal of Nutrition*, October, 1975, pp. 1286–1290.

Vergroesen, Antoine J. "Physiological Effects of Dietary Linoleic Acid." *Nutrition Reviews*, January, 1977, pp. 1–5.

### Minerals

Hughes, A., and Tonks, R. S. "Platelets, Magnesium, and Myocardial Infarction." *Lancet*, May 15, 1965, pp. 1044–1046.

Sacchetti, G. et al. "Effect of Manganese Ions on Human Platelet Aggregation *In Vitro*." *Experientia*, May, 1974, pp. 374–375.

### Stroke

Al-Mefty, O. et al. "Transient Ischemic Attacks Due to Increased Platelet Aggregation and Adhesiveness." *Journal of Neurosurgery*, April, 1979, pp. 449–453.

Barnett, H. J. M. et al. "Randomized Trial of Therapy with Platelet Antiaggregants for Threatened Stroke. 2: Observations on the Pathogenesis and Natural History of Threatened Stroke." *Canadian Medical Association Journal*, March 8, 1980, pp. 535–539.

Kalendovsky, Z.; Austin, J.; and Steele, P. "Increased Platelet Aggregability in Young Patients with Stroke." *Archives of Neurology*, January, 1975, pp. 13–20.

## Sucrose

Mehta, J.; Mehta, P.; and Conti, C. R. "Platelet Function Studies in Coronary Heart Disease. IX. Increased Platelet Prostaglandin Generation and Abnormal Platelet Sensitivity to Prostacyclin and Endoperoxide Analog in Angina Pectoris." *American Journal of Cardiology*, December, 1980, pp. 943–947.

Szanto, Stephen, and Yudkin, John. "The Effect of Dietary Sucrose on Blood Lipids, Serum Insulin, Platelet Adhesiveness and Body Weight in Human Volunteers." *Postgraduate Medical Journal*, vol. 45, no. 225, pp. 602–607.

Yudkin, John; Szanto, Stephen; and Kakkar, V. V. "Sugar Intake, Serum Insulin and Platelet Adhesiveness in Men Without Peripheral Vascular Disease." *Postgraduate Medical Journal*, vol. 45, no. 527, pp. 608–611.

## Vitamin $B_6$

"Is Vitamin $B_6$ an Antithrombic Agent?" *Lancet*, June 13, 1981, pp. 1299–1300.

Kornecki, E., and Feinburg, H. "Mechanism of Inhibition of Thrombin-Induced Platelet Aggregation by Pyridoxal Phosphate." *Biochemical and Biophysical Research Communications*, October, 1979, pp. 963–968.

## Vitamin C

Bordia, A. K. "The Effect of Vitamin C on Blood Lipids, Fibrinolytic Activity and Platelet Adhesiveness in Patients with Coronary Artery Disease." *Atherosclerosis*, vol. 35, 1980, pp. 181–187.

"Low Vitamin C Tied to Platelet Clumping Seen in Diabetes." *Family Practice News*, September, 1978, p. 31.

## Vitamin E

Steiner, M., and Anastasi, J. "Vitamin E: An Inhibitor of the Platelet Release Reaction." *Journal of Clinical Investigation*, March, 1976, pp. 732–737.

A painter exposed to toxic metals from paint, especially cadmium, finds his blood pressure on the rise. A dietary program with special emphasis on adding supplements of vitamin C, zinc, and selenium continues to drop his pressure so that within a relatively short period of time it is perfectly normal.

# 16 A CASE OF CADMIUM-RELATED HIGH BLOOD PRESSURE

"I've been told my blood pressure is too high. The last doctor I talked to said I'd better go on blood pressure pills to cut down my risk of stroke, heart attack, and kidney damage. But I thought I'd check around a little first, because I've got an idea it's my work that's causing the trouble."

A glance at Mr. Barra's hands gave a clue to his occupation. Although scrubbed and clean, they were rough, with traces of at least three different colors of paint scattered here and there.

"You're a painter?"

"The hands give me away every time. I do industrial-commercial painting: bridges, factories, things like that. No residential jobs at all for years."

"Different sorts of paints, aren't they?"

"Quite a bit. We do a lot of metal and concrete, and the paints vary for each use."

"Do you know what's in them?"

"That's another problem. We can't always find out everything that goes into each paint without a lot of hassle. Besides, I didn't realize it might be causing me any problems until my blood pressure started going up, and I started checking around."

"How high has your blood pressure been? When did it start to go up?"

"It must have been at least three years ago, although I ignored it at the time. I had it taken at one of those shopping mall health fairs. It was 'something' over a hundred, I don't remember what the top number was. The person who measured it checked twice, then wrote me out a slip advising me to see a doctor. I thought it was just a fluke. I'd been working extra hard and just had a hassle with one of the kids."

"Then what?"

"Well, about six months later, I was at a different shopping mall, and there was the same lady taking blood pressures. So I wandered over to say hello. She found out it was high again. This time"—he searched through his wallet—"I figured I'd write it down." He pointed to the first entry on the smudged card.

"156/100. That is higher than it should be, especially at age 43."

"It's not any better at age 46 either. Look at the last few readings."

I turned to the back of his card. The last few entries, made at increasingly regular intervals, read 168/104, 180/110, 172/106.

"It's supposed to be 140/90, isn't it?"

"That's actually the upper limit that most doctors like to see, especially in younger people."

"You know, I've tried everything I could on my own to get it down. When that didn't work, I checked with a local doctor and had all the regular tests done—blood, urine, even kidney x-rays. All negative. That's why I think it might be something from the job."

"What have you done to try to get your blood pressure down?"

## Cut Back on Salt

Mr. Barra smiled. "My wife's a real bear about our diets. No sugar anywhere in the house, no refined flour. When my blood pressure first started to go up, she got rid of all the salt, too, which she hadn't done before because there's no high blood pressure in either of our families. Lately, she's started adding small amounts of that potassium chloride type of salt substitute they have in the grocery stores, because she read potassium helps blood pressure go down. Is that safe?"

"Yes, particularly in small quantities. But you have to be careful in cases of kidney or heart disease, and with infants and small children."

"None of those at our house."

"How about caffeine, coffee, tea, cola drinks, chocolate?"

"Never have any of that at home. Betty got after me to stop the occasional cup I was having at work.

"That's not all. The last two-and-a-half years, since this thing started, we don't see much beef or pork around the house. Fish, chicken, and not so much of that. Betty read that vegetarians usually have much lower blood pressure. I told her I wouldn't be a vegetarian unless it was a matter of life or death. She's really gotten creative about nonmeat cooking, though, as my blood pressure wouldn't come down."

"Do you check your blood pressure at home?"

"Yeah, we learned to do that. It's in these records." He handed me a packet of photocopies. I put them aside for a moment.

"Thank you. I want to ask you about exercise, first, before I look at these."

"Never has been a problem there. Betty and I met on a tennis court. Except when the kids were small, we've played tennis about twice a week since we were married. When we can't find an indoor court when it's raining, we usually go swimming, or skiing in the winter. But we're really amateur tennis nuts."

I looked over my notes. "No added salt, using salt substitute; no sugar, refined flour, or caffeine; more vegetables and fruits; good exercise. . . . No family history of high blood pressure. . . . You've certainly done everything possible to get your blood pressure under control. In fact it's a surprise it's high in the first place. Oh, I almost forgot to ask. Do you take any vitamins?"

"Vitamin C, one gram a day, and vitamin E, but only 200

international units. Betty said occasionally it causes high blood pressure, so I cut it out entirely for six months. It didn't make any difference. Still, I only take a little, just to be cautious."

"Excuse me a minute." I picked up his photocopied records. As Mr. Barra said, he'd had all the usual tests done, and all were negative.

"It's not unusual for tests for causes of high blood pressure to be negative, you know," I observed. "Textbooks say that in a majority of cases, a specific cause can't be found. However, even when the cause is unknown, usually measures such as you've taken are a substantial help in controlling the problem, sometimes completely. Of course, they work best in mild to moderate cases, but yours is certainly still that."

"So what else can I do?"

"There are a few vitamins, minerals, and other supplements you could add . . . but before we do anything, let's get your checkup done, and any tests that might be helpful."

Three weeks later, Mr. Barra was back for the results of his checkup and tests.

"As I mentioned when you were here last, your physical examination was excellent. Most of your tests were negative, too, with the exception of your mineral analysis."

"What did that show?"

"Remember I asked you to turn in a specimen of pubic hair, rather than head hair?"

"Yeah, you said something about contamination."

"Right. Workers who might be exposed to airborne metals—welders, machinists, painters, aircraft workers, auto body repairmen—sometimes get metals in their head hair that aren't absorbed into their bodies in similar quantities. As pubic hair isn't exposed, it's a better specimen location, especially for toxic metal exposure."

"What did mine show?"

# High Cadmium and Lead

"Much higher than usual levels of lead, cobalt, and cadmium. The cadmium level is especially high."

"Does cadmium cause high blood pressure? Or the lead or cobalt?"

"Cadmium is most suspect. Evidence from experimental animals is very solid about cadmium-caused high blood pressure. In people, the evidence is conflicting, but some investigators are convinced."

"What do you think?"

"I've seen blood pressure go lower as high cadmium levels are reduced, so I know it's true in some cases. By the way"—I checked my notes—"you're not a smoker, are you?"

"No, that was my father. Why?"

"Studies have shown that smokers inhale considerably more cadmium than nonsmokers."

"It's absorbed through the lungs?"

"According to studies, cadmium is absorbed through the lungs better than from food or water."

Mr. Barra thought for a minute. "I certainly do breathe in more paint and paint fumes than I eat. And I know some of our paints have cadmium in them."

"So it's possible you're right about your blood pressure being related to your work. Excess cadmium could be the main problem. Though it's not proven in humans, selenium and zinc are protective against cadmium in animals. You have both these minerals low on your test."

"I don't have to quit work, do I?"

"Probably not . . . but remember we don't even know for sure that it's the cadmium that's doing it. We'll only know if your blood pressure goes down with specific treatment."

"How long will that take?"

"Can't say for sure. Probably at least six months to start seeing change, and up to two years for solid improvement."

"I'd rather not take drugs to lower the blood pressure if I don't have to, but is it safe to let my blood pressure stay where it is that much longer?"

"At the level it's been, at your age, and given your physical condition, probably. Besides, both you and I will monitor it to make sure it doesn't get worse. Lastly, as I think we have a specific cause to work on, it makes sense to do it, at least for a while."

"So how do we counteract the cadmium?"

## More Zinc and Vitamin C

"We not only try to counteract it, we get rid of it. Extra zinc will force it slowly out of your system. I know you'll still have some exposure, but you can try to minimize that at work, now that you know specifically what the problem might be.

"Please get zinc gluconate with 50 milligrams of zinc per tablet, and take one tablet, three times a day. That is a relatively high zinc dose to take for a long period of time, so we'll have to check your HDL cholesterol and blood count periodically. Zinc can adversely affect them, as well as occasionally cause irregular heartbeats in persons who are low in copper. Yours was quite normal, but if it weren't, extra copper would prevent zinc side effects.

"Secondly, vitamin C. In general, vitamin C detoxifies most heavy metals, such as lead, which you also have too much of. In animals, it's known to protect against cadmium toxicity. Please use as much as you can without causing yourself excess intestinal gas or diarrhea. If you can take as much as five or six grams three times a day, that will be good. It'll be necessary to use some extra B complex with at least 100 milligrams of vitamin $B_6$ to make sure there's not even a remote possibility of those levels of vitamin C causing a kidney stone.

"Lastly, selenium, 100 micrograms daily. In animal research, selenium helps protect against cadimum toxicity."

"Is that it?"

"For specific anti-cadmium treatment, yes. On other grounds, I'd like you to use a tablespoon of linseed oil daily, and raise the vitamin E to 400 international units. A small amount of research shows that essential fatty acids such as those in linseed oil can lower blood pressure a few points. But as far as is known, this isn't associated with counteracting cadimum."

Six months later, Mr. Barra's "average" blood pressure had dropped to 154/96. At 12 months, it was 142/90, and by 18 months 134/80, a very normal number. His hair cadimum also dropped to a much more acceptable level. As his blood pressure hadn't dropped during the previous two years, we concluded that the cadmium must have been the problem.

We cut back on the quantities of each supplement, but continued zinc and vitamin C at relatively high levels to try to prevent recurrence.

## Minerals That Interact with Each Other

The interaction of zinc and copper is becoming well-known, as are those of other nutrients. Sometimes they cause unwanted side effects (although not nearly as often as do drugs). Often such interactions can be put to good use. Zinc's ability to force out cadmium is a good example.

Similarities in the basic structure of certain minerals make such interactions possible. Because of this, lithium, sodium, and potassium can be used to manipulate each other. The same is true of zinc, copper, calcium, magnesium, and cobalt, another "group" of similarly structured minerals that can be expected to exert influence on companion minerals.

Of course, this isn't an absolute rule. Some elements interact for other reasons. But when side effects, especially mysterious ones, do occur, similar minerals are the first to be looked at. Fortunately for us, with careful study and application, these interactions can be used to our benefit.

### REFERENCES

**Cadmium**

Glauser, S. C.; Bello, C. T.; and Glauser, E. M. "Blood-Cadmium Levels in Normotensive and Untreated Hypertensive Humans." *Lancet*, April 3, 1976, pp. 717–718.

Ostergaard, Karen. "Cadmium and Hypertension." *Lancet*, March 26, 1977, pp. 677–678.

Perry, H. Mitchell, Jr.; Erlanger, Margaret; and Perry, Elizabeth F. "Hypertension following Chronic, Very Low Dose Cadmium Feeding." *Proceedings of the Society for Experimental Biology and Medicine,* vol. 156, 1977, pp. 173–176.

Skoryna, Stanley C. et al. "Prevention of Gastrointestinal Absorption of Excessive Trace Elements Intake." Paper presented at University of Missouri's 6th Annual Conference on Trace Substances in Environmental Health, June 13–15, 1972.

Thind, Gurdarshan S.; Fischer, Grace M.; and Flowers, Nancy C. "Trace Elements in Human Arterial Hypertension." *Physiologist,* August, 1976, p. 388.

Underwood, Eric J. *Trace Elements in Human and Animal Nutrition.* Academic Press, 1977, pp. 243–257.

## Essential Fatty Acids

Rao, R. Harsha; Rao, U. Brahmaji; and Srikantia, S. G. "Effect of Polyunsaturate-Rich Vegetable Oils on Blood Pressure in Essential Hypertension." *Clinical and Experimental Hypertension,* vol. 3, no. 1, 1981, pp. 27–38.

Vergroesen, A. J. et al. "The Influence of Increased Dietary Linoleate on Essential Hypertension in Man." *Acta Biologica Et Medica Germanica,* vol. 37, 1978, pp. 879–883.

A misinterpretation of the results of a hair mineral analysis leads to much confusion about calcium needs in the diet. The role and value of using the hair mineral test in nutritional-biochemical medicine is discussed and clarified.

# 17 A CASE OF CALCIUM CONFUSION

"I've been trying to cut back on the calcium and magnesium in my diet for three years, and I'm getting nowhere. In fact, my problem's getting worse. That's mostly why I'm here, to find out what I can do. I really don't have any illnesses or anything."

My visitor that morning was a young woman apparently in her late twenties or early thirties. She had on a floor-length flower print dress, and was carrying a copy of a book about nutrition.

"Why would you be trying to cut back on the calcium or magnesium in your diet? Most of the time we need more, not less."

"I suppose I should explain. I've been studying about good health for a few years, and of course diet is an important part of that. Three years ago, I found out I could get a mineral analysis done on a hair specimen on my own. I did, and was surprised to find out my calcium and magnesium were a little high. Well, I'd been taking two dolomite tablets a day for a month or two before that, so I cut those out. I didn't feel any different, but I read there aren't any symptoms from a little too much calcium or magnesium.

"About a year and a half later, I had another mineral test done, and was really surprised that the calcium and magnesium were even higher than before. The analysis report said they were too high, but then said that didn't necessarily *mean* they were too high. I didn't want to get toxic or anything, so I quit drinking milk, stopped eating yogurt and cheese, and even stopped eating soybeans because I read they were high in calcium and magnesium."

"What did you eat instead of cheese, yogurt, and milk, if you used to eat a lot of them?"

"Well, not beef or pork much, because I know red meats aren't so good for health. I substituted more sunflower seeds, chicken, fertilized eggs, almonds . . . things like that so I'd get more protein since I stopped milk and cheese. I used to eat Cheddar a lot for extra protein.

## Muscle and Menstrual Cramps

"Anyway, I've been doing that for about the last year and a half. Even though I haven't had any illness, I started getting muscle cramps when I exercised about three months ago. I tried taking potassium supplements, but it didn't help. I've been having so much cramping, I've temporarily cut down on my exercise. I'm kind of upset about that."

"Did you try taking any extra calcium for the cramps?"

"No. I thought I'd try another hair mineral test first. I did that two months ago. I was really surprised when the test showed calcium and magnesium higher than ever. I noticed the test said again that high calcium and magnesium didn't necessarily *mean* high calcium. I don't understand how my calcium could be normal if the test says it's too high. After all, why is it too high on the test if it really isn't? What good is testing, then? Don't I have too much calcium?"

"No, you don't. Actually you have way too little. That's what your muscle cramps are telling you."

"You know, I've been having menstrual cramps for the first time in my life, too. I mentioned that to my gynecologist. He just laughed and said it was time I got married and had a baby; that always stopped menstrual cramps. I know I'm 30 but I just haven't met the right person yet. I don't want to get married to anyone just because of my age."

I nodded agreement. "Your menstrual cramps probably come from lack of calcium and magnesium. By the way, do you have copies of your mineral analyses?"

"Yes, I thought you might want to see them, so I brought them in." She handed me three copies.

Her first mineral analysis showed calcium at 930 parts per million (ppm), magnesium at 85 ppm. The second, taken approximately 18 months ago, reported calcium at 2,100 ppm, magnesium at 440. The third, some two months ago, gave calcium at 3,200 ppm, magnesium at 1,000 ppm. All of the numbers were higher than the laboratory normal, and progressively so.

"Looks like a fairly clear-cut case of too little calcium in your diet," I said.

"Is the magnesium short, too?"

"Possibly. But I can't say for sure. The calcium is probably the controlling factor."

"I believe you . . . particularly since my menstrual cramps are worse, and my muscle cramps with exercise haven't gone away. But could you please explain why? I like to understand what's going on, and this is a real puzzle."

"I can see that you do. I'm glad you're interested in keeping yourself healthy—in the long run that's the best way to avoid illness."

## Hair Tests Can Be Confusing

"For a number of years, doctors working with mineral analysis have observed that some minerals on the hair analysis seem to show a false elevation—that is, the test reports high numbers when they're really not.

"I guess I should explain that a little further: Actually, the calcium and magnesium are higher than usual in your hair, but deficient in your entire body.

"Jeffrey Bland, Ph.D., of the University of Puget Sound, did a study which explained the reason for this clinical observation. He had two study groups: one on a diet with less calcium than phosphorus; the second with the same amounts of calcium and phosphorus. He did blood serum and hair tests for levels of calcium, magnesium, and phosphorus.

"He found that in the group eating the diet with less calcium, the hair contained, on the average, 952 ppm of calcium and 155 ppm of magnesium. In the group with *more* calcium in the diet, the hair contained on the average 303 ppm of calcium and 43 ppm of magnesium. That is definitely a significant difference. You can see that the low-calcium diet produced higher levels of calcium and magnesium in the hair. Oddly enough, the difference in the serum wasn't significant.

"Professor Bland explains that a low-calcium diet causes the parathyroid glands to become somewhat overactive, in order to help maintain normal levels of calcium in the blood. That is called secondary hyperparathyroidism, and means overactivity of the parathyroid glands not due to actual parathyroid disease. When that happens, calcium is drawn from the bones to put into the blood, and less is excreted by the kidneys. Apparently, at the same time more calcium and magnesium are deposited in soft tissues such as hair, and the levels are found to be higher than normal— instead of lower than normal as might be expected with a low-calcium diet. That's apparently what's happened in your case, secondary hyperparathyroidism."

"Can't we run a test for parathyroid hormone, to be sure?"

"There is a new test for parathyroid hormone, but it's extremely expensive and usually not necessary in cases like yours."

## The Calcium Challenge

"So switching away from milk, cheese, yogurt, and other dairy products wasn't such a good idea, was it?"

"I didn't say that. It was probably half a good idea—drinking milk of any sort past weaning doesn't seem to be part of nature's plan. But unfortunately, the foods you said you switched to for replacement protein happened to have a high phosphorus to calcium ratio. High phosphorus also stimulates parathyroid hormone, and further aggravates a low-calcium problem."

"So even though they're really healthy foods, they were out of balance for me. Should I stop them?"

"No. As you said, they are healthy foods. Just cut back some and put in other foods higher in calcium than phosphorus, like green leafy vegetables."

"What about fish?"

"Many fish products are high in calcium, but even higher in phosphorus. Make sure to look up these and other foods for calcium and phosphorus content. The absolute amount of calcium is important, but the calcium to phosphorus ratio is equally important. High calcium isn't very helpful if phosphorus is high. In general, most animal products except milk and some dairy products are just as high in phosphorus, or higher, as they are in calcium. Most green vegetables are the opposite—higher in calcium than phosphorus."

"Should I go back to milk and dairy products?"

"I'd rather you try a little yogurt or cheese."

"I guess I'd better take some calcium, too, then."

"I think you'd better. I'd suggest you use 1,500 milligrams of calcium, as well as 300 milligrams of magnesium and 1,200 international units of vitamin D to help the calcium along. All of this for at least a few months or longer, until your hair mineral test is normal again. You should be able to get back to exercising fairly soon, and get rid of the menstrual cramps without having a baby."

"I hope so. When should I do another hair mineral test?"

"That's up to you, but give it at least six months. It usually takes at least that long."

Her muscle cramping disappeared in just a few weeks, and menstrual cramps after three cycles. The mineral analysis in six months, although showing lower levels of calcium and magnesium, was not yet normal. Normalization of the mineral test took a year.

## Hair Tests Need Careful Interpretation

This case illustrates one of the many hazards interpreting the meaning of a hair mineral analysis. It's possible to take enough supplementary calcium and magnesium to produce a truly high reading, but it also takes considerably more than two daily dolomite tablets in most cases. Without supplementing the diet, it's very difficult to produce that high calcium reading, and virtually impossible in the case of magnesium.

Hair analysis for minerals, when properly performed at the laboratory, is useful for exactly one thing: telling us what levels of minerals are present in the hair. What that information means for the rest of the body, and what recommendations should be based on it, is not, at present, an exact science.

That's not to say hair mineral analysis is useless. In conjunction with a medical history, physical examination, and other laboratory determinations, it's quite valuable. Actually, that's the case for most laboratory test results, not just the hair mineral analysis. Very few lab tests are useful in isolation.

Hair analysis is the best test available for detecting toxic minerals in the body. Elements such as lead, mercury, cadmium, and nickel are stored away in bones, teeth, and hair. Blood levels of these minerals show only current exposure; urine tests disclose what the body is disposing of, and without stimulus, disposal is often slow. Hair analysis can disclose toxic mineral exposure when blood and urine analyses don't.

For other minerals, the value of hair mineral testing is not as clear-cut. Since I've looked at more than 10,000 of those determinations by now, I think I know what to do with the information in most cases. I'll be the first to admit, however, that what isn't known about the mineral analysis is more than what is known. It's often useful to do follow-up testing on blood or urine specimens to bring out the meaning of a hair mineral analysis.

A high zinc level, for example, usually indicates a need for zinc supplementation, but not always. In a minority of cases, it really means excess zinc in the body. Follow-up urine testing will almost always answer the question raised by such an abnormal hair mineral test. Supplemental zinc shouldn't automatically be recommended, as excess zinc can be toxic.

Besides incomplete knowledge of the meaning of all mineral levels on hair tests, another problem is the performance of the test itself. In 1982, the Hair Analysis Standardization Board issued recommended guidelines in an effort to establish uniformity of testing procedures. Due to intraindustry jealousies and rivalries, those guidelines have not yet been adopted by even a majority of testing laboratories. The sooner a uniform set of procedures or performance specifications is adopted by the entire industry (whether proposed by the Board or not), the sooner more physicians and interested members of the public will develop more confidence in the procedure.

Despite its drawbacks, hair mineral analysis is an invaluable part of an overall health evaluation. It can disclose unsuspected problems with mineral assimilation and it can give important information about possible mineral needs which should be considered. It's also beginning to provide clues to the status of a few hormones. Critical condemnation of hair mineral analysis because of its misuse by some people is certainly no reason to throw out such a potentially useful tool.

## REFERENCE

**Calcium-Phosphorus Ratio**
Bland, Jeffrey. "Dietary Calcium, Phosphorous and Their Relationships to Bone Formation and Parathyroid Activity." *Journal of the John Bastyr College of Naturopathic Medicine*, May 1, 1979, pp. 3–7.

**Canker sores are often linked to food allergy. In this case, a woman in her early fifties finds that her allergy to the eggs she eats every morning for breakfast is the cause of her perpetual problem.**

# A CASE OF CANKER SORES 18

"I've really had it with these canker sores," Mrs. Townsley declared. "There must be vitamins to get rid of them. I've tried enough things, but nothing seems to work very well."

Mrs. Townsley was in for a checkup. She'd recently moved to Washington with her husband, who accompanied her to my office. She appeared to be in her early fifties, a little overweight, but not unwell.

"How long have you had them?"

"I can't remember when I didn't. I remember when I was six years old, in the first grade, several of us had sores at the same time. They told us it was a virus going around or something like that. I had 27 canker sores, more than anyone else. Actually, they do go away for weeks to months at a time, but they always come back. When I was a teenager I thought I was over them for two years, but as soon as I got to college . . . wham! Canker sores again."

"That's for sure," Mr. Townsley said. "Almost broke up a great romance. I was afraid she had something really contagious.

213

Wouldn't kiss her for nearly a year after we started going together seriously."

"Even when I didn't have canker sores! At first I thought he was shy, gentlemanly, but he avoided me when no gentleman would. I was really hurt."

Mr. Townsley looked embarrassed. "We finally talked about it. She told me nobody had died from kissing her. More practically, she took me to her doctor, who explained she'd had tests for herpes virus several times, always negative. He said canker sores didn't appear to be very contagious, especially when they were healed."

"I wouldn't have put up with all that if I hadn't been very fond of him." Mrs. Townsley smiled. "Imagine taking your boyfriend to the doctor to make sure it's OK to kiss you."

"Luckily, when we talked to the doctor, my wife didn't have any canker sores. I'm happy to say, despite all her troubles, I haven't had a canker sore once in 30 years."

"Wish I could say the same."

"So you've been checked for herpes virus?"

"When I was in college, and a time or two since. One dentist a few years back, just wanting to be sure, said testing might have improved. But the results were negative again."

## Helped by Acidophilus

"What else have you done?"

"I've had tests for other germs—negative except for normal mouth bacteria. I've tried a variety of antibiotics, capsules, and mouthwashes. None of them worked at all. The most effective thing I've found so far, but it doesn't work all the time, is acidophilus."

"How do you use acidophilus?"

"When I feel a canker sore coming on, I take a dozen capsules a day and rinse my mouth out with acidophilus mixed with water. Years ago I read about using acidophilus, but I couldn't remember any instructions on how to take it, so I just tried. Funny thing: Sometimes it seems to take the sores away before they really start, and other times it doesn't make any difference. For a while I took acidophilus all the time. I did seem to have fewer sores, but then I got another bad attack, lots of them, and got discouraged."

"Is there any scientific basis explaining why acidophilus might help?" Mr. Townsley asked. "Sure sounds weird."

"If you mean step-by-step biochemical evidence, no. But it's been observed to work often, and it's harmless. Sometimes results are quite good. As your wife noted though, acidophilus doesn't help every time."

"One doctor said I had . . . aphthous stomatitis, I think it was. That's just canker sores in Greek or Latin, isn't it?"

"Yes."

"Well, they hurt just as bad in English, let me tell you."

"Do you have any canker sores now?"

"No, darn it. My car always runs perfectly when I take it to the shop, too."

"That's OK. By now I'm sure you know what you have. Perhaps they'll be there another time."

"I hope not too many other times. Isn't there anything I can do?"

"Let me get the rest of your health history and do your checkup. Maybe we can find some clues."

"I've been really very well except for canker sores."

"Have you ever been in the hospital?"

"For my children."

"Nothing else?"

"You were in for your gallbladder, Ann," Mr. Townsley said.

"That doesn't have anything to do with canker sores, Harry."

"I do need health background information, though. Sometimes things that don't seem relevant turn out to be. What happened?"

"When I was 44, I had my gallbladder out. Runs in the family: My mother, her sister, and one of my sisters have all had their gallbladders out."

I made a note. "Any other hospitalizations or surgery?"

"No. . . . Well, I did have my tonsils and adenoids out when I was four. Kept having ear infections. Didn't have any after that."

"Do you take any medications?"

"No, just vitamins."

"Any allergies?"

"No."

"Any illnesses in the family besides gallbladder disease?"

"Diabetes. My mother's mother."

"Any heart attacks, strokes, cancer . . . any other serious or chronic diseases in the family?"

Mrs. Townsley thought for a few seconds. "No, unless you consider chronic sinusitis serious. My father and his brother both have that."

The rest of Mrs. Townsley's health history was negative. Her checkup was physically normal.

## Egg Allergy Suspected

"What do you think, doctor?" Mr. Townsley asked. "Ann sometimes makes a joke of these sores, but they really are a problem."

"I understand. For now, I think she should stop eating eggs, pork, and onions; take some allergy tests; and see what happens."

Mr. and Mrs. Townsley looked at each other. "Are you implying that eggs cause canker sores?" Mrs. Townsley asked.

"You've misunderstood me. This applies specifically to you. I think eggs very likely cause some of your canker sore problem, not necessarily anyone else's."

Mr. Townsley crossed his arms and sat back. "How did you arrive at that conclusion?"

"I haven't for sure. So far, I'm just guessing. Canker sores frequently are an allergic problem. Your most likely allergen is eggs."

"I have eggs nearly every morning for breakfast," Mrs. Townsley said. "I feel fine afterwards. What makes you think I'm allergic to them? Why do you think I'm allergic anyway? I've never had any allergies—no wheezing, hay fever, itching, or hives. Is it because my father has sinus problems?"

"That's a clue, but not the main one. Let me answer your questions one at a time. I think you have allergies because of your past gallbladder problem and because of your aphthous stomatitis, or canker sores. Also, there's your recurrent earaches as a child. Recurrent ear infection in children is most frequently set off by allergy."

"But the tonsillectomy cured that," Mrs. Townsley broke in.

"Took away those symptoms, anyway. Unfortunately, the allergy or allergies probably remained. Your canker sores and gallbladder problems are probably evidence of that."

"Canker sores I'll accept, but allergic gallbladder? That sounds unreal. You mean my mother, aunt, and sister could have avoided gallbladder surgery by not eating eggs?"

'Eggs and a lot of other things. Don't misunderstand me: Eggs are very good food. I usually recommend them, except for those who are allergic. I know allergic gallbladder sounds strange. I thought so too when I first read a report by Dr. James C. Breneman about it. I thought I'd try it out, though, and was amazed. The overwhelming majority of persons with gallbladder problems are very allergic. Dr. Breneman found 93 percent of his study group to be egg allergic; I've found he was completely correct. Egg allergy is almost always present, along with a varying list of allergies to other foods."

"So, because of recurrent childhood earaches and gallbladder problems ten years ago, you think I'm allergic?"

"Don't forget canker sores most of your life. Dr. Breneman's book lists them as a common allergic problem."

"Who's Dr. Breneman?"

"At the time his book was published, he was a member of the board of regents, American College of Allergists, and chairman of their Food Allergy Committee."

"Let's try it out, Ann. You've got nothing to lose but your canker sores."

"And some blood. You use blood tests for allergy, don't you, Doctor?"

"At present, yes, The RAST test. It's the best I've found, so far."

"One of my cousins is really allergic," Mr. Townsley said. "His doctor says RAST tests aren't that good."

"It depends on the type of procedure followed, what lab is doing them. When RAST tests first became available, I took specimens from several people at the same time, sent them to different labs, and got vastly different results. One result worked very well in practice; the other didn't. After further evaluation, I've settled on one type of RAST procedure."

"You feel it's always accurate?"

"No lab test is perfect; RAST testing isn't perfect, either. In clinical practice, it's the most accurate test I've seen, except for those done by doctors trained in clinical ecology. I don't have that training."

"I've read about that: fasting and challenge testing, that sort of thing," Mrs. Townsley said. "I don't think I can handle fasting right now. I'll get the blood tests done."

Mrs. Townsley's test showed distinct allergy to eggs, wheat, oranges, pork, honey, and brewer's yeast. Once she dropped those items from her diet, along with all vitamin products containing brewer's yeast, her recurrent canker sores cleared up. She's not had one in the three years since then.

# Canker Sores Linked to Food Allergy

Canker sores are one of the many common manifestations of food allergy. Following the lead of Dr. Breneman, I always make sure to check for allergy, and find it frequently.

Canker sores aren't an overwhelmingly allergic condition, though. Investigators have shown that physical injury which doesn't lead to canker sores in most people will definitely set off sores in chronic sore-formers. They recommend commonsense measures such as not brushing the teeth too hard, using softer toothbrushes, and avoiding hard or sharp foods.

It's also been shown that nutrient deficiencies can lead to repeated canker sores. In one series of tests reported in the *Journal of the American Medical Association,* that was the case 14 percent of the time. Deficiencies in iron, $B_{12}$, and folate were at the top of the list. Some had more than one nutrient deficiency. In my experience 14 percent is a bit low; I've often had individuals tell me that canker sores cleared up when they cleaned up their diets and took general vitamin and mineral supplementation.

More stubborn and extensive cases of canker sores, like Mrs. Townsley's, have a high percentage of allergic involvement.

## REFERENCES

**Allergy**

Breneman, J. C. *Basics of Food Allergy.* Charles C Thomas, 1978.

Wilson, C. W. M. "Food Sensitivities, Taste Changes, Aphthous Ulcers and Atopic Symptoms in Allergic Disease." *Annals of Allergy,* May, 1980, pp. 302–307.

**Vitamin and Iron Deficiency**

"Aphthous Stomatitis Is Linked to Mechanical Injuries, Iron and Vitamin Deficiencies, and Certain HLA Types." *Journal of the American Medical Association,* February 12, 1982, pp. 774–775.

An abnormal Pap smear leads to worry and concern about a diagnosis of cervical dysplasia and a recommendation for surgery. The Pill is believed to be the cause. Change to a good, healthy diet along with supplements, especially folate and vitamin A, completely eliminates the problem and thus avoids the surgery.

# 19  A CASE OF CERVICAL DYSPLASIA

Sandra Gallegos looked very worried. "I've had an abnormal Pap smear two times in a row, and I just know the birth-control pills I was taking had something to do with it. Now they're talking about some kind of surgery. I don't want any surgery done unless it's absolutely necessary. I thought maybe vitamins would help, or something."

"Have you been told you have cancer?"

"No, not necessarily. The doctor said it might be turning into cancer, or the early stages, but he couldn't say positively. Here . . ." She reached into her purse and handed me copies of two laboratory reports.

Both were reports of Pap smears. The first, dated just a little over six months previously, was marked "mild dysplasia." The second, three months ago, showed "moderate dysplasia."

"Neither one of these is cancer for sure," I observed. "Dysplasia means abnormal change or abnormal development, but not necessarily a cancer. Also, there's another stage—'severe'—between these and the stage considered cancerous."

"I know. That's the reason they want me to have surgery done; I think it's a biopsy and something called conization, where they take out a piece of the cervix."

"I don't understand. . . ."

"I didn't mention I just saw my gynecologist last week for another Pap smear. I don't have a copy of that one yet but I got a call from the nurse. She said it was still 'moderate,' but the doctor called the pathologist who said it looked worse than the last time, even though he didn't change the rating on it. So the doctor said it would be better to have surgery before it turns into a cancer for sure. So I called over here and you just happened to have a cancellation. . . . Is there anything I can do except surgery?"

"Can't say yet, I really need more details. Have you had any examinations done other than a Pap smear?"

"The doctor had me come back for a colposcope exam. He said it was negative."

"Good." I made a note.

"Do you have any other problems with your health, as far as you know?"

"No."

"Is there any cancer in your family?"

"None at all. I've really checked in the last six months, but no one can remember any relatives with cancer. That's another reason I think the birth-control pills must have had something to do with this."

"Another reason? What's the first one?"

"They made me sick when I started using them. We switched around some, finally found a lower-dose type I could tolerate, but I still felt bad from it occasionally."

"When did you start taking birth-control pills?"

"When I was 20."

"How old are you now?"

"Twenty-six."

"Are you still taking the birth-control pills?"

"No, I got really nervous and quit after that second Pap smear came back with 'moderate' dysplasia. I was hoping the Pap smear last week would be better since I'd stopped. The doctor said he didn't think the Pill had anything to do with it one way or the other, but I might as well stop anyway."

"So you haven't had them for . . . three months?"

"Right."

"Are you taking any other medications?"

"No."

"Vitamins?"

"No."

"What do you eat every day? How about breakfast?"

## Too Busy to Cook

She looked embarrassed. "That's another reason I thought I'd check about vitamins and things. I haven't been eating very well . . . I've been busy at my job. I live alone, don't have much time for cooking."

"You still didn't tell me about breakfast."

"I usually skip breakfast. When I get to work, I have a cup of coffee or two. Sometimes someone brings in donuts or rolls."

"Do you eat lunch?"

"Yes, I'm really starved by then. Usually I'm out with clients. I'm assistant to the owner of an interior design studio. I have a small steak with mushrooms, or fish. Usually cottage cheese. Sometimes soup with lunch, or by itself."

"Salad or vegetables?"

"Sometimes salad, but not every day."

"When do you eat next?"

"I have more coffee and maybe an apple or an orange in the afternoon. Dinners are just what I can find: hamburger, fries, and a diet soft drink; fish and chips; frozen dinners. That's when I'm by myself. I don't have much time to cook; a lot of times I work late. When I'm out socially, I usually eat light at lunch."

I looked over my notes. "Do you usually have vegetables with meals? How about nuts, seeds?"

"I stay away from nuts and seeds because of the calories. I do eat salads occasionally, and there are vegetables in the frozen dinners, but I have to admit I've never been much of a vegetable eater. It's gotten worse since I left home where Mom isn't after me all the time about it."

"Carrots, celery?"

"No."

"You do have some diet problems here. Perhaps it has something to do with your main problem. But let's go over the rest of your health history, and do an examination first."

Aside from the usual childhood mumps and measles, Ms. Gallegos's health history was negative. As she said, there was no cancer in her family anywhere. Two grandparents had high blood pressure, and a cousin had asthma. Other than birth-control pills and aspirin, she'd taken no medication in the past few years. She didn't smoke, drank alcohol only socially, mostly on weekends.

Since stopping her birth-control pills three months before, her menstrual periods had become extremely heavy. They were on time, but "much heavier than I've ever had, especially the last two. The last one was eight rather than five days."

Her checkup was almost normal, with minor indications of a need for zinc, vitamin A, and essential fatty acids, but no observable disease.

I left the examination room while she got dressed. When I came back, she asked what I meant about her diet possibly being related to her abnormal Pap smears.

"Remember, I can't say for sure. But there have been a few research indications that the extra hormones of pregnancy and the hormones in birth-control pills can lead to abnormalities of the cells of the uterine cervix (where the Pap smear is taken) that are totally correctable by folate."

She looked puzzled. "Folate? That's a vitamin, isn't it?"

"Yes. It's usually grouped with B complex vitamins. It's been known for a long time that birth-control pills can lead to folate deficiencies, as well as other B vitamin problems, especially $B_6$. The evidence is just starting to come in about folate and cervical problems.

"How that fits you particularly, though, is that your diet has been remarkably poor in sources of folate. The best are raw deep green leafy vegetables—raw, and uncooked because heating or freezing always destroys some folate. Spinach, beet greens, kale, endive, and turnip greens are all good sources. So are broccoli, asparagus, liver, wheat germ, lima beans, and black-eyed peas."

"I hardly touch any of those, so should I take folate?"

## More Vitamin A Needed

"That's not all. There are also reports that vitamin A deficiency may predispose to cancer formation, and that vitamin A can prevent certain types of tumors in animals. Interestingly enough, one of those types is cervical cancer in hamsters. Of course hamsters aren't people, and such findings may not be relevant, but can you guess what else your diet's low in?"

"Vitamin A."

"Remember you mentioned your last two menstrual periods were much heavier? Two South African researchers have reported that vitamin A is extremely effective treatment for very heavy menstrual periods when there are no obvious problems like fibroids or endometrial cancer. I've found they were right; it works in practice, so that may be a clue in your case, too.

"Now . . . the best food sources of vitamin A are . . ."

". . . carrots, liver, dark green leafy vegetables. I remember that from Mother."

"Also broccoli, sweet potatoes, squash. . . . Sounds rather like the folate list, doesn't it?"

Ms. Gallegos looked considerably more cheerful. "So folate and vitamin A might cure my cancer?"

"No, no, there's no evidence to say they cure cancer. Besides, we can't even say you've got cancer, just 'dysplasia,' which is getting worse and might eventually turn into cancer. But then some cases have gotten better on their own after looking bad for a while."

"Probably after eating a lot of spinach and carrots." She laughed. "But seriously, with my diet the way it's been, particularly bad in those two vitamins . . ."

"Yes, there is enough research data to at least suggest this might be your problem. Since surgery isn't mandatory right away, if you promise to check in with your gynecologist regularly, it is reasonable to try diet and vitamins."

"Well, he did say the same as you—that sometimes even 'severe' dysplasia gets better, as he put it, 'spontaneously,' with no treatment. How much folate and vitamin A do I need?"

"First, food. If you can talk yourself into a good diet, even if you don't have time to cook, you could possibly prevent this sort of problem without many supplemental vitamins. Have you heard of the 'Yogi Bear' or 'Caveman' type of diet? It's ideal for younger single persons who don't like to cook, or don't have the time."

"Yogi Bear? I think I remember from TV when I was a kid . . . nuts, seeds, berries, . . . that kind of thing."

"Sure. Raw vegetables, nuts, seeds, fruit, berries . . . none of that needs cooking, just a refrigerator. Add in cheeses, whole grain breads, a little milk if it doesn't give you gas. Then all you might need to cook would be meat, maybe liver, fish, chicken, and perhaps potatoes or beans. All in all, very healthful, lots of vitamins and minerals, and not too much work. If you get bored, you can get more fancy or eat out—good food, of course.

"Now, about specific vitamins. I don't want to write an entire list until we see your various test results, but I agree you should start folate and vitamin A now. Folate is unfortunately not available in doses larger than one milligram even on prescription. If you get them in a health food store, they're 0.8 milligrams (800 micrograms) at the largest, even though there's never been toxicity recorded. On the other hand, if you're going to Vancouver soon . . ."

"I'll make a trip."

"Fine. You can get 5 milligram tablets over the counter. Please use one, three times a day, for now. Vitamin A, 60,000 international units daily for two months, then drop off to 25,000 international units daily. To back up the folate, B complex '50,' one tablet two times a day. And for general good health, vitamin C, one gram daily, and vitamin E, 400 international units daily.

"But most important: Please fix your diet!"

Two months later, Sandra Gallegos had both a Pap smear and colposcopy at her gynecologist's. Both examinations were perfectly normal. She's continued to have regular examinations for four years since; the problem of dysplasia has not returned. She's now married, but continues on what she calls a "modified Yogi Bear" diet program, as both she and her husband work full-time, and neither likes to cook much.

According to the most critical reviewers, the evidence is not conclusive to suggest that folate may prevent some cervical cancer, or that vitamin A prevents tumors. Since folate is generally considered safe, I recommend at least one milligram daily to anyone taking birth-control pills, pregnant or soon to be, or anyone taking estrogenic hormones of any type. As vitamin A in very high doses might be toxic, don't take more than 25,000 international units a day for any extended period. Or take even less and eat carrots.

## Vitamins Can Reverse Cervical Dysplasia

Since this treatment was recommended for Sandra Gallegos, C. E. Butterworth, M.D., and associates, researchers at the University of Alabama, have reported that folate does in fact reverse cervical dysplasia in women who've been using oral contraceptives. The amount of folate used was 10 milligrams daily.

In addition to folate and vitamin A, it appears vitamin C may also protect against cervical cancer. In a diet-comparison study, conducted by Sylvia Wassertheil-Smoller, Ph.D., and associates at Albert Einstein Medical College, women with cervical dysplasia were found to eat significantly less vitamin C than women (of similar age, race, and number of children) without cervical dysplasia. Although these results are considered preliminary, I expect the effect will be confirmed, as vitamin C has been found to be cancer protective in many other circumstances.

The largest dosage tablet of folate available in the United States, even on prescription, is only one milligram. That makes it a real nuisance for free citizens of the United States to take an adequate dose for cervical dysplasia reversion, and virtually impossible to use larger quantities sometimes useful in other conditions, including gout, where up to 400 to 600 milligrams daily is sometimes helpful. Yet folate is generally considered safe.

In Canada, folate is available in one, 5, 10, and 25 milligram dosages (the latter only in some areas, and along with vitamin $B_{12}$). If there's ever time, I think I'll write a paper entitled "The Geographic Effect of the 49th Parallel on Folate Metabolism." One might conclude there is such a geographic effect, since Canadians living north of the 49th parallel in British Columbia (and elsewhere) are "allowed" to obtain and swallow folate much more conveniently and in larger doses than people living south of the 49th parallel in Washington State, where I live, and elsewhere. Or maybe it's the cold.

Seriously though, it's time for federal regulaton of contraband high-dosage nontoxic folate to be removed. The original "thought" (if we can call it that) behind restricting folate availability was that folate can mask the effects of degeneration of the spinal cord (caused by vitamin $B_{12}$ deficiency) and make it harder to diagnose. Why an obscure bureaucrat thought American physicians were less perceptive than Canadian physicians, who are "forced" to make this diagnosis without folate regulation, isn't known.

Instead of keeping higher-dose folate away from everyone even on prescription, because of the remote possibility of a missed diagnosis (a situation similar to keeping everyone after class because one student misbehaves), it would seem more reasonable (if it's really necessary) to put a warning label on higher doses of folate. Something like "folate can hide signs of vitamin $B_{12}$ deficiency." Warning labels appear to be sufficient for a toxic substance like tobacco; surely folate isn't more dangerous. Or perhaps, as is done by one Canadian manufacturer, vitamin $B_{12}$ can be added to higher doses of folate.

Whatever the solution, folate should be deregulated. As accumulating research shows the usefulness of folate, its unavailability in anything but small-quantity tablets is increasingly ridiculous.

# REFERENCES

**Folate**

Butterworth, C. E., Jr. et al. "Improvement in Cervical Dysplasia Associated with Folic Acid Therapy in Users of Oral Contraceptives." *American Journal of Clinical Nutrition*, January, 1982, pp. 73–82.

Kitay, David Z., and Wentz, W. Budd. "Cervical Cytology in Folic Acid Deficiency of Pregnancy." *American Journal of Obstetrics and Gynecology*, August 1, 1969, pp. 931–938.

Lindenbaum, John; Whitehead, Nancy; and Reyner, Franklin. "Oral Contraceptive Hormones, Folate Metabolism, and the Cervical Epithelium." *American Journal of Clinical Nutrition*, April, 1975, pp. 346–353.

Perloff, Betty P., and Butrum, Ritva R. "Folacin in Selected Foods." *Journal of the American Dietetic Association*, February, 1977, pp 163–167.

Roe, Daphne A. "Nutritional Effects of Oral Contraceptives." In *Drug-Induced Nutritional Deficiencies*. Avi Publishing, 1976, p. 222.

Whitehead, Nancy; Reyner, Franklin; and Lindenbaum, John. "Megaloblastic Changes in the Cervical Epithelium: Association with Oral Contraceptive Therapy and Reversal with Folic Acid." *Journal of the American Medical Association*, December 17, 1973, pp. 1421–1424.


**Vitamin A**

Chu, Elizabeth W., and Malmgren, Richard A. "An Inhibitory Effect of Vitamin A on the Induction of Tumors of Forestomach and Cervix in the Syrian Hamster by Carcinogenic Polycyclic Hydrocarbons." *Cancer Research*, July, 1965, pp. 884–894.

Lithgow, D. M., and Politzer, W. M. "Vitamin A in the Treatment of Menorrhagia." *South American Medical Journal*, February 12, 1977, pp. 191–193.

Romney, Seymour L. et al. "Retinoids and the Prevention of Cervical Dysplasias." *American Journal of Obstetrics and Gynecology*, December 15, 1981, pp. 890–894.

**Vitamin A and Cancer**

Basu, T. K. "Vitamin A and Cancer of Epithelial Origin." *Journal of Human Nutrition*, February, 1979, pp. 24–31.

Shamberger, Raymond J. "Inhibitory Effect of Vitamin A on Carcinogenesis." *Journal of the National Cancer Institute*, September, 1971, pp. 667–673.

"Vitamin A, Tumor Initiation and Tumor Promotion." *Nutrition Reviews*, May, 1979, pp. 153–156.

**Vitamin C**

Wassertheil-Smoller, Sylvia et al. "Dietary Vitamin C and Uterine/Cervical Dysplasia." *American Journal of Epidemiology*, November, 1981, pp. 714–724.

**One heart attack does not necessarily lead to another. A good diet, plus supplements of lecithin, oil, and vitamins C and E, is suggested as a preventive measure. The importance of "high-density cholesterol" is discussed.**

# 20  A CASE OF CHOLESTEROL IMBALANCE

Homer Gibson didn't appear pleased. He walked slowly from the waiting room to my office, prodded by his wife, Mary, whom I'd known for several years. Even though he'd not been in before, I thought I knew what we'd be talking about. Several months ago, at one of her infrequent visits, Mary Gibson had appeared depressed and very tired. She reported that Homer had "finally had his heart attack" after several years of intermittent chest pains. We'd discussed what could be done to prevent recurrence; she left looking grimly determined.

"What can I help you with today?" I asked as the Gibsons sat down.

"You could not keep us waiting half an hour past the appointment time. That'd be a help," Mr Gibson replied.

"Homer, keep a civil tongue," his wife admonished. "You promised you'd listen."

"Sometimes explanations take extra time," I said. "And sometimes people don't want to leave when the appointment time is over. Unfortunately, we've had a little of each today. It's a good thing there weren't any emergencies, too."

"Never mind Homer. He's just grumpy because it isn't raining today and he'd rather be playing golf."

"First sunny day in two weeks. My luck," Mr. Gibson grumbled.

"What's your score?"

"Let's talk about my dense cholesterol. That's what I'm here for."

"Your dense cholesterol?"

"My doctor says that's probably why I had heart trouble. Not enough dense cholesterol, or something like that. Some new-fangled test."

"High-density cholesterol, Homer."

"Yeah. For years they've been telling me too much cholesterol was bad—now they tell me I had a heart attack because I didn't have enough."

Mary Gibson sighed. "I already explained that to him, Doctor. He's just being stubborn."

"So you've had a low HDL cholesterol test?"

"His highest reading has been 27. One time it was 19. Trouble is, I've had a hard time talking his doctor into doing the test. He said even checking the total cholesterol was mostly useless, because lowering cholesterol with drugs didn't seem to prevent heart trouble."

"That's true. One recent series of reports demonstrated that a commonly prescribed cholesterol-lowering drug was associated with increased overall mortality, some 20 to 25 percent, even though the incidence of heart attacks appeared to be less."

"I don't need lower cholesterol, anyway," Mr. Gibson said. "It's more of those dense ones I need. Got the overall cholesterol controlled a few years back by cutting down animal fats. Cholesterol came down from the 400s to around 300. Doctor told me that was OK for my age. I'm 74, you know."

## Two Years of "Nagging"

"He makes it sound easy, like he did it all himself. It took me two solid years—"

"Of nagging," Mr. Gibson cut in.

"For your own good. Two solid years to get him to change his ways. And I still couldn't get him to take one solitary vitamin pill. He treated them like poison."

"Bad enough giving up deep-fried shrimp," Mr. Gibson complained. "But I did it. I thought between that, taking those dynamite tablets whenever I had a little pain, and playing golf every day it didn't rain, for exercise, that would be enough. Besides, my doctor says if you eat a well-balanced diet you don't need any vitamins."

"No, just dynamite pills instead," Mrs. Gibson observed sourly.

"Dynamite pills?"

"That's what he calls nitroglycerine tablets."

"Oh. Are you still using them?"

"Nope. Haven't had any chest pains since the heart attack. Thought it cured me, but my doctor says it happens sometimes, and I could still have trouble."

"Homer, let the doctor tell you about vitamins."

"Before vitamins, shouldn't we talk about diet in general? That's always more important than supplements. There are several good diet programs. For example, the Pritikin . . ."

Mr. Gibson's face clouded. "I told Mary I've made all the diet changes I'm going to. This time I'll try her vitamin pills. Give up this, give up that . . ."

Mrs. Gibson looked a little distressed, and gave me a warning look. "Let's just go over vitamins and things you said would help HDL cholesterol. We'll talk about diet at home. You did say certain vitamins would raise HDL levels when I was here last, didn't you?"

"Yes."

"Homer, show him your report from last week."

Mr. Gibson reached into his pocket, pulling out a copy of a lab slip. He passed it to me.

"Total cholesterol 293, HDL cholesterol 25. Not so good."

"That's what my doctor said. Seems he believes in dense cholesterols now. He said there weren't any drugs for it, though."

"Reports indicate that the greater the proportion of HDL cholesterol to the total cholesterol, the more protection there is against atherosclerosis. It doesn't guarantee no further heart attacks, but does lessen the risk.

"Your test at present shows relatively high risk. Total cholesterol 293, HDL 25. Gives you a ratio of 11.7. That's high risk."

"So how do I get more high-densities? That's what I'm supposed to need."

"That's true, but as far as I'm concerned you could use less total cholesterol, too. If you haven't been taking any vitamins or other supplements at all, that's possible."

"Until now, he wouldn't take a one, Doctor. It took a heart attack before he'd listen to me."

"OK, Mary, you made your point. Let's get on with it. What do I do?"

I got out a notepad. "Using these supplements, nutritionally oriented physicians have been helping people with atherosclerosis, including heart disease, for literally decades before anyone ever heard of HDL cholesterol. Now that HDL tests are available, it's been shown that one of the ways supplements help is by raising HDL levels, as well as lowering total cholesterol."

"Doctors should pay more attention to the patients and how they do rather than having to have scientific laboratory explanations every time. Sometimes it takes science too long to catch up," Mrs. Gibson observed.

## Start with Lecithin

"Let's start with lecithin. Please use three of the 19-grain capsules, twice daily. As long ago as 1943, and several times since, lecithin has been shown to lower overall cholesterol levels. Yet a 1980 report, which showed the same thing, said this overall reduction was 'unexpected.' Another report shows that lecithin raises HDL cholesterol, too, while lowering LDL cholesterol.

"Secondly, vitamin E, 800 international units daily. Vitamin E has been shown to raise HDL cholesterol from 100 percent to over 300 percent.

"Third, vitamin C, two grams, twice daily. This helps raise high-density cholesterol; some reports say it lowers the total.

"Lastly, sunflower or safflower oil, one tablespoon daily. Linseed oil is even better, if you don't mind the taste. It's also available in capsules. Oils lower overall cholesterol but haven't yet been shown to raise HDL levels. They shouldn't be taken without vitamin E."

I handed Mr. Gibson the note. He looked it over, and got up to go.

"Don't you have any questions, Homer?" Mrs. Gibson asked.

"I said I'd take your pills, didn't I? Well here's the list, and I got the explanation. Now, let's go, and not make anyone else late. Besides, the golf course is waiting."

"Please check back in six weeks for follow-up cholesterol and HDL tests," I said, but Mr. Gibson was gone.

"He will," replied Mrs. Gibson, and hurried after him.

Four months later, Mr. Gibson's total cholesterol was 214 and his HDL cholesterol was 56, giving him a ratio of 3.8, much better than his previous 11.7 ratio. He can't be guaranteed no further heart attacks, but he's definitely lowered his risk to the "less-than-average" category.

One addition had to be made to his program, a pancreatic enzyme supplement, which appeared to aid in the digestion and absorption of his fat- and oil-soluble vitamins and supplements.

## Cholesterol Can Be Lowered through Diet Alone

If Mr. Gibson had wanted to talk about diet and HDL cholesterol, he would have heard that it's frequently possible to reduce total cholesterol and normalize the ratio of total cholesterol to HDL cholesterol through food alone. Although nutritional biochemistry makes extensive use of dietary supplementation, the basic principle of optimum diet first, supplementation later, always applies.

What Mr. Gibson would have heard about is fish and vegetables. Renewed research interest in the relationship of diet to disease, including atherosclerotic disease, has produced a number of studies showing that vegetarianism and exclusion of food of animal origin is associated with lower overall blood fats and an improved cholesterol to HDL cholesterol ratio. The animal-origin food group which appears to be an important exception is fish.

Probably because of their content of important unsaturated oils, fish appears to be protective against cardiovascular disease. One recent study, by Ann Fehily, Ph.D., and associates, demonstrated that increasing quantities of fish in the diet are associated with increasing levels of HDL cholesterol, and decreasing quantities of LDL cholesterol (low-density lipoprotein cholesterol). Higher levels of LDL are associated with greater risk for cardiovascular disease.

Although vegetarianism is one important way of lowering cardiovascular disease risk, population-group studies have shown that it's distinctly possible to eat very few vegetables and still have low cardiovascular risk. A diet heavy in fish and fish oils appears to be one way; research work among Greenland Eskimos, who live on such a diet, has attracted considerable attention. It's been shown they have comparatively much less cardiovascular disease, yet they certainly aren't vegetarians. Investigators have identified one component of fish oils, eicosapentaenoic acid, as probably exerting a strong protective effect. Although I didn't need to ask Mr. Gibson to use it, eicosapentaenoic acid, identified as "EPA," is available as a dietary supplement.

Many surveys of diet and health have demonstrated an association between vegetarianism and reduced cardiovascular disease risk. A group associated with the Framingham Study of cardiovascular disease investigated some of the reasons why. Comparing vegetarians to controls of the same age and sex, they found that the vegetarians had lower levels of total cholesterol, LDL cholesterol, triglycerides, and even slightly lower levels of HDL cholesterol. Even though the HDL cholesterol was slightly lower, the total cholesterol was proportionately much lower, producing a significantly lower cholesterol to HDL cholesterol ratio.

These investigators also found that both dairy products and eggs, significant parts of some vegetarian diets, were associated with slightly higher total cholesterol and LDL cholesterol levels. Their statistics also demonstrated that body weight in and of itself was not correlated with higher levels of cholesterol. One interpretation of this last finding, which seems to contradict the perennial instruction to lose weight, would be that it's not fatness itself that's a problem, but what type of foods the individual used (in excess) to become fat.

Mrs. Gibson has heard all of this before. I suspect that Mr. Gibson, despite his reluctance, is gradually being persuaded to eat more fish and vegetables, as well as continue his diet supplements.

# REFERENCES

**Cholesterol**

Adlersburg, D., and Sobotka, H. "Effect of Prolonged Lecithin Feeding on Hypercholesterolemia." *Journal of the Mount Sinai Hospital*, March–April, 1943, pp. 955–956.

Childs, Marian T. et al. "The Contrasting Effects of a Dietary Soya Lecithin Product and Corn Oil on Lipoprotein Lipids in Normolipidemic and Familial Hypercholesterolemic Subjects." *Atherosclerosis*, vol. 38, 1981, pp. 217–228.

Fehily, Ann M. et al. "Dietary Determinants of Lipoproteins, Total Cholesterol, Viscosity, Fibrinogen, and Blood Pressure." *American Journal of Clinical Nutrition*, November, 1982, pp. 890–896.

Hermann, William J.; Ward, Karen; and Faucett, James. "The Effect of Tocopherol on High-Density Lipoprotein Cholesterol." *American Journal of Clinical Pathology*, November, 1979, pp. 848–852.

Horsey, Jennifer; Livesley, Brian; and Dickerson, J. W. T. "Ischaemic Heart Disease and Aged Patients: Effects of Ascorbic Acid on Lipoproteins." *Journal of Human Nutrition*, vol. 35, no. 1, 1981, pp. 53–58.

Tompkins, Ronald K., and Parkin, Lillie G. "Effects of Long-Term Ingestion of Soya Phospholipids on Serum Lipids in

Humans." *American Journal of Surgery,* September, 1980, pp. 360–364.

**Clofibrate**
Oliver, M. F. et al. "W.H.O. Cooperative Trial on Primary Prevention of Ischaemic Heart Disease Using Clofibrate to Lower Serum Cholesterol: Mortality Follow-up." *Lancet,* August 23, 1980, pp. 379–385.
Silverman, Harold M., and Simon, Gilbert I. *The Pill Book.* Bantam Books, 1979, pp. 64–66.

**Heart Disease**
Hancock, E. William. "Coronary Artery Disease—Epidemiology and Prevention." In Section 1: Cardiovascular Medicine, *Scientific American Medicine.* Scientific American, pp. 1–8.

**Linoleic Acid**
Vergroesen, Antoine J. "Physiological Effects of Dietary Linoleic Acid." *Nutrition Reviews,* January, 1977, pp. 1–5.

**Vegetarianism**
Cooper, Richard S. et al. "The Selective Lipid-Lowering Effect of Vegetarianism on Low Density Lipoproteins in a Crossover Experiment." *Atherosclerosis,* vol. 44, 1982, pp. 293–305.
Nestel, Paul; Billington, Timothy; and Smith, Brian. "Low Density and High Density Lipoprotein Kinetics and Sterol Balance in Vegetarians." *Metabolism,* October, 1981, pp. 941–945.
Sacks, Frank M. et al. "Plasma Lipids and Lipoproteins in Vegetarians and Controls." *New England Journal of Medicine,* May 29, 1975, pp. 1148–1151.

**Vitamin E**
Shute, Evan V. "Alpha Tocopherol In Cardiovascular Disease." *Summary,* December, 1973, pp. 5–9.
————."Vitamin E." *Journal of Applied Nutrition,* Winter, 1973, pp. 25–39.

A routine nutritional checkup leads to the discovery that bad circulation may be due to poor digestion. Intravenous therapy of high doses of vitamin C plus other nutrients is eventually the most effective treatment.

# 21    A CASE OF POOR CIRCULATION

Inez Cerillo was in for what she called a "routine maintenance and preventive" check. We'd completed her health history and were nearly done with her checkup when we got to her feet.

"What are you looking for?" she asked.

"Various things. Warts, corns, calluses . . . right now I'm trying to find your pulses."

"Pulses in my feet?"

"Sure. Just a routine check to make sure enough blood's getting through."

"Must be. My feet haven't dropped off yet."

"Do they get cold or bluish?"

"Always have had a tendency to cold hands and feet. My husband calls me "old refrigerator foot." But it's on and off, and nothing new. I always thought it was 'nerves.' When I was a teenager nearly forty years ago, I got cold hands and feet on every date."

"You're right—that kind of cold hands and feet is usually due to overactivity of the sympathetic nervous system. Deliberate relaxation will take it away.

"But that's not what I mean. Have you noticed any steady, all-the-time coolness in your feet? Do they get colder or whiter than they used to when you go out in the cold?"

"Can't say they do. Is there a problem?"

I continued to check a minute or two. "Don't really know yet. I can feel a very faint pulse on the top of your right foot, here, and none on the left. I don't feel any pulses in the usual alternative places, either, like behind your ankles."

Mrs. Cerillo looked concerned. "What does that mean?"

"Maybe nothing. We'll have to check further. First let's look for the pulses behind your knees and in the groin area."

The pulse behind her right knee was nearly normal, but the left side seemed decreased. Both groin pulses were normal. I checked her feet again while she made sure that there was no pressure on the back of her leg to stop or slow blood flow.

"Still nothing on the left?"

"Afraid not."

"I've been thinking while you were checking. My left leg below the knee has seemed a little more tired than the right when I go for walks. But it doesn't hurt. Isn't it supposed to hurt if the blood isn't getting through?"

"When it gets bad. Besides, checking with the fingers for a pulse is a good 'screening test,' but it isn't conclusive. The next thing to do before really getting concerned is to check the blood flow in the entire leg, including surface pulsing vessels and deeper ones that can't be felt with the fingers. Also, to make sure the blood vessels aren't simply constricted by the nervous system."

"Is that one of those artery-grams? My aunt, the one with diabetes, had that. Dye in the artery to her leg, then x-rays."

"Arteriograms are one way to check blood flow. They're very important in surgical situations. Another way to check is with ultrasound, called a Doppler examination. I use a third type of procedure, plethysmography."

"Say again?"

"Plethysmography. Cuffs like blood pressure cuffs are placed around certain locations on the leg, including the thigh, calf, and one of the toes. Each cuff contains a transducer which measures the pulse in the entire extremity at that point, surface and deep. The measurement is recorded as a pulse wave through standard electrocardiogram equipment."

"So sometimes the pulse wave for the whole leg or whole ankle is normal even if you can't find it with your fingers?"

"Sometimes. Also, the person being tested is given a rapidly acting blood vessel dilator to relieve spasm in the artery. If there is any spasm, the test becomes more normal."

"Meaning it's not a blockage in the artery, then?"

"Can't be much of one if blood flow becomes normal or nearly so with dilation."

"I hope that's me. When do I have that done?"

"Later this week, if you can." Since we'd finished her examination, we went over other tests before she left for the laboratory.

Mrs. Cerillo was back in three weeks looking grim and determined. She handed me a sheet of paper. "Will these do for starters?" she asked.

The paper listed several vitamin and mineral supplements, including vitamin C powder, "body-tolerance" dose; vitamin E, 2,000 international units; lecithin, 2 tablespoons; zinc, 100 milligrams; selenium, 100 micrograms; B complex; and calcium pangamate, 100 milligrams.

"Are you sure you need to see me? Looks like you're doing fine on your own."

"No, I'm not. If I were, that plethysmogram would have been normal. I talked it over with the medical technologist. It doesn't take much to see the pulse wave was nearly flat in my left toes, and reduced in my left calf. Even the right side was diminished compared to the normal standard. The blood vessel dilator didn't help the pulses much—it only made me dizzy."

I looked at her medical record. "Those are the problem areas, all right. With some adjustments here and there, this list of supplements should help. You've really been doing some reading."

"No point waiting around. What annoys me most is that I've

eaten hardly any junk food for years. No sugar in the house, hardly anything canned, whole grains. . . . Of course I wasn't taking many vitamins, but I didn't have any symptoms of anything. A person shouldn't have to take a ton of vitamins just to stay normal, should she?'"

"With no symptoms, not a ton, no. Some vitamins C, E, perhaps a multiple vitamin and mineral supplement. . . . Although with worsening soil mineral depletion, insecticides, overly long food storage, gas-ripening, artificially added ingredients—not to mention air pollution, water pollution and industrial chemicals pervading the food chain, perhaps a bit more would be wise.

"But back to your case. From the appearance of your mineral analysis, you haven't been absorbing many of the nutrients from the good diet you've been following. Calcium, magnesium, iron, copper, manganese, zinc, chromium, selenium . . . all low."

Mrs. Cerillo looked surprised. "But I don't have any symptoms of bad digestion. No gas, bloating, constipation, burping, nothing. My digestion's just fine."

"This mineral analysis suggests it isn't. Every once in a while we find someone with no digestive symptoms whose tests prove hypochlorhydria, or low stomach acidity, lack of pancreatic enzymes, food allergies, or one of the other causes of poor absorption."

"Will I need to take all those minerals, too?"

"Yes, plus whatever it takes to get them absorbed. Fortunately, most of them can be taken in 'multiple' form. As you're taking extra zinc to help the circulation, we'll have to be careful it's balanced with copper."

"Yes, I read about that, too."

Mrs. Cerillo subsequently proved to have a moderate deficit in stomach acid production. In addition to the list she'd prepared for herself, I added an average adult dose of hydrochloric acid capsules, vitamin $B_{12}$ by injection, the minerals she was low on, and 1½ tablespoons of sunflower oil as an essential fatty acid precursor.

Unfortunately, it didn't work. After ten months, we had to decide what to do next.

"My pulses are as bad as ever," Mrs. Cerillo reported. "I've been practicing finding them on my husband ever since the first time I was here. His are beautiful, mine nowhere. I still don't have any symptoms except a little tiredness in the left calf, but then I didn't have any in the first place. My plethysmogram's scarcely any better. And my mineral analysis is showing only a slow improvement."

I looked at the mineral analysis. "It is slow, but definite. You are absorbing things better."

"But at this rate it could take years. It's been nearly a year now. My husband's pushing me to take chelation therapy. It cleared up a case of angina for one of our neighbors. Angina's supposed to be caused by blocked arteries around the heart, and he's read chelation is supposed to clear that. He figures it'll work on my legs, too."

"Chelation frequently helps circulatory problems, although whether it does so by clearing blood vessels or by altering the handling of calcium is uncertain. I can refer you to a colleague who does chelation therapy if you'd like."

"I'm a little uneasy about that. I've read that the chelating agent used is a synthetic drug, possibly dangerous. I've been trying to avoid synthetic drugs."

"Given by qualified doctors, it's usually quite safe. However, there's an alternative you could try first."

"What's that? I thought I'd tried everything: good diet, loads of vitamins, minerals, vigorous exercise every day, aerobic dance classes. . . . "

"It's vitamin C again, but intravenously, 30 to 50 grams at a time in a solution with B vitamins, calcium, magnesium, and other nutrients."

"Why should it work intravenously if it didn't work when I swallowed it?"

"Can't say for sure, but I've seen it happen before. Remember, you do have an absorptive defect. It's been at least partly corrected with hydrochloric acid supplements, but that may not be the entire answer. Also, like the drug used in chelation therapy, vitamin C is a chelating agent. A weaker one, but it still does a chelating job."

"Including affecting calcium metabolism?"

"Definitely. We have to be careful with intravenous vitamin C, so not too much calcium is removed.

"One other thing to remember ... you could give what you're already doing some more time. You're not having symptoms right now. There's no rush."

Mrs. Cerillo thought for a minute. "No, let's go ahead and try it. I want to get my arteries cleared as soon as possible, as long as it's reasonably safe. I'm getting more nervous. I can't help but think that other arteries elsewhere might be partly blocked, too."

Mrs. Cerillo came in for intravenous high-dose vitamin C twice weekly. To our surprise, three weeks later we both could find a pulse in her left foot, although it was slight. The pulses on the right were stronger. By eleven weeks, the pulses on both sides were normal. Another plethysmogram confirmed what our fingers had found: Her pulse waves were nearly perfect. We stopped the intravenous treatments, and cut down on her oral supplements.

Two years later, the pulses in her feet were still normal. Her mineral levels were nearly normal, indicating a slow continuing improvement in nutrient absorption.

Not everyone responds as rapidly to intravenous high-dose vitamin C as Mrs. Cerillo did. However, most don't need intravenous therapy, as oral vitamin C and other supplements are usually effective. Probably her absorptive defect was a little more complicated than low stomach acidity, although the usual tests showed no other causes. Whatever the ultimate explanation, we agreed that she had definitely accomplished valuable preventive maintenance, finding and solving a health problem before it gave her painful and possibly disabling trouble.

# Nature Needs a Little Help Sometimes

Nature's plan was not for us to take nutrients intravenously. Whenever possible, I try to use diet and oral supplementation. It's not only closest to nature's design, but also inherently safer than injections.

However, sometimes shots, both intramuscular and intravenous, are the only way to get nutrients into the body in adequate quantities, and in time. The best example of this is vitamin $B_{12}$, usually in cases of low or no stomach acidity, but occasionally when absorption appears normal. Despite scientific proof that microscopic quantities of vitamin $B_{12}$ given infrequently by mouth or by injection are enough, experience has taught me to believe the hundreds of people who've told me that larger amounts injected once or twice weekly are necessary for optimum well-being.

The idea that atherosclerosis may be reversible is starting to spread, although very slowly. In 1979 a newspaper for physicians reported that atherosclerosis reversal had been demonstrated in man "for the first time." The effect was achieved with drugs. The idea that diet and nutritional supplements might be even more effective does not appear to be under investigation. Yet, 30 years ago, a Canadian physician using a single vitamin proved it was sometimes possible.

G. C. Willis, M.D., and associates took arteriograms (x-ray pictures of arteries using a dye) of individuals with atherosclerosis of the leg arteries. They then asked them to take 500 milligrams of vitamin C three times daily, a small dose by today's standards, for several months. Following this, the arteriograms were repeated. In six of ten cases, some areas of atherosclerosis were measurably smaller. No diet changes or other supplements were used.

Recently, it's been shown that chromium can reverse atherosclerosis in experimental animals. Indications are that it will work for humans as well. In 1968, two ophthalmologists, using direct observation of the arteries of the retina, concluded that iodide was a powerful agent to reverse atherosclerosis. There's every reason to suspect that many other individual nutrients, if studied, would show the same effect. However (once again), overall diet change to a "new traditional" pattern, plus supplementation with all nutrients deficient and extra quantities of those known to be helpful, is always the preferred route.

Chelation therapy is another alternative to surgery for treatment of atherosclerosis. Starting as simply a series of intravenous infusions of the drug ethylenediaminetetraacetic acid (EDTA), chelation therapy has grown to include attention to diet, and vitamins and minerals as well. Although ignored and put down by established medical organizations, physicians who practice chelation therapy have helped many individuals with atherosclerosis and serious symptoms regain their health without surgery. Many practitioners of chelation therapy are members of the American Academy of Medical Preventics, whose headquarters is in Beverly Hills, California.

It's been my observation that a disproportionately large number of individuals with atherosclerosis at a relatively young age have problems with nutrient malabsorption, as did Inez Cerillo. Certainly not all do, though.

Most people who have cold hands and feet assume it's due to poor circulation, but that's not the case. Compromised circulation to the hands is an extremely rare phenomenon. As noted, when both hands and feet are cold, it's a "nerve problem."

Infrequently, atherosclerotic disease is so advanced when an individual comes to my office that I concur with a recommendation for surgery. (Atherosclerosis shouldn't be confused with heart valve damage and disease, which at present can't be corrected with nutritional or biochemical means.) After surgery, though, it obviously makes no sense to do nothing and allow the process to recur all over again. By diet change and other nutritional-biochemical means, a repetition of the same problem can always be prevented.

Of course, prevention of the problem in the first place is always the best course. Attention to diet, exercise, mental health, and sometimes (as in Inez Cerillo's case) an occasional nutritional-biochemical checkup can almost always achieve this goal.

## REFERENCES

**Atherosclerosis**

"MD Offers Proof Atherosclerosis Is Reversible." *Medical World News*, November 26, 1979, pp. 29, 33.

Willis, G. C. "The Reversibility of Atherosclerosis." *Canadian Medical Association Journal*, July 15, 1957, pp. 106–109.

Willis, G. C.; Light, A.W.; and Gow, W. S. "Serial Arteriography in Atherosclerosis." *Canadian Medical Association Journal,* December, 1954, pp. 562–568.

Walker, Morton, and Gordon, Garry F. *The Chelation Answer.* M. Evans, 1982.

**Chelation Therapy**

Casdorph, H. Richard. "EDTA Chelation Therapy, Efficacy In Arteriosclerotic Heart Disease." *Journal of Holistic Medicine,* Spring/Summer, 1981, pp. 53–59.

Cranton, Elmer M., and Frackelton, James P. "Current Status of EDTA Chelation Therapy in Occlusive Arterial Disease." *Journal of Holistic Medicine,* Spring/Summer, 1982, pp. 24–33.

**Chromium**

Abraham, Abraham S.: Sonnenblick, Moshe; and Eini, Maya. "The Action of Chromium on Serum Lipids and on Atherosclerosis in Cholesterol-Fed Rabbits." *Atherosclerosis,* vol. 42, 1982, pp. 185–195.

———. "The Effect of Chromium on Cholesterol-Induced Atherosclerosis in Rabbits." *Atherosclerosis,* vol. 41, 1982, pp. 371–379.

Abraham, Abraham S. et al. "The Effect of Chromium on Established Atherosclerotic Plaques in Rabbits." *American Journal of Clinical Nutrition,* November, 1980, pp. 2294–2298.

Newman, Howard A. I. et al. "Serum Chromium and Angiographically Determined Coronary Artery Disease." *Clinical Chemistry,* vol. 24, no. 4, 1978, pp. 541–544.

Vobecky, Josef, and Shapcott, Dennis. "Ischemic Heart Disease and Elements in Water." Letter in *Canadian Medical Association Journal,* November 22, 1975, pp. 922, 925.

**A persistent eye irritation clears up in four days following the use of specially prepared eyedrops containing sodium ascorbate.**

# A CASE OF ULCERATED CORNEA    **22**

Henry Thompson didn't come to the office often. He worked hard, watched his diet, took supplements, and got plenty of exercise, generally keeping himself well. In fact, the only times I'd seen him were for physical exams, which he scheduled every two years as part of his personal health-maintenance program. So, when I saw his name on my schedule, I guessed that more than a little was the matter.

When he arrived, he had a patch over his right eye. "I know you're not an eye doctor," he said, "but I've been working with an ophthalmologist on this for nearly three months, and it isn't getting any better. He sent me to another ophthalmologist for an opinion, but that doctor couldn't help. I have an ulceration on my cornea that just won't heal."

"What caused it?"

"I don't know. The doctor isn't certain, either. He says it could be from an injury, or perhaps an infection. Sometimes it seems to be almost gone, and then it gets worse again. It hurts all the time, so he told me to put this patch on. That relieves the pain a lot."

Mr. Thompson had just come from a visit to the eye doctor's. He still had a trace of a fluorescent dye in his eye used to better demonstrate ulcers and abrasions. It was apparent that there was an ulceration. Other than this, and a bit of a bloodshot appearance, I couldn't find anything else. (I should insert here, as Mr. Thompson noted, that I am not an eye specialist and have no special equipment for the diagnosis of eye disease. Except for extremely simple eye problems, I always refer patients to specialists for more complete diagnostic work.)

"Well, what do you think?" Mr. Thompson asked.

"I think it's worth at least a try," I said. "Let me put together some solution for you for eyedrops. This isn't a standard item at the stores. It's sodium ascorbate solution."

"What's sodium ascorbate?"

"It's a form of vitamin C, buffered so it's nonacidic. Regular ascorbic acid would sting and burn. Also, I use a sterile, intravenous-type solution, so it's safe to put in your eye. Lastly, I find certain strengths work best, so I put it together myself. It's not difficult. I start with a standard solution available commercially."

"Does it really work?"

"Like most other remedies, it doesn't work 100 percent of the time—especially when we don't know what we're treating. But I've found it works much better than 50 percent of the time for things like allergic conjunctivitis, corneal ulcerations, viral infections, and other superficial eye problems."

"Well—I don't know about all that, but I hope it works for me."

Mr. Thompson took the sodium ascorbate solution, with instructions to put one or two drops in his eye several times daily. Characteristically, he didn't return to the office, but phoned in three weeks later to report that his eye had healed in four days—he'd just waited before calling to make sure it stayed that way.

# Sodium Ascorbate Eyedrops Really Work

Most of the cases in this and my previous book describe diagnoses and treatments taken from the work of clinical pioneers and research scientists in nutritional biochemistry, adapted to the needs of each individual. References listed (which represent only a very small percentage of everything in my files) are to the data developed, collected, and published by these workers.

Occasionally, a treatment is my own (or at least I think it is). Sodium ascorbate eyedrops is one of these as I've not been able to find any previous references on the subject. This case was first published in *Prevention* in July of 1978. Since that time, I've had further opportunity to recommend the treatment, and have been very pleased with the continuing good results.

Sodium ascorbate eyedrops are good for more than corneal ulcerations. They're excellent against allergic conjunctivitis and superficial viral infections. They're not as useful or effective as antibiotics for most bacterial infections.

Since 1978, I've received sufficient inquiries regarding sodium ascorbate eyedrops that it became necessary to compose a form letter response, which follows:

*Dear Doctor:*

*The formula for sodium ascorbate eyedrops is simply sodium ascorbate and distilled water to a concentration of 125 milligrams per cc. I have used commercially available sodium ascorbate for intravenous use by one particular pharmaceutical company, but any commercially available sodium ascorbate will do.*

*In cases where results are encouraging, but not complete, I sometimes will increase the concentration to 250 milligrams per cc and frequently the results are better.*

*As yet, I have not run into any side effects in the last five years through the use of this, although I suppose that they are possible. If reactions do happen, I would be more suspicious of the preservative used in the intravenous preparations than the sodium ascorbate itself.*

*I have found this quite helpful in allergic conjunctivitis, viral conjunctivitis, and various problems with corneal ulceration of unknown etiology. It does not seem to be particularly helpful in bacterial conjunctivitis.*

Feedback I've gotten about this type of treatment has been very encouraging. Apparently, it's effective enough for physicians who try it to continue its use.

Since this letter was written, a preservative-free sodium ascorbate for intravenous use has become available.

Severe menstrual cramping is an often painful and frustrating experience, one that in this case sent a young woman to bed a few days each month. A combined treatment of diet plus spinal manipulation by a qualified professional completely relieved her of her discomfort.

# A CASE OF SEVERE CRAMPS 23

Karen Sharpless didn't appear ill at all. She came in energetically, smiled, and sat down on the edge of the chair. "I feel fine right now," she said. "Usually I'm very well. It's this once-a-month thing that's getting to me. Before this last medication, I was spending two days a month in bed, half due to pain, and half because of being all doped up with painkillers. The other three days of my period weren't so great, either. I was getting around, but in pain. That's no way to hold a job. At least this medicine"—she handed me a bottle—"keeps the pain down a lot. How does it work?"

I looked at the medication label. It was a drug first introduced for arthritis pain relief, but in recent years found helpful for menstrual cramping, and widely prescribed. "That is an anti-inflammatory medication. Drugs like this cut down on pain by interfering with prostaglandin metabolism. It's known that prostaglandins are involved with inflammation and pain. However, prostaglandins of various types also influence smooth-muscle contraction and relaxation. The theory is that menstrual cramps occur when there's overproduction of the type of prostaglandins that lead to muscle contraction, causing pain."

Karen looked puzzled. "You said prostaglandins? I thought only men had a prostate gland."

"You're right, only men do. Don't let the name confuse you. Prostaglandins are natural, hormonelike molecules found in nearly every tissue of the body. They're named as they are because they were first isolated from prostate gland secretions, but they're found everywhere, including in the uterus, where they definitely affect contraction and relaxation."

"So this drug works by interfering with the ones that cause contractions?"

"That's the theory."

"Whatever, it does work enough to get me out of bed. My husband said if it works, why fool around coming here—just take it. But I'd rather not take a drug if I don't have to. I was told this one doesn't have many side effects, which is good, but I still like to have a natural alternative. Is there one?"

"Frequently. In fact, most of the time. You're right, though. Compared with many drugs, this one causes fewer troubles. So, if you needed to use it while waiting for something else to work, it'd be OK."

"Waiting for something else to work?"

"Natural treatment can take two to three months to become effective."

"Oh. I was hoping for something sooner. But I guess I shouldn't be so impatient. I've had these cramps since I started my menstrual periods, except for a few months."

## Ten Years of Discomfort

"Very bad? Enough to put you to bed?"

"After my periods became regular. That was when I was 15. I'm 25 now."

"What happend for those few months?"

"I was taking birth-control pills."

"Why did you stop?"

"I didn't like the idea of taking a chemical all the time. Then they came out with those warning labels. Also, they kind of made me sick."

"How did they make you sick?"

"Kind of a nagging nausea. Not enough to make me throw up, but like seasick. Also, I retained a little fluid. The only good thing was the cramps stopped while I was taking them."

"Speaking of fluid retention, do you have that before menstrual periods now?"

"Yes, a little, but I just ignore it. It's nothing like my sister has. She puts on nearly ten pounds."

"How about depression, nervousness, acne, or headaches before periods?"

"Maybe a little nervous, but not bad. I just take [she named an over-the-counter remedy]. It helps enough."

"Do you have any other problems with your health?"

"No, except for those cramps I feel fine. I don't want to give you the impression I'm a complainer. Those pills do help. I'm just looking for an alternative if possible, and besides, it's time for my checkup. I haven't had a Pap smear for nearly two years, or a full checkup for three or four years or so. I'd like to try to prevent other problems, too."

I asked her questions about a long list of other symptoms. She reported none, except for a little low back pain on rare occasions. She'd had no surgery, took no other medications, had no allergies and no major illness in the past. Her mother and sister had both had intense menstrual cramping, which went away, as is usual, after their first pregnancies. "But I don't want to get pregnant just to get rid of cramps!" she exclaimed.

Her diet was spotty, with some good foods but also sugar and refined foods. I mentioned that we'd best discuss that later on.

# Dry, Flaky Skin

Karen's checkup was generally normal, with two minor exceptions. Her skin was dry, a little flaky. I mentioned it to her.

"Oh, yes, that's just me. I didn't think to say anything; it's just dry skin. I use cream or lotion. Is that some kind of problem?"

"Not in itself, but it might be indicative. By the way, do you get much gas or bloating in your abdomen?"

"I get a little bloating before periods, but not otherwise. I do get some gas on and off—a lot sometimes—not much otherwise."

The second finding was tenderness over two sacral vertebrae. She jumped a little when they were pressed, but tolerated pressure over all the other vertebrae with no problems.

"What does that mean?" she asked.

"Usually that the vertebrae are a little out of line. Sometimes, in the sacral (very low back) area, this can make a difference to menstrual cramping. You should check with a chiropractor or osteopath."

"That really makes a difference to menstrual cramping?"

"It could in your case. It certainly doesn't in everyone with menstrual cramps, only those with vertebral misalignment. That's a fraction, not everyone. But it looks like you're in that fraction."

"My father sees an osteopath for adjustments. He swears by him. I'll go tomorrow, if I can. My period's due, and it's usually on time. Do you think it'll help the pain?"

"Probably, but I can't tell you how much. Occasionally, it gets rid of the pain completely. But in your case, I think at best it'll be partial."

"Why's that?"

"Because of the severity. Also, it appears you might have higher than usual biochemical need for one or more nutrients."

"Which ones?"

"Essential fatty acids, and possibly other fat-soluble vitamins. Or perhaps you're not absorbing them, or there might not be enough in your diet, or maybe your system doesn't handle them right."

"What makes you think I might have trouble with fatty acids?"

"I can't be sure, but your dry skin could be an indicator. Dry, flaky skin can be caused by other things, too, but as essential fatty acids are *usually* very helpful as part of treatment for menstrual cramping, as well as dry skin, it's likely you need them."

# Linked to Prostaglandins

"Do fatty acids help relieve cramps for women who don't have dry skin?"

"Usually."

"They sound pretty important, then. Why do they work?"

"It's probably those prostaglandins again. Essential fatty acids are vitamins that are precursors of prostaglandins. That is, our bodies turn them into prostaglandins."

"How can that help? I thought you said prostaglandins cause the pain problem, and inhibiting them relieves it."

"Remember there are different types of prostaglandins. Some cause contraction, some relaxation. Theoretically, if essential fatty acids are combined with certain other vitamins and minerals, they'll turn into the right kind of prostaglandins—the kind that help with relaxation instead of causing pain."

"What do you mean, theoretically? I thought you said it usually works."

"Usually does, in clinical practice. What I mean is, there's still speculation about *why* it works. It's not actually been proven step by step on a molecular basis."

"But it usually works in practice?"

"Most of the time."

# A Regimen to Follow

"So what should I do?"

"Most important, eat foods that are good sources of essential fatty acids, as well as the other nutritional supplements I'll write down for you. Your diet was rather short of those. But the foods may not work alone. You may require higher than usual amounts for genetic reasons, or you may not be absorbing some of the nutrients. So you'll need supplemental sources, too, at least to start with, and possibly indefinitely. You'll just have to see how it goes. We should run tests for pancreatic enzymes, as they're often low in people who don't absorb fats or oils well."

"What supplements should I use?"

I wrote her a list as follows:

- Flaxseed oil (linseed oil): one gram, two times a day
- Vitamin $B_6$: 100 milligrams, three times a day
- B complex vitamins: 50-milligram formula, two times a day
- Dolomite: three tablets, three times a day
- Zinc: 50 milligrams daily
- Vitamin E: 400 international units daily
- Vitamin C: one gram, two times a day.

She looked at the list for a minute. "Gee, maybe I should just keep on taking the pain reliever. This is sure a lot of pills, comparatively. Do I really need all of them?"

"Possibly not. Sometimes people do prefer to take one drug in preference to several vitamins, as it seems easier. There are several reasons for all of this, though.

"First, the flaxseed oil, vitamin $B_6$, zinc, and vitamin C are all known to be modifiers of prostaglandin metabolism. I can't tell which ones your body doesn't have enough of or isn't absorbing or properly metabolizing. So, to start, I want you to use relatively large amounts of each. Almost undoubtedly, the quantities can be cut back later.

"Sunflower, safflower, or flaxseed oil sometimes help prostaglandin metabolism, but occasionally primrose oil is the only type effective.

"Vitamin E is good as a supplement for nearly everyone, as a detoxifier and antipollutant, but there's a more particular reason for it here. Whenever unsaturated fats are used as supplements, they should always be accompanied by some vitamin E, to prevent any possibility of long-term cell damage from the unsaturated fat.

"Dolomite has been known for years to have a beneficial

effect on menstrual cramping. Whether it affects prostaglandins, I don't know, but I've observed that this list works better with it than without it.

"The B complex is to back up the vitamin B$_6$. Whenever large amounts are used, it's a good idea to have the rest of the B vitamins available at the same time, even though the amounts don't need to be quite as large."

She nodded. "It all seems reasonable enough. Thanks for explaining it, though; I like to know as much as I can about what I'm doing. I really didn't mean it about taking a pain pill, instead. I want to do this with things that belong in my system, if I can." She got up to go. "What tests do I need?"

"Particularly, pancreatic enzyme tests and a mineral analysis, to help judge whether you're assimilating nutrients. General screening tests, also."

## Digestive Enzymes Low

She was back four months later. As she sat down, I checked her record. "It appears your pancreatic enzymes were low," I said.

"Oh, yes. I called in to your nurse a few days after the test was done. She told me to get some pancreatin. You know, I was so surprised. I haven't had any gas or bloating since, except once or twice, and my bowels are more regular. Aren't I kind of young to have low digestive enzymes?"

"No, you're not too young to have low-level digestive enzymes. That problem turns up in two- and three-year-olds sometimes. For some reason, a lot of physicians believe that pancreatic function must either be totally gone, or it must be normal. That's not so: There are all stages in between. You are in an in-between state. Your lowered enzyme secretion probably was keeping you from assimilating nutrients at optimum levels. Speaking of that, how are the cramps?"

"I didn't have any last time. That was my fourth period since I've been here. The first one was right after I was here, so I didn't figure any of the supplements would help that quickly. But the pain was noticeably less; I went to the osteopath, as you suggested, and he gave me three adjustments. I could go longer between taking the pain pills.

"My second period was about 50 percent better; the third I didn't have to take any pain pills though I hurt a little; and this last one, that I just finished, was pain free. I sure hope it keeps up. How long do I have to take these supplements?"

"The more food you eat with those nutrients in them, the fewer supplements you'll need, although I suspect you'll need a little supplementation for quite a while. For example, remember what you said about how birth-control pills affected you? Women who have that problem usually have relatively weaker vitamin $B_6$-dependent enzyme systems. Make sure to take extra $B_6$ if and when you get pregnant, as a precaution.

"Try cutting everything back after three pain-free periods. You can increase again if you need to. But don't stop the pancreatin. I'm sure you'll need it for a while to aid digestion and assimilation. It wouldn't hurt to check back with your osteopath, either, if any pain returns."

By concentrating on whole, unprocessed foods with emphasis on those containing the highest amounts of the nutrients in the supplements she needed, Karen was able to cut back to 500 milligrams of flaxseed oil, one B complex tablet, two dolomite tablets, and 20 milligrams of zinc. After a year, she remained pain free. For good health, she continued her vitamins C and E at the same levels.

## Manipulative Therapy Has Its Place

Nearly all the cases in this book concern dietary and supplemental treatments designed to have a beneficial effect on body chemistry, and thus on various symptoms. I don't want to create the impression, though, here or anywhere else, that biochemical alterations will solve all health problems. They won't. Sometimes a surgeon is needed, or a good psychologist. Acupuncture can help a lot. Many other techniques of health care are useful; even drugs and radiation have their place, although it's a lot less than presently imagined by those who use them routinely.

Manipulative therapy, performed properly by an osteopathic or chiropractic practitioner, has a major place in everyday health care. I've seen case after case of unnecessary pain and suffering, sometimes prolonged for years, that's been entirely corrected with a series of spinal manipulations. Some individuals have been evaluated by major referral centers and university hospitals on one or more occasions before finally attaining symptom relief through manipulative therapy.

While manipulative therapy isn't always helpful for relief of menstrual cramps, it's very useful in some cases.

## REFERENCES

**Prostaglandins**

Horrobin, D. F., and Campbell, A. "Sjogren's Syndrome and the Sicca Syndrome: The Role of Prostaglandin $E_1$ Deficiency. Treatment with Essential Fatty Acids and Vitamin C." *Medical Hypotheses*, vol. 6, 1980, pp. 225–232.

Horrobin, David F., and Mandu, Mehar S. "Possible Role of Prostaglandin $E_1$ in the Affective Disorders and in Alcoholism." *British Medical Journal*, June 7, 1980, pp. 1363–1366.

A 48-year-old woman and her niece who have suffered the pain of fibrocystic breast disease for years find complete relief following slightly different treatment programs. Here's a good example of two important principals of nutritional medicine. First, that each of us is biochemically a different person; and second, that there may be more than one way to treat the same condition.

# 24 TWO CASES OF CYSTIC MASTITIS

Mrs. Delores Lundgren was 48 years old, and very worried. "I really don't know what to do," she said. "One doctor said I should have my breasts removed because I might get cancer. Another one said I did have more risk, but it wasn't all that much more, so I should wait to see. My regular doctor agrees with that, and says I should just have mammography x-rays every six months to find any problem early, and then have surgery. But I've already had 10 or 12 x-rays, and I'm really worried that all those x-rays will start to cause cancer. I just don't know what to do."

"What sort of problem do you have?"

"Most of the doctors call it fibrocystic disease. One called it cystic mastitis, but I understand that's all the same thing, isn't it?"

"Yes. How long have you had it?"

"Really bad, about seven or eight years. But I've actually had trouble with my breasts all my adult life. When I was a teenager and in my twenties, I got tenderness in my breasts before menstrual periods. But a lot of women get that—that's normal, isn't it?"

"No, it's not normal or even necessary. It's just a sad commentary on the nutritional status of so many of us that this abnormality is thought of as normal. But, please excuse the editorial—go on."

"Well, for nearly 20 years, I've had to wear a bra to bed. At first, it was mostly before periods. Then, when I was in my early thirties, I started getting some small lumps. I was really scared when they first appeared—I thought I had breast cancer. But the doctor said it was just fibrocystic disease; a lot of women had that; I shouldn't worry."

## "I Had to Wear a Bra All the Time"

"When I started getting more lumps, my breasts became painful to the touch. I had to wear a bra practically full-time. I got so bad before menstrual periods that my doctor gave me water pills to drain the fluid. Those helped a little, but I didn't like using them.

"Just after I turned 40, I started getting those big, really painful lumps. I've had to have two of them removed surgically—they were both benign cysts—and any number of them drained with needles. So far it's all been noncancerous, but my breasts have been painful for years. Sometimes, I can barely stand to touch myself, and my husband can't even come near me.

"My mother has had the same problem for years, too. After her periods stopped, it seemed to subside. But, last year, she had to have one breast removed for cancer. After that is when that surgeon told me I should just have my breasts removed, to prevent cancer. That's when I decided I'd look for something else. That seemed to me to be like committing suicide to prevent dying of old age!"

I agreed that I wouldn't go along with the recommendation for surgery, either. "I know you've had lots of examinations," I said, "but since this is the first time you've been here, I'd like to examine you myself."

"I expected that. Where do I go?"

I showed Mrs. Lundgren to the examination room. When she was ready, I went to check.

Both her breasts were painful and tender. She winced whenever touched. The tissue felt hard; there were numerous lumps, large and small, making up most of the hard consistency. The left side was worse than the right, but both were quite bad.

"It's too bad you couldn't have gotten after this ten or more years ago, before it really got bad," I said. "You have a much more severe case than most. Most early cases and many moderate cases can be cleared up completely—reverted to normal. But don't be discouraged. Even in severe cases, treatment usually brings substantial relief.

"Diet is a part of the treatment. So is a certain group of vitamins and mineral supplements. Without a basically good diet, even the best supplemental program can't work as well.

"Of course, diet and oral vitamin supplements do take a while to work. There is a method that'll get things started much more quickly. I don't know exactly why it works the way it does, but I do know it works well. I learned it from a wise old doctor who's been doing clinical research with minerals for years.

"In less severe cases, diet and oral supplementation are frequently sufficient. In your case, the method recommended by Dr. John Myers, a Baltimore, Maryland, physician, should be followed."

## Two Vital Elements

"Two of the elements particularly important in the treatment of fibrocystic disease are iodine and magnesium. Sometimes they have to be given in a special way. The iodine is painted on intravaginally because it's believed to be absorbed faster there. Then the magnesium is immediately injected intravenously."

"How often does that have to be done?"

"It depends on how you do. Sometimes once, sometimes more often. We'll need to recheck to see."

"Is that all?"

"No, there is a list of supplements to be taken. I'll give you that after your first treatment."

"Do I get the treatment today?"

"Please make an appointment to return for that. I'm sorry, but we're out of time today, except that I want to mention one thing: your basic diet. That absolutely has to be changed if you're going to stay as well as you can."

"My sister's been saying that for years. No sugar, right?"

"Yes, and more than that. No refined sugar, no white bread, or refined flour products. On the positive side, as much of your diet as possible should be fresh, raw foods. Frozen foods (when necessary) instead of canned or packaged. Eliminate artificial flavors, colors, and preservatives. I know it'll take a little while to make this change, but it's important that you do it as soon as you can. Have a long talk with your sister; I'm sure she'll be quite a help.

"In medicine, there are hardly ever any guarantees, but I can tell you that this system has worked well for everyone else I've used it for."

"I'll be back," she said, and went off to make her appointment.

When Mrs. Lundgren returned she first received the treatments described above. I then asked her to get dressed and return to my office.

As she came in, she observed, "You know, when I got that injection, I felt very warm all over, particularly in my throat and pelvic area. Is that supposed to happen?"

"That's quite frequent. It's really not a problem."

"I just wanted to make sure."

"Have you started changing your diet over?"

"Yes, and my husband's grumbling, too."

## After the Treatment, Supplements

"I'm sure he'll feel better for it in the long run. Now, I'd like to go over a list of supplements I'd like you to take.

"First, vitamin $B_6$. To start I'd like you to use 100 milligrams three times daily."

"You didn't mention that before. What's that do?"

"I'll try to explain each item as we go through. The vitamin $B_6$ helps to modulate the production of a hormone called prolactin, which is frequently out of proportion in women with premenstrual problems. It also helps to counteract the effects of high levels of undetoxified estrogen usually present in fibrocystic disease.

"Secondly, B complex vitamins, a '50' formula three times daily. This is to back up the high dose of vitamin $B_6$.

"Next, iodine . . ."

"Will kelp tablets do?"

"If you want to take 500 or 600 of them a day, which I certainly can't recommend. For now, you need a prescription form of iodine."

"Please give me the prescription. That sounds more convenient."

I wrote the prescription. "The iodine appears to reduce the overproduction of estrogen. It also has its own effect on breast tissue. That's why Dr. Myers recommends putting it on directly in a relatively large quantity.

"Magnesium is next. For now, I'd like you to get 135 milligrams of chelated tablets, and take one twice a day. Later, to stay in balance with calcium, I'll probably ask you to switch to dolomite tablets. I'm not sure exactly what magnesium does, although Dr. Myers had found it an essential part of the treatment. Of course, magnesium and vitamin $B_6$ work together in many enzymatic systems.

"Two things left. Please get essential fatty acid capsules, approximately 400 milligrams each, and use three a day. These make iodine much more available in the bloodstream.

"Lastly, vitamin E, 600 international units daily. This is to help protect against problems that might potentially be caused by taking essential fatty acids over a period of time."

# Improvement Noticed

Mrs. Lundgren returned in a week. I had her go into the examination room once more.

It was evident that her treatment was working already. Her

breasts were definitely softer, no longer having the rock-hard consistency. Although there was still tenderness, it was lessened and took more pressure to bring it out. Many of the cystic lumps were slightly smaller.

Mrs. Lundgren was enthusiastic. "My breasts don't feel tense anymore. The pain is much less. I can tell something's working inside—my breasts have just felt different all week."

I recommended that she have the iodine and magnesium treatment again and that she continue the follow-up visits.

It took eight months (since Mrs. Lundgren had a relatively severe case), but her fibrocystic problem resolved almost completely.

Her breasts became soft and pain free. She no longer needed to wear a bra to bed. She had no further premenstrual problems. Of course, she had some small residual lumpy areas scattered through both breasts, probably scarring that will remain.

I asked her to continue on small quantities of all the supplements to prevent recurrences. Of course, she'd become convinced of the value of a good diet, which reduced her need for supplements.

As I'd mentioned to Mrs. Lundgren, a case as severe as hers is totally unnecessary in view of what's known about the prevention of breast problems—even though that information is far from complete. In fact, in my experience, even "a little case" of fibrocystic disease is almost always preventable.

## Cystic Mastitis Runs in the Family

"My aunt, Dolores Lundgren, was in to see you four or five years ago about a breast problem. She told me you helped it go away with a weird treatment: iodine internally, magnesium shots, and a list of several vitamins. Well, I have the problem, too, and Aunt Dolores and my mother have been after me to get in here and get something done about it before I'm really bad, like Aunt Dolores."

I thought for a moment. "Oh yes, Mrs. Lundgren. She hasn't

been in for two or three years, now. She did have a bad case of cystic mastitis. I hope she's still doing well."

"Very well. That's why I'm here. Actually Aunt Dolores told me I should go to the library to read about what to do, but some of her treatment, especially the iodine and the shots, sounded like something maybe a little dangerous, or I couldn't do it for myself, so I just decided to come in."

"That's just as well. If you've done extensive reading, it becomes clear that some vitamins are quite safe to take on your own, even in somewhat large doses. But others are safer to check first with someone who works with them all the time. Also, even though a problem appears the same, and treatment may be very similar, everyone's different, and may need variations, additions, or subtractions to a basic program. Let's go ahead and get the facts in your case."

Melanie Samuels was 26. She'd first started noticing a slight lumpiness to her breasts immediately before menstrual periods, when she was a college sophomore.

"Before then, I'd had a little breast pain and some fluid retention before periods since high school, but no big deal. The lumpy feeling bothered me a little, but it always went away right after my monthly period started, so I just ignored it. I was really busy in college, anyway, taking all my classes, working nearly full-time, too."

"Staying up late a lot at night?"

"Yes, but not much partying, mostly studying. Had to keep my grades up to land the job I have now."

"What do you do?"

"Copy editor for a small newspaper. Doesn't sound like much, but even those jobs are hard to get."

I made a note. "So what happened to your breast lump problem after college?"

"It got better for a year or two. Just a little lumpiness. I almost convinced myself it was stress and tension, like the doctor said."

"Doctor?"

"Oh, that's right, I forgot to mention it. By the end of my senior year, it got so bad I went in to see a doctor at the school health service. I was having a little pain all month, and the lumpiness wasn't going away completely after periods started, anymore.

"She examined me, said I did have a few more cysts than usual, and had me get a mammogram. It was 'normal'—just cysts, no cancer.

"She told me many women had a little cystic mastitis; it wasn't usually a problem. I just needed to be checked from time to time, maybe a mammogram, as the risk of breast cancer was slightly higher. She also explained that she'd noticed a lot of college women had aggravations due to the stress of school, like some women skip periods or get irregular. I did get better for two years after graduation, as I said, so I figured she was right."

"Let's see: That brings you to age 24, and you're 26 now. What's happened the last two years?"

"It's just like between my sophomore and senior years in college: slowly, steadily worsening, starting two years ago, and really getting bad over the past six months. The cysts are there all the time, although less after menstrual periods. I'm sore and tender the week before, with no pressure, and hurt with pressure otherwise."

"Any more stress in your life?"

"No, actually, things have settled down a lot this year. I'm into this job; it'll be a year or two before I try for a better one. Socially, things are no more or less a hassle than they've been for three or four years."

"Living on your own?"

"Yes, for now."

"Doing your own cooking?"

"If you can call it that. I do eat out a lot, since I'm single, and"—she hesitated—"sometimes skip meals or get into fast food since I'm often working late. Food just isn't the most important thing in my life."

"I can understand that. Why don't you tell me what you do eat?"

"Well, it's not the best. . . ." She hesitated again.

"That doesn't matter. Remember, we're not here to pass

judgment on your behavior, only to collect accurate facts on anything that might affect your health. I'm not going to tell you what you're eating is 'good' or 'bad,' but only my opinion of how it may affect your health. What you do with that information is your choice."

She relaxed a little. "Well, I did get rid of all the refined sugar. Mother's been telling me that for years, since I was a teenager, but I had to do my own thing, you know, like a lot of kids. I've done some reading since, though, and decided it wasn't such a good idea. I even quit putting it in my coffee. That was the hardest. I use none at all, now."

The rest of her diet included black coffee or cereal and milk or nothing for breakfast; a salad, usually lettuce, tomatoes, cucumbers with no dressing ("calories, you know") for lunch, and coffee; sometimes beef, potatoes or rice, and cooked vegetables for dinner ("when I'm out") or cheeseburger and coffee, or a taco and coffee ("when I'm working late, or going home tired").

"I've got the 'basic four groups' they taught me in school covered, mostly," she said. "Meat, vegetables, milk and dairy, cereal and starch."

"No bread?"

"Hardly any. Rice or potato when I'm out. Sometimes cereal in the morning."

"Brown rice?"

"No, white."

"Nuts or seeds?"

"No . . . calories, again."

"Salad oils?"

"No."

"Seafoods?"

"No."

"Do you take any vitamins?"

"B complex and vitamin C, 'stress' vitamins. My mother said those might be the most important."

I looked at my notes, then asked a few more questions to fill in her background health history. Once this was complete, I asked her to go to the examination room for a checkup.

"Is it necessary to do an entire checkup?" she asked.

"Not absolutely, but I prefer to do one to start for two reasons. First, even though you are concerned about a particular problem, I'm just as concerned about your overall health from the point of view of diet, vitamins, minerals, as well as other environmental influences. Secondly, sometimes things which show up in one area of the body mean something to another area, such as the problem area."

"OK. Just thought I'd ask."

Her checkup was generally OK, with only a few minor abnormalities. Her skin, particularly the lower legs, was dry and a little flaky. She had a minor case of dandruff, and much more earwax than usual. Her nails showed signs of need for zinc.

As it was right before her menstrual period, her breasts were in what she called "the worst shape." She had numerous small tender cystic areas scattered throughout, but fortunately no large cysts.

As we finished her checkup, she asked, "Aren't you going to do the iodine thing now? My aunt said you started right away with her."

"That's true, but remember everyone's case is different. In milder cases (and even though it might not feel that way, yours is milder) frequently 'oral therapy,' diet, and vitamins are enough. Also, there are some peculiarities of your diet and checkup which give clues about what might be going on."

"Really? Well, I'm just as glad not to come in once weekly for iodine treatment and shots. You can always use that later if the first treatment doesn't work, can't you?"

"Exactly."

"So what do I do?"

"To start with, please stop all coffee and anything else with caffeine in it. Chocolate, cola drinks, tea, cocoa, even pain pills with caffeine. You didn't mention it, but have you been drinking more coffee lately, say the last two years?"

"Well, yes, now that you mention it. It's kind of a 'thing' where I work, coffeepot going all the time, particularly at late hours. Typical newspaper office."

"And were you drinking lots of coffee when you were in college?"

"Not so much as a freshman; I actually didn't like the taste. But now that you mention it, I used more and more from my second year on, as my work load got heavier. Studying for tests, staying up . . . you know."

"Have you seen any of the reports on caffeine and breast cysts?"

"Vaguely. But I figured that if caffeine were the entire cause, then most of the women I know should have the same problem, and most of them don't."

"It appears that not everyone is susceptible to caffeine in the same way. Some women can use caffeine and not get cysts. Like many other things, it's individual."

"But in my case . . ."

"It would be best to eliminate the caffeine."

"OK, what else? Iodine?"

"Maybe a little. But in your case there are two other factors that may be even more important. The first is vitamin E; the second, essential fatty acids."

"Vitamin E? Most of the things I read, on the newspaper wire, you know, say that vitamin E is just a fad. Supposedly responsible nutritionists say that, too."

"That's really too bad. Those of us who work with nutrient therapy have seen the results for years. As far back as 1965 an article appeared in the *New England Journal of Medicine* reporting on vitamin E for cystic mastitis.

"However, the most convincing evidence was published by researchers from Johns Hopkins University. Using a placebo (fake pill) versus vitamin E, they showed that vitamin E produced changes in women's hormones, correcting an abnormal progesterone-to-estradiol ratio usually found in cystic mastitis. They even said this might reduce the risk of cancer.

"Another study, in Great Britain this time, showed that a specific source of essential fatty acids produced a highly significant improvement in breast pain and lumpiness.

"How this applies in your case is that your checkup shows signs of need for essential fatty acids—dry skin, dandruff, excess earwax. Your diet doesn't have many sources of essential fatty acids, such as salad oils, unroasted nuts or seeds, or whole grains. Of course these are all excellent sources of vitamin E, as the two are usually found together in nature.

"Lastly, you show signs of need for zinc, which affects the body's ability to make use of essential fatty acids."

"So I've been using too much caffeine, and not eating foods with essential fatty acids or vitamin E, and all these things can affect breast cysts?"

"Right. Also, you haven't had much iodine intake. That's mostly from seafoods, supplements like kelp, and of course iodized salt. And in your particular case, you need zinc, which wasn't important for your aunt."

I wrote out a note, which said:

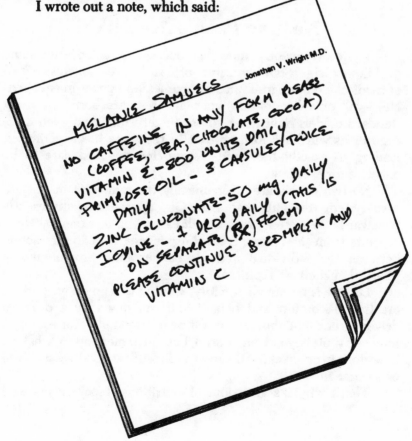

"Try this, before we go on to the type of treatment your aunt needed. It's effective but a hassle to do. Remember, if you can alter your diet to include sources of these nutrients, you may not need as much supplementation in a few months."

Six months later, Ms. Samuels had no problem at all with cystic mastitis. She reported the large majority had gone in the first 90 days, and, with diet alterations, she was beginning to cut down her list of supplements.

Her treatment was different than her aunt's, even though for the same problem, once again showing two principles of nutritional medicine: First, each of us is a biochemically different person; and second, that there may be more than one way to take care of the same condition.

## No Two People Are Alike

There's frequently more than one way to achieve the same goal in medicine. Standardization of health care—an elusive goal of medical societies, insurance companies, and government agencies—will only be possible when all of us are born in exactly standard models right down to our fingerprints. And even then, each of us will have to have exactly the same life experiences, leading to exactly the same disease, for standard care to be effective for everyone.

No two people are biochemically the same, yet our health care system treats us that way. Our approach seems exactly backwards. We often treat the disease as if it were somehow separate from the person, instead of viewing it as an interaction between the individual and his or her total environment—physical, mental, and spiritual.

Disease is not an alien entity, waiting to leap on each of us, creating discomfort and pain. Being run down by a drunken driver, struck by lightening, or hit by a stray bullet, for example, may be events beyond our control, but much more often, what we have done in our lives has the most to do with whether we stay well or become ill.

That's why it's an axiom of nutritional biochemistry and

holistic medicine in general that we work with the total individual who happens to have symptoms and diseases.

In our century, much of the disharmonic interaction between individuals and their overall environment—sometimes called disease—is due to a processed chemicalized food supply to which our bodies aren't adapted. Many of us are underinformed about proper nutrition—partly through disinterest, partly because we don't realize how important it is to health, and partly because of misinformation spread by persons who supposedly are authorities. Had either Dolores Lundgren or Melanie Samuels known about the importance of essential fatty acids, had they been aware of food sources of vitamin E, and had Melanie Samuels acted on her knowledge of the ill effects of caffeine on health, both might never have developed their disease at all.

But it's not just them. Many of the people with whom I work could have prevented their symptoms or diseases. The reason they're in my office is because their bodies are refusing to go along with a maladapted diet any longer.

Caffeine elimination has received remarkably widespread publicity as one means of treating cystic mastitis, or fibrocystic breast disease. For many women, stopping all coffee, tea, chocolate, cocoa, and caffeine-containing colas and medications is so effective that no other measures are needed.

Vitamin E has also been found useful (by itself) in treating cystic mastitis. Research done at Johns Hopkins University, by G. S. Sundaram, M.D., and associates, not only demonstrated a favorable clinical effect, but also identified a biochemical change associated with vitamin E treatment which altered the ratio of progesterone to estradiol—two important female hormones believed responsible for the development of cysts. (Research like that appears to have finally put an end to the ancient myth promoted by critics of nutritional therapy—that vitamin E is "a vitamin in search of a deficiency.")

I often hear from women who've solved their own breast problems just by taking vitamin E and eliminating caffeine.

Somehow, the involvement of iodine deficiency in cystic mastitis and possibly breast cancer has been overlooked, despite a remarkable series of experiments by Bernard Eskin, M.D., and his associates at the Medical College of Pennsylvania. Although Dr. Myers was probably the first to demonstrate that iodine is an extremely useful therapeutic agent in clinical practice, Dr. Eskin has done the methodical research necessary to nail down the importance of iodine.

Dr. Eskin's work has been done with rats; the type of scientific work he's doing generally precludes using people. Despite that, it appears that his results apply to women as well.

In one experiment, Dr. Eskin's group found that iodine deficiency caused mild atrophy of breast tissue. When sex hormones were given to iodine-deficient animals, tissue changes closely resembling those observed in fibrocystic disease in humans were observed under the microscope. Iodine-deficient diets, plus an iodine-blocking agent, also produced mild cystic changes, but giving sex hormones to this group produced cystic tissue most closely resembling human disease.

In another experiment, Dr. Eskin and his co-workers demonstrated that giving older animals an iodine-blocking agent alone also caused breast tissue changes, again similar to human fibrocystic disease.

He points out in a paper published in the *Journal of the American Medical Association* that breast cancer is generally accepted to occur four times as often in breasts with dysplasia (more severe cystic changes) than in normal breasts. He also notes that breast cancer occurs more frequently in association with hypothyroidism or underactivity of the thyroid gland. Iodine deficiency is a direct cause of that problem, too. (However, Dr. Eskin was able to prove that iodine deficiency independently leads to breast changes, and not indirectly through causing hypothyroidism.)

Population-group studies have also uncovered an association between low-iodine areas of the world and a higher incidence of breast cancer. Large areas of the United States, in fact, are included in the iodine-deficient regions of the world. Adding iodine to salt has not entirely solved that problem. In addition, many people with high blood pressure have been cutting down on dietary salt and thereby cutting back on iodine as well.

# Evidence Links Lack of Iodine
# with Breast Cancer

Despite the clear experimental evidence linking iodine and fibrocystic disease (cystic mastitis) in animals, and the strong circumstantial link between iodine, fibrocystic disease, and breast cancer in humans, the evidence cannot be interpreted to say that iodine deficiency alone causes breast cancer. It does appear sufficient, however, to support a conclusion that iodine deficiency may be a major risk factor for both fibrocystic disease and breast cancer, and that adequate iodine nutrition might substantially reduce that risk.

Dietary change and additional supplementation with vitamin E, essential fatty acids, and iodine usually is the only treatment needed to correct cystic mastitis. Only in the most severe cases, as in Mrs. Lundgren, is more than oral iodine required.

The treatment procedure I used in her case originated with Dr. Myers. Physicians interested in the topical application of iodine and the total program can write to me directly for complete details.

Regarding oral doses of iodine, I find that supplements can go as high as 200 to 300 milligrams (in the iodine form) daily, at least initially, for best results. The prescription-only calcium iodide mentioned in Mrs. Lundgren's case has been discontinued. What remains are niacinamide and iodide tablets containing 135 milligrams of iodide each as well as potassium iodide (SSKI) and other liquid iodine or iodide preparations. So far I've used only the first two. Niacinamide can help prevent potential iodine side effects, which explains its presence in the tablets. The tablets also have a completely unnecessary coating of artificial color, which fortunately rinses off easily.

High doses of iodine can affect thyroid function adversely on occasion, although I've yet to see it happen to any woman with cystic mastitis I've treated. Likewise, I've seen no iodine allergy in women with cystic mastitis, although that's possible, too. The worst has been a beginning acnelike rash in two individuals, which subsided promptly on cutting back the dose. Since higher doses require a doctor's prescription, your doctor can help you monitor for side effects.

The average amount of iodine in a kelp tablet is 0.15 milligrams (some have 0.225 milligrams). At this dose, it would require 1,333 to 2,000 kelp tablets daily to provide 200 to 300 milligrams of iodine. Obviously, for many reasons, I don't recommend taking this quantity. In milder cases of cystic mastitis, less iodine is required. I've had several women tell me that supplementing with several kelp tablets daily is noticeably helpful.

Capsules of primrose oil are available now. One British study has shown that primrose oil is independently capable of improving cystic mastitis. It's much more effective than linseed oil or any other source of essential fatty acids; I've been recommending it in the more difficult cases. However, it's also substantially more expensive, and frequently a less effective oil does as well when cystic mastitis isn't severe.

If you have breast disease in your family, the regular inclusion of iodine-containing foods (almost exclusively seafoods) in your diet would be wise. If they're not to your taste, then iodine supplemented from kelp, for example, may be advisable. Although an overdose with iodine is possible, it's extremely unusual with the small amounts found in kelp.

If you already have cystic mastitis, and caffeine elimination plus vitamin E and essential fatty acids haven't gotten rid of it, you might consider the iodine treatment received by Mrs. Lundgren. But that technique really requires the aid of a physician familiar with the treatment.

# REFERENCES

**Caffeine Consumption**
     Check, William. "Benign Breast Lumps May Regress with Change in Diet." *Journal of the American Medical Association,* March 23, 1979, p. 1221.

**Evening Primrose Oil**
     Pashby, N. L. et al. "A Clinical Trial of Evening Primrose Oil (Efamol) in Mastalgia." Paper presented at the British Surgical Research Society meeting, July, 1981.

**General Breast Cancer Information**

Fredericks, Carlton F. *Breast Cancer, A Nutritional Approach.* Grosset & Dunlap, 1977.

**Hormones and Lipoproteins**

Sundaram, G. S. et al. "Serum Hormones and Lipoproteins in Benign Breast Disease." *Cancer Research,* September, 1981, pp. 3814–3816.

**Iodine Deficiency**

Aquino, Thomas L., and Eskin, Bernard A. "Rat Breast Structure in Altered Iodine Metabolism." *Archives of Pathology,* November, 1979, pp. 280–285.

Eskin, Bernard A. et al. "Mammary Gland Dysplasia in Iodine Deficiency." *Journal of the American Medical Association,* May 22, 1967, pp. 115–119.

Krouse, Theodore B.; Eskin, Bernard A.; and Mobini, Jabal. "Age-Related Changes Resembling Fibrocystic Disease in Iodine-Blocked Rat Breasts." *Archives of Pathology and Laboratory Medicine,* November, 1979, pp. 631–634.

Schutte, Karl H., and Myers, John A. *Metabolic Aspects of Health.* Discovery Press, 1979.

Staoel, B. V. "Dietary Iodine and Risk of Breast, Endometrial and Ovarian Cancer." *Lancet,* April 24, 1976, pp. 890–891.

**Vitamin E**

Abrams, Archie A. "Use of Vitamin E in Chronic Mastitis." *New England Journal of Medicine,* May 20, 1965, pp. 1080–1081.

London, Robert S. et al. "Endocrine Parameters and a-Tocopherol Therapy of Patients with Mammary Dysplasia." *Cancer Research,* September, 1981, pp. 3811–3813.

During the past few years, a man suffering from worsening depression and insomnia undertakes an exercise and high-protein diet program. His new shape-up routine may have interfered with the absorption of the amino acid, tryptophan. The addition of tryptophan, niacinamide supplements, and reduction of vitamin $B_6$ eliminate his depression and insomnia altogether.

# 25 A CASE OF WORSENING DEPRESSION

"I've always been a little on the depressed side," Mr. Hinshaw said. "Thought it was pretty natural, considering the way the world is. When I got a little older, I found it wasn't just the world. It was me, too. Finding that out didn't make my depressions less bad, but easier to live with somehow. Trouble is, the last year or two, it's been a lot worse."

"Have you been able to identify any changes the last two years that might have something to do with it?"

"Well, yes and no. The only real change is that I've been working on getting back into shape. Otherwise, my life's been about the same, no big upsets. A few hassles with the kids, no worse than the usual teenage growing-up stuff. No problems with my wife. The job's the same as it's been for years. I did get a promotion, but the stress level's the same. Really, I think it's my body chemistry, not outside stress."

"How bad is your depression?

"Don't get me wrong, I'm not thinking of suicide or anything like that. But I don't enjoy anything much anymore, or want to do things like I used to. Haven't been golfing in months, and I don't care. For years we've been to the movies every once in a while. Now I don't feel like going at all. Some parts of my job should be a challenge; instead I just get through them. I don't think that's right; I wasn't this bad three or four years ago."

"Have you tried to do anything about it?"

"Yeah, I went to a psychiatrist a few times about a year ago. He agreed I was depressed, all right, and wanted to put me on a drug for it. He said that more and more psychiatrists are recognizing depression as being a problem in brain biochemistry, and there are some pretty effective drugs that work by changing brain chemistry."

"That's true."

Mr. Hinshaw looked surprised. "You don't recommend drugs, do you?"

"Only if nothing else works and it's a serious situation."

He relaxed a little. "That's what I thought. That's why I'm here. The psychiatrist agreed with me about stresses. In my case, he said, I just didn't have anything going on to make my usual depressive tendency so much worse now. We went into my background for a few sessions, too, but didn't find any real clues. So, he suggested the brain chemistry problem and a drug to change it."

## Insomnia Also Worse

"You have any trouble sleeping?"

"Yeah, had that a long time, too. It's also been worse the last couple years. Most of the time, I can't get to sleep; sometimes I wake up and stay awake. The psychiatrist said something about insomnia being a 'hallmark of depression.' The two get worse together."

"Very frequently. Makes very good sense biochemically."

"Before you tell me to take tryptophan, I should tell you I tried it for three months steady, and it doesn't work for me."

"What made you think I'd suggest tryptophan?"

Mr. Hinshaw smiled a little, for the first time. "I've done

some reading about brain chemistry since I left the psychiatrist's, to see what I could do on my own. I read where one of you nutrition doctors said if a person had both depression and insomnia, tryptophan might be the answer. So I tried it. Didn't work."

"How much did you take?"

"Total of two grams: one gram twice a day, with some food."

"What sort of food?"

"Either a regular meal, or milk, cheese, egg, or something like that. I read you're supposed to take your vitamins with meals."

"Tell me what you eat every day, please. Start with breakfast."

## Plenty of Protein

Mr. Hinshaw patted his stomach. "Remember I said the only real change in the last two years was working on getting into shape? I've lost . . . let's see . . . 42 pounds. Down from 210 to 168. I read up on diet and health; cut out all the sugar; went on a high-protein diet; started exercising, swimming, and running. It's ironic. I'm trying to improve my health, and physically I'm much better, but mentally worse. Can't figure it out, because I figured I had a touch of that low blood sugar thing, and a high-protein diet is supposed to help, as well as get weight off."

"It does help low blood sugar, usually. But please go over what it is you're eating."

"Breakfast: two eggs, sausage (the no-nitrate kind), half a piece of toast, no jam or butter, decaffeinated coffee. Lunch: cottage cheese salad, or steak and salad, sometimes. Dinner: beef, fish, chicken, pork, salad, spinach, asparagus, olives, cabbage. I've been staying away from bread, potatoes, and starchy vegetables."

"Do you have any snacks?"

"Yes, I was going to mention that next. I'd noticed I was getting especially tired before lunch and in the late afternoon, and I figured it was low blood sugar. So I have cheese, a hard-boiled egg, peanuts, or a protein snack of some sort between meals, and usually when I get hungry in the evening or before bedtime.

"It's worked for getting weight off. Like I said, 42 pounds. With that and all the exercise I'm getting, I should be bursting with good health. I read that exercise is supposed to be good for mental health, too."

"Usually it is. Don't stop exercising now."

"I don't know, I was thinking maybe I should. Mentally I'm much worse, not sleeping as well either, which doesn't help. Diet and exercise have been my only big changes the last two years. More and more I'm thinking it's not a coincidence. Maybe there is something to this 'fat and jolly' thing. I wasn't exactly happy-go-lucky before, but at least I was a lot less depressed."

"Are you taking any vitamins?"

"A few. Vitamin C, two grams a day; vitamin E, 400 international units; B complex, one of those '50 of everything' formulas, twice a day. A multiple mineral. That's all."

I jotted down his list. "You've really done well on weight reduction and exercise, getting into shape. You should be congratulated. But I think you may be right; your dietary pattern may be aggravating your depression and insomnia tendencies. Before we go further into it, though, I need to get more of your health background and check things physically."

I completed my usual series of questions and found nothing unusual in Mr. Hinshaw's examination. I asked him to get routine biochemical testing done.

"I know it'll take two or three weeks to get those tests back," Mr. Hinshaw said. "Isn't there something I can try in the meantime?"

## Start with Tryptophan

"Certainly. I was just about to write it down. Actually those tests are mostly for screening any health-maintenance reasons. We may find something with a bearing on depression, but I think that may be clear already."

"Really?"

"Possibly. You may be right about your diet. Before making another entire change, I want you to try taking tryptophan."

"Tryptophan? I already tried that, remember? For three months. It didn't work."

"I know. Unfortunately, the way you took it, it probably didn't have a chance to help you. The tryptophan has to get into your brain to help you sleep and to help relieve depression. In animal work, Drs. Fernstrom and Wurtman of MIT have demonstrated that a meal containing only carbohydrate causes a rise in blood and brain tryptophan. A meal that contains both protein and carbohydrate causes a rise in blood tryptophan, but no rise at all in brain tryptophan."

"But protein has tryptophan in it; carbohydrate doesn't. How does that work?"

"Dr. Fernstrom explains it by pointing out that injected or internally secreted insulin causes a marked rise in blood tryptophan, which then penetrates the brain. Eating carbohydrate, which stimulates internal insulin, will set off this chain of events."

## Effectiveness Blocked

"Doesn't eating anything, even protein, set off insulin secretion?"

"Yes, but not as rapidly or as much as carbohydrate does. However, that isn't the whole story. Dr. Fernstrom explains that tryptophan is carried into the brain by the same system that transports certain other amino acids—tyrosine, phenylalanine, isoleucine, leucine, and valine. In proteins, tryptophan is always in the smaller quantity; any of those other amino acids is present in greater quantity, and as a group in much greater quantity. So when protein is eaten, tryptophan does rise in the blood, but those other amino acids rise, too."

"So since they all get into the brain in the same way, the other amino acids block out the tryptophan?"

"That's Dr. Fernstrom's explanation. He supported it further by using protein without those amino acids but with tryptophan. Then both blood and brain tryptophan levels rose."

"So you think that when I took the tryptophan with protein, I blocked its effectiveness?"

"That's my theory."

"Has this been proven in humans?"

"Not in the same way. Unfortunately, the experimental animals had to be killed to test the brain levels of amino acids."

"I see."

"However, in clinical practice, I've observed that tryptophan does work better when taken with carbohydrate, and no protein for one-and-a-half hours before or after."

"Why do you think it'll work for me?"

"You said you've had some depression and insomnia most of your life, worsened when you started on the high-protein diet. That could mean you normally have more problems with tryptophan metabolism than most people. High protein could aggravate your usual problem by blocking tryptophan from getting into your brain even more than usual.

"In human experiments, tryptophan has been found to decrease the length of time it takes to get to sleep and the number of awake periods. Unlike sleeping pills, it doesn't distort normal sleep physiology, short- or long-term, even after withdrawal.

"Tryptophan has been widely used for depression. One test showed it to be just as effective as a commonly prescribed antidepressant."

## On the Right Track

"So you were on the right track when you read that tryptophan helps depression and insomnia. Because of the way you took it, you might not have given it an adequate chance. Please try two grams of tryptophan twice daily, with no protein for at least one-and-a-half hours before or after. Also, please take 500 milligrams of niacinamide twice a day, and temporarily eliminate any vitamin $B_6$."

"Eliminate $B_6$? Why? I've been taking extra B complex on purpose."

"Theoretically, extra vitamin $B_6$ can lead to such rapid

breakdown of tryptophan before it gets to the brain that there might not be enough left to do any good."

"And the niacinamide?"

"For the opposite reason. An animal experiment shows that niacinamide raises brain tryptophan levels by slowing tryptophan breakdown."

"So B$_6$ speeds up tryptophan breakdown, and niacinamide slows it? Sort of like an accelerator and a brake?"

"Sort of. This research is all in its early stages, and many further wrinkles may be found. Since it's relatively safe, and much safer than taking drugs, please try it."

"Beats being depressed, too. What about my diet?"

"Perhaps you should start to deemphasize the heavy protein, but let's talk about that when your tests are back."

"OK, but it sounds like high-protein diets may not be as good as they're said to be, doesn't it?"

"Not at all. For some people, they're just the thing to do. Even if we're correct in our case, all we've done is found that high protein isn't so good for you, personally. Remember, biochemically everyone's different. No one program is correct for everyone."

Mr. Hinshaw found that with tryptophan, niacinamide, and not more than 10 milligrams of B$_6$ daily, his depression and insomnia were gone. He subsequently switched to a high-complex-carbohydrate diet, watching his calories much more carefully to control weight, as well as continuing to exercise. After that diet change, he was able to reduce his tryptophan to one gram twice daily, taken with niacinamide (500 milligrams), and no protein for 90 minutes before or after.

# Brain Chemistry Depends on Good Nutrition

In 1974, Richard J. Wurtman, M.D., and John D. Fernstrom, Ph.D., of MIT wrote: "One wonders why something as important as brain neurotransmitter levels should be subject to the vagaries of what one chooses to eat for breakfast." In the relatively few years since 1974, the accumulated evidence is much stronger. It appears that brain chemistry, like the chemistry of the rest of our bodies, is dependent not only on what we eat for breakfast, but also lunch, dinner, and all the snacks in between.

As reported in 1982 by the prestigious journal *Science:* "Research on whether food and nutrients affect human behavior is gaining serious attention these days. [On November 9, 1982,] the Center for Brain Sciences and Metabolism at the Massachusetts Institute of Technology (MIT) held a meeting to bring together reputable investigators who are studying this subject. 'To my knowledge, this is the first meeting on this subject that was not held by and for the true believers,' says Richard Wurtman of MIT, who was the conference organizer."

One wonders why something as important as the effects of diet on brain and body chemistry has been overlooked and even denied by "reputable investigators" for so long. Until very recently, physicians who dared to suggest in public or in print that diet might affect behavior were condemned as quacks and charlatans. A phenomenon appears to be repeating itself: Now that "reputable investigators" are belatedly awakened to the facts, no apologies will be offered to those who've been condemned in the past for reporting them. Pioneers in the investigation (and treatment) of the effects of diet on behavior will be ignored, as "reputable investigators" claim credit for "responsible scientific investigation" of the field.

Research and publication on the effects of diet on behavior have been available since the 1920s, and before. The best compilation and listing of hundreds of such references is available in the book *Diet, Crime, and Delinquency* by Alexander Schauss, director of the Institute for Biosocial Research, Tacoma, Washington. This volume is a goldmine of information, most of it developed by researchers and clinicians who would be very surprised to find themselves called "true believers."

Research papers reported by those "reputable investigators" at the MIT conference included work on tryptophan and sleep, carbohydrate and mental performance, carbohydrate and hyperactivity, tryptophan and pain, and tyrosine and depression. Another surprised investigator was Bonnie Spring, M.D., of Harvard University, who found that changes in mental performance could be found after a single meal. "The fact that we could detect an effect after one meal is surprising," she said.

Commenting on the conference, Dr. Wurtman is reported to have said: "There is no longer any real controversy over whether nutrients can affect behavior."

Well, better late than never. Now, if we can get "reputable investigators" (certified, of course, as "nontrue believers") to admit that nutrients affect the rest of body chemistry as well, those of us in nutritional biochemistry can use less time, energy, and money on defending ourselves—and all of us, reputable and irreputable together, can get on with the job of effective health care.

One further brief note: The question of whether vitamin $B_6$ should or should not be used with tryptophan is still unsettled, and may not be decided for a long time. I've worked with some individuals who must use vitamin $B_6$ with tryptophan to achieve the desired effect, and an equal number who must keep $B_6$ intake low or tryptophan doesn't help. The most practical approach at present is to try it both ways and decide for oneself which is best.


# REFERENCES

**Diet**

Fernstrom, John D. "Effects of the Diet on Brain Neurotransmitters." *Metabolism*, February, 1977, pp. 207–223.

Kolata, Gina. "Food Affects Human Behavior." *Science*, December 17, 1982, pp. 1209–1210.

Schauss, Alexander. *Diet, Crime, and Delinquency*. Parker House, 1980.

Wurtman, Richard J., and Fernstrom, John D. "Effects of the Diet on Brain Neurotransmitters." *Nutrition Reviews*, July, 1974, pp. 193–200.

**Food Chemistry**
Meyer, Lillian Hoagland. "Proteins in Foods." In *Food Chemistry*. Reinhold Publishing, 1960, p. 114.

**Nutrition**
Guthrie, Helen Andrews. *Introductory Nutrition*. C. V. Mosby, 1979.

**Tryptophan**
Badawy, A. A.-B., and Evans, M. "Tryptophan Plus a Pyrrolase Inhibitor for Depression." *Lancet*, November 1, 1975, p. 869.

Chouinard, Guy et al. "Tryptophan-Nicotinamide Combination in the Treatment of Newly Admitted Depressed Patients." *Communications in Psychopharmacology*, vol. 2, no. 4, 1978, pp. 311–317.

Hartmann, Ernest. "L-Tryptophan: A Rational Hypnotic with Clinical Potential." *American Journal of Psychiatry*, April, 1977, pp. 366–370.

Kline, N. S., and Shah, B. K. "Comparable Therapeutic Efficacy of Tryptophan and Imipramine: Average Therapeutic Ratings Versus 'True' Equivalence. An Important Difference." *Current Therapeutic Research*, July, 1973, pp. 484–487.

Winston, Frank. "Treatment of Unipolar Depression." *Lancet*, November 1, 1975, pp. 868–869.

---

For a note on the "tryptophan scare" of 1989–1990, see Appendix D.

**A 47-year-old man with a family history of diabetic complications discovered that he has developed a mild case of diabetes. To avoid the complications that afflicted the rest of his family, he modifies his diet to a more natural one and takes a variety of supplements. His signs of diabetes disappear.**

# 26  A CASE OF DIABETIC COMPLICATIONS

"I'm determined to find a way to prevent the rest of this 'family curse.' Maybe I can't, but now that I know I'm not immune, I'm really going to fight it."

About a year before, Sam Jenkins was "just not feeling right, nothing specific, just not good." Knowing his family history, he'd visited his doctor and requested a glucose tolerance test. "I got it done after a little argument, and sure enough, I have a mild case of diabetes.

"I really wasn't surprised. My father has diabetes, had two cataract surgeries. His mother had diabetes, and went blind with eye hemorrhages as well as cataracts. Both of my father's brothers have diabetes, and had heart attacks in their fifties. One died. On the other side of the family, I have an aunt with diabetes and high blood pressure, both grandparents had 'old-age' diabetes, a great uncle had cataracts, and one cousin my age has had a heart attack already. Not exactly good odds, I know."

I agreed, and wrote his family history as fast as I could, to keep up. When done, I asked, "What about your mother? You didn't mention her. Is she in good health?"

"Far as we can tell. She says she won't go to a doctor unless she's dying, but she's remarkable for 70. Farsighted as ever, up working early, always busy. After I left home, she went into this health-food thing in a big way; she's been at it for 30 years now. She couldn't talk Dad or the rest of the family into it, but now they're thinking maybe she was on to something after all."

I glanced at Mr. Jenkins's records; he was 47.

"You're a bit young for maturity-onset diabetes," I said. "Sometimes that indicates a greater chance of complications: There are more years left for them to develop. What have you done about laboratory tests so far?"

"As soon as I found out about the diabetes, I had a complete checkup.

"My blood pressure was high-normal, and I did a treadmill electrocardiogram. I was OK, which I was glad to hear with all those heart attacks in the family.

"I had my cholesterol level checked and it was normal, but the triglycerides were on the high side. I asked by doctor what to do about all this. He said I wasn't bad enough to need insulin or any diabetes pills; they could always be used later if necessary.

"I asked about preventing complications like the rest of my family's had—heart attacks, cataracts, high blood pressure, and so on—with diet and maybe vitamins. He said to cut down on sugar and salt, get more exercise, and that's all I could do."

"That's a start, anyway."

"Actually, I've never been much of a sugar or salt eater. I listened to Mother a little over the years. But I haven't spent any time working positively on my health. I kept putting it off, you know, hoping it wouldn't happen to me.

"I'm a general contractor, nothing big, but I've worked hard 10, 12, and more hours a day, six days a week until lately to build the business, and figured I didn't have time to work on much else. But last year I decided I'd best work on my health some, or I might not be able to enjoy what I've worked for.

"This last year, I've worked on getting my diet in order. It's a gradual process; can't do something like that overnight. I talked with Mother, and I did a lot of reading.

"I knew that most doctors don't know much about nutrition, but I was really surprised at all the varying opinions among all the experts. Seems like if you read five books you get six different answers."

## Medicine Is Not an Exact Science

"That's true. Medicine isn't an exact science, and neither is nutrition. People are all different; circumstances change. There are too many variables. I don't mean to say scientific methods aren't relevant in medicine; of course they are. But as an individual, you have to decide what applies to you, what works in your particular circumstances."

"That's why I'm here. I hope I've got the diet partly under control, but I'm not sure. I'm not taking vitamins yet, even though Mother's been telling me to. I've done some reading, but figured I wanted to talk to a few experts first before putting together a list. My main concern is my vision, and after that heart attacks and strokes. I know that those are all diabetic complications. I want to prevent them all. Are there any vitamins I can take to stop cataracts?"

"Probably, but before we get to that, I want to go back to diabetes prevention itself. If you can prevent the diabetes, you can prevent a lot of complications, can't you?"

Mr. Jenkins looked puzzled. "But I've already got diabetes. How can I prevent what I've got?"

"Diabetes is like many other health problems. Doctors agree that if your blood sugar is too high; if you have various complications such as retinal hemorrhage, kidney failure, peripheral vascular disease, and so on, that these are all indicative of diabetes, signs of diabetes, but what diabetes is itself isn't known exactly."

"I thought diabetes meant you didn't have enough insulin, so your blood sugar just goes up."

"That seems to be a large part of what's called juvenile or

insulin-dependent diabetes, where the cells in the pancreas don't produce enough insulin, and it has to be injected. Particularly in children, those cells appear to die. Even then, though, there's the question of what makes them die. But did you know that doctors such as James Anderson at the University of Kentucky or John Douglass in southern California have been able to help diabetics who were taking insulin discontinue it with appropriate diet?"

"I think I read about that. Isn't that called a stone-age diet?"

## Getting Back to Prehistoric Basics

"That's one of the terms that has been used. Dr. Anderson calls his approach a high-complex-carbohydrate diet. Another California researcher, Nathan Pritikin, has achieved the same results in a similar fashion. What all of these approaches have in common is the elimination of as much as possible of all of the changes that have occurred in our diets due to food processing and refining. Getting out sugar is a big part, but returning as much as possible to what our prehistoric ancestors ate is a basic principle."

"How does that apply to me? Today, I'm not going to take up cave living; I build houses. I have to go to the grocery store. I can't shoot a wild boar for lunch."

"I know. Perhaps I'm being too theoretical, but I'm trying to make the point that you probably don't have a disease to be cured, but a maladaptation to be prevented. Human bodies in general are not adapted to the sorts of foods that are generally available since food processing and refining got started.

"To prevent diabetes, I'd like you not to think that you've got a disease that has to be cured or controlled, but instead that you've got a body to keep healthy with foods suited to it. When you go to the store or eat out, ask yourself if you could have eaten the food 100,000 years ago. That way you can quit worrying about various expert theories, and make your own decisions easily. I know that isn't always possible, depending on where you are, and that food supplies just don't have the nutrients in them that they might have had years ago. That's where food supplements, vitamins, and minerals comes in. But you can eat that way at home.

"Also, don't forget exercise. Prehistoric man got lots more than we do. Modern studies have shown that exercise improves blood sugar tests."

"So you're saying I can throw out the books, and just make like a caveman when I eat? If a food could have been eaten by a caveman, OK, and if not, forget it. Is that it?"

"As much as possible. As you said—five books, six different opinions. It's my opinion that much so-called diabetes isn't disease at all, but maladaptation, like trying to grow corn in Antarctica. There's nothing the matter with the corn; the environment isn't right. Likewise, there's probably nothing wrong with you. It's your nutritional environment. Remember, I'm not saying all diabetes is that way. But I'm sure a large part is, especially maturity-onset diabetes."

# Role of Bioflavonoids

"Now about your specific concerns. Let's start with cataracts. There's very firm scientific evidence from experimentation that a basic problem in diabetic cataracts is overactivity of an enzyme called aldose reductase, present in the lens of the eye. That enzyme links simple sugars from the blood into more complex molecules in the lens. In diabetes, too many of these complex molecules are made, leading to cataracts. Researchers have found that substances called bioflavonoids can inhibit aldose reductase, probably preventing cataracts."

"Probably? Not for sure?"

"For sure inhibiting aldose reductase, which should stop cataracts. Remember, something can only be called sure after carefully controlled work in humans. That would be difficult to do—would you volunteer for an experiment knowing you might get a cataract that might well have been prevented?"

"I guess not."

"There are ways around that, but they've not been done yet. However, the experimental work is good enough that Dr. Mark Altschule, recommends taking bioflavonoids for cataract prevention."

"Any hazards?"

"None that anyone knows. Bioflavonoids are natural to the body, don't appear harmful. No overdose has ever been reported."

"How much?"

"A gram a day should be enough. Bioflavonoids are probably helpful in preventing hemorrhage from small blood vessels. They've been known for years to prevent capillary fragility."

"What about heart attacks, strokes, and retinal hemorrhage?"

"Studies have shown that diets high in natural fiber, roughage—more vegetarian in character—tend to be associated with lower incidence of heart attack and stroke."

"Didn't cavemen and prehistoric man eat a lot of meat?"

"It's thought that some did, but much of a prehistoric diet was roots, vegetables, berries, seeds. Also don't forget that most modern meat supplies are very different from wild game. The animals are largely grain fed, fatty, and bred so that they're very different from their wild ancestors. Some vegetable foods are selectively bred and altered, too, but not as greatly."

## Platelets Are Important to Blood Clotting

"Aside from general theory, scientific research has provided further particular details about possible causes of diabetic complications. It's been found that in diabetics, blood elements called platelets tend to clump together too quickly."

"Doesn't that lead to clotting?"

"Yes. Platelets are part of the natural clotting system. In diabetes, since the platelets clump too quickly, it's thought that they contribute to the various vascular complications such as bleeding into the retina, thrombosis in coronary arteries, and blockage of small blood vessels elsewhere."

"My cousin who had the heart attack is taking a drug that's

supposed to help prevent heart attacks by interfering with his platelets. Does that work?"

"A controlled study has shown that it does. But there are at least eight natural substances I know of that have also been shown to inhibit platelet clumping. Two have been studied specifically in diabetes; all the others have been studied with human platelets. All slow platelet clumping or aggregation."

"What are those?"

"Vitamins C, E, $B_6$, linoleic acid, onions, garlic, bromelain, and mackerel."

"Mackerel? The fish?"

"Yes. Actually, the researchers who found that a diet high in mackerel inhibited platelet aggregation attributed its effect to an essential fatty acid found in it called eicosapentaenoic acid."

"No wonder you said mackerel."

"But the point is, why use a drug if a vitamin, an onion, or even mackerel will work instead?"

"Have those been studied in humans like the drug has?"

"No. Unfortunately, broad-scale studies with nutrients still aren't being done as they are with drugs."

"So how do I know if it'll work on me, or if I even have a platelet problem?"

"Simple. We can just measure your own platelet aggregation time. If it's normal, no problem. If your platelets clump too quickly, you can add one or more of the items above and see what happens to your platelet aggregation time."

"I haven't had that checked. I haven't eaten, just in case I need any tests."

"Good. I usually have that test done after fasting, as elevated blood fats could affect platelet function."

"Any other tests I should have done?"

"You've had most of the important ones: cholesterol, triglycerides, treadmill EKG. By the way, did you have the HDL-cholesterol done?"

"Yes, I'd forgotten. It was normal, too."

"How about a hemoglobin Alc?"

"What's that for?"

"It's a way to monitor diabetes in addition to the blood sugar test. It reflects elevations of the blood sugar over a period of time."

"Sort of a summary?"

"Yes. The blood sugar measures more short-term control."

"Anything else?"

"A mineral analysis. There are several minerals that are related to blood sugar and diabetes control. It's wise to find out which ones you might need. By the way, you did have the multiphasic screening type of blood testing for kidney, liver, and other organ function, as well as a urinalysis?"

"Yes. That was all normal."

We talked a little further about diabetes prevention and control. After Mr. Jenkins's checkup, which was normal, he left to have his tests done.

His platelet aggregation time was, indeed, too fast. In order to see what would help to normalize it, he chose to add vitamin C (three grams daily) and vitamin E (800 international units daily) to his diet. After a month, platelet aggregation was improved but not yet normalized. He then added B vitamins, including 50 milligrams of vitamin $B_6$, and two tablespoons of cod-liver oil daily. Following this, his platelet aggregation time became normal.

His mineral analysis showed, as is frequent in diabetes, deficiencies in chromium, manganese, and zinc. I recommended he use supplements, as well as food sources of these minerals, and taper off the supplements as the levels normalized.

In view of his family history of cataracts as well as diabetes, he decided to continue to use one gram of bioflavonoids daily as a preventive measure.

Obviously, Mr. Jenkins could not eat a 100 percent caveman-type diet. As he pointed out, it just isn't available today. However, he's as strict as he can be, and his tests no longer show any signs of diabetes. He intends to continue monitoring his biochemical tests from time to time, to help him prevent as many problems as possible.

Whether he's "cured" diabetes, or simply cleared up a maladaptation, is of course debatable. But as you can see, I think it's the latter.

# Chromium Helps Normalize Blood Sugar

It's difficult to overemphasize the importance of returning as much as possible to the diet best suited to our bodies. That's what I call the "new traditional" diet. As Mr. Jenkins pointed out, we can't shoot wild boar for lunch, or duplicate the human diet of 100,000 years ago. But if all of us could come as close as possible by eating whole fruits, vegetables, nuts, and seeds, for example, a great deal of disease could be prevented. Besides diabetes, many other diseases of civilization, noted in "The Case for a 'New Traditional' Diet," may not be diseases at all—but maladaptation to our present nutritional environment.

Unlike our ancestors, we eat processed foods. Food refining literally "processes away" the majority of many nutrients found in whole foods. Although all the nutrients lost are important to health, research has shown that chromium, a mineral present in only trace quantities even before food processing, may be of major importance in preventing maturity-onset diabetes; it is significantly lost during the refining process. Research pioneered by Walter Mertz, M.D., director of the USDA's Human Nutrition Laboratory in Beltsville, Maryland, has shown that chromium is a key component of a nutrient complex called the glucose tolerance factor, which can improve the body's sensitivity to insulin.

In Type II or maturity-onset diabetes (noninsulin-dependent diabetes mellitus) there's usually plenty of insulin being secreted, a situation unlike Type I or juvenile diabetes, where there's not enough insulin. In many Type II diabetics, there's actually too much insulin. Insulin is a message carrier that orders the blood sugar to go down. In juvenile diabetes, there isn't any message, so the blood sugar rises. In maturity-onset diabetes, there are often too many messages, but no one's receiving them. Again, blood sugar rises.

Starting with experimental animals, Dr. Mertz and others

demonstrated that supplementation with brewer's yeast, a rich source of chromium containing the glucose tolerance factor, could significantly improve blood sugar metabolism. Other evidence developed since their work shows that it does so by improving sensitivity to insulin.

Work with noninsulin-dependent diabetics has confirmed these findings. Both brewer's yeast (nine grams daily) and trivalent chromium (150 to 1,000 micrograms daily) have been shown to significantly improve blood sugar metabolism when taken for several weeks to months. As a side benefit (a term that occurs much more frequently than side effect in nutritional biochemistry), it's also been found that brewer's yeast and chromium supplementation lower elevated total cholesterol and total lipids, and significantly raise the levels of HDL cholesterol—the beneficial or protective fraction of cholesterol.

As valuable as supplemental chromium appears to be in the treatment of maturity-onset diabetes, it's obvious it might not be needed at all as a supplement if it weren't refined out of our diets in the first place. It's rather a sick joke (pun intended) that we pay to have chromium removed from our diets, then pay again for it to be put into tablets to correct the problem caused by taking it out originally. It would be cheaper (not to mention healthier) to not abuse our bodies from the beginning.

Exactly the same thing can be said for all the other nutrients processed away by civilized methods of food refining. If you want to stay as healthy as possible, and haven't done it yet, now is the best time to put yourself on a whole-food "new traditional" diet.

# REFERENCES

**Bioflavonoids**
Altschule, Mark D. *Nutritional Factors in General Medicine.* Charles C Thomas, 1978.

**Chromium**
Freiberg, M. et al. "Effects of Brewer's Yeast on Glucose Tolerance." *Diabetes*, vol. 24, 1975, p. 433.

Glinsmann, Walter H., and Mertz, Walter. "Effect of Trivalent Chromium on Glucose Tolerance." *Metabolism*, June, 1966, pp. 510–520.

Levine, Robert A.; Streeten, David H. P.; and Doisy, Richard J. "Effects of Oral Chromium Supplementation on the Glucose Tolerance of Elderly Human Subjects." *Metabolism*, February, 1968, pp. 114–125.

Mertz, Walter. "Chromium—An Overview." In Shapcott, D., and Hubert, J., eds. *Chromium in Nutrition and Metabolism.* Elsevier/North Holland Biomedical Press, 1979.

Offenbacher, Esther G., and Pi-Sunyer, F. Xavier. "Beneficial Effect of Chromium-rich Yeast on Glucose Tolerance and Blood Lipids in Elderly Subjects." *Diabetes*, November, 1980, pp. 919–925.

Riales, Rebecca, and Albrink, Margaret, J. "Effect of Chromium Chloride Supplementation on Glucose Tolerance and Serum Lipids Including High-Density Lipoprotein of Adult Men." *American Journal of Clinical Nutrition*, December, 1981, pp. 2670–2678.

## Diabetic Cataracts
Varma, S. D.; Mizuno, A.; and Kinoshita, J. H. "Diabetic Cataracts and Flavonoids." *Science*, January 14, 1977, pp. 205–206.

## Diet
Douglass, John M. "Raw Diet and Insulin Requirements." Letter to *Annals of Internal Medicine*, January, 1975, pp. 61–62.

Kantor, Yoram et al. "Improved Glucose Tolerance and Insulin Response in Obese and Diabetic Patients on a Fiber-Enriched Diet." *Israel Journal of Medical Sciences*, January, 1980, pp. 1–6.

Kiehm, Tae G.; Anderson, James W.; and Ward, Kyleen. "Beneficial Effects of a High Carbohydrate, High Fiber Diet on Hyperglycemic Diabetic Men." *American Journal of Clinical Nutrition*, August, 1976, pp. 895–899.

Pritikin, Nathan. *The Pritikin Program for Diet & Exercise.* Grosset & Dunlap, 1979.

### General Diabetes Information

"Blood Test May Start New Era in Diabetes Therapy Evaluation." *Journal of the American Medical Association,* February 28, 1977, pp. 347–348, 850, 856.

"Diabetes Research Is Greatly Expanding." *Journal of the American Medical Association,* August 8, 1980, pp. 549–550.

Krupp, Marcus A., and Chatton, Milton J. *Current Medical Diagnosis & Treatment, 1978.* Lange Medical Publications, 1978.

Lewis, Dale and Camp, Bill, eds. *The Self-Care Newsletter for Diabetics.* Sunbeam Books, 1983.

### Platelet Aggregation

Anturane Reinfarction Trial Research Group. "Sulfinpyrazone in the Prevention of Cardiac Death After Myocardial Infarction." *New England Journal of Medicine,* February 9, 1978, pp. 289–295.

Bordia, Arun. "Effect of Garlic on Human Platelet Aggregation *In Vitro.*" *Atherosclerosis,* August, 1978, pp. 355–360.

Creter, Draga; Pavlotzky, Fira; and Savir, Hanna. "Effect of Vitamin E on Platelet Aggregation in Diabetic Retinopathy." *Acta Haematologica,* vol. 62, 1979, pp. 74–77.

Fleischman, Alan I. et al. "Beneficial Effect of Increased Dietary Linoleate Upon *In Vivo* Platelet Function in Man." *Journal of Nutrition,* October, 1975, pp. 1286–1290.

Heinicke, R. M.; van der Wal, Linda; and Yokoyama, M. "Effect of Bromelain (Ananase) on Human Platelet Aggregation." *Experientia,* July, 1972, pp. 844–845.

Jakubowski, J. A., and Ardlie, N. G. "Modification of Human Platelet Function by a Diet Enriched in Saturated or Polyunsaturated Fat." *Atherosclerosis,* November, 1978, pp. 335–344.

Kwaan, H. C. et al. "Increased Platelet Aggregation in

Diabetes Mellitus." *Journal of Laboratory and Clinical Medicine,* August, 1972, pp. 236–246.

"Low Vitamin C Tied to Platelet Clumping Seen in Diabetics." *Family Practice News,* September 1, 1978, p. 31.

Makheja, Amar N.; Vanderhoeck, Jack Y.; and Bailey, J. Martyn. "Inhibition of Platelet Aggregation and Thromboxane Synthesis by Onion and Garlic." *Lancet,* April 7, 1979, p. 781.

Siess, W. et al. "Platelet-Membrane Fatty Acids, Platelet Aggregation, and Thromboxane Formation During a Mackerel Diet." *Lancet,* March 1, 1980, pp. 441–444.

Steiner, Manfred, and Anastasi, John. "Vitamin E: An Inhibitor of the Platelet Release Reaction." *Journal of Clinical Investigation,* March, 1976, pp. 732–737.

Subbarao, Kuchibhotla; Kuchibhotla, Jaya; and Green, David. "Pyridoxine-Induced Inhibition of Platelet Aggregation and the Release Reaction." Abstract of the 50th Scientific Sessions for Nurses, American Society for the Study of Arteriosclerosis, part 2, vol. 56, no. 4; American Heart Association Monograph no. 57, pp. iii–77.

A 67-year-old man suffering for the past several years from diabetes develops a leg ulcer which refuses to heal. A new high-fiber diet, exercise, and supplement program heal the ulcer and eliminate the need for his anti-diabetes prescription.

# A CASE OF DIABETIC LEG ULCER

# 27

The base of the ulcer crater glistened wet and pink, with a trace of yellow matter, surrounded by a ragged, pale edge of skin. Irregularly shaped, it measured approximately 1¼ inches by ¾ inch at its widest points. Located just above the left ankle, it lay along the inside of the leg, within 2 inches of the prominence of bone.

All around the ulcer the skin appeared unhealthy, thin, shiny, alternately reddened and pale white, with bluish mottling here and there. Almost all the hair was gone, leaving but a wisp or two.

"Looks terrible, doesn't it?" asked Mr. Lehrman. "And look at my other leg and my feet. The skin looks like it could go anytime. Rebecca says I should do something soon or I'll end up an amputee like her grandfather. He had diabetes, too."

"Actually, it looks like you've been taking care of the ulcer quite well. Clean, not infected . . ."

"I don't want to take care of the ulcer. It's getting rid of it I'd like. But thank you, I'm doing the best I can. Rebecca's done the most. We change the dressings several times a day. I see the doctor twice a month. He gives me things to put on. He suggested surgery; I said I'd rather wait. If this won't heal, why should surgery heal? He says sometimes it does. But I decided to come here first." As he talked, we replaced the ulcer dressing with layers of fresh gauze, taped over an application of vitamin E.

Mr. Saul Lehrman was 67. His diabetes had been discovered at age 60, at a routine checkup.

"Nothing specific, working too hard, not feeling good at the time. Can't say I was surprised. My mother developed diabetes in her sixties . . . never seemed to bother her. Maybe that's why I didn't take it seriously. I did cut out the sugar, mostly. Rebecca kept telling me I should be really strict, eat right, get some exercise, take my vitamins, or this would catch up with me. She was right."

Mr. Lehrman's diabetes had gradually become worse. Two years after his initial diagnosis, he started taking "pills for diabetes" on prescription. For a while they appeared to help. But then his blood sugar readings rose once more, and his doctor recommended insulin.

"When my blood sugar started to go up again I was on the maximum number of antidiabetes pills. I'd been putting a lot of stress on myself, working long hours. I turned the whole business over to my son, took a long vacation, started in on regular exercise. Apparently that helped; my blood sugar stabilized and my doctor stopped talking insulin so much. I cut out absolutely all the sugar, too."

However, 18 months later, the skin on the inside of his left lower leg had begun to break down and ulcerate. "My doctor was surprised," Mr. Lehrman observed. "He said ulcers don't usually happen unless the diabetes is bad enough to require insulin. Then he took another look at my blood sugar readings the few months before, and said stabilized yes, but good control, no. Years before, I had injured my leg badly in exactly that place. He agreed that's maybe why the ulcer started there."

# Applied Vitamin E

"The ulcer was quite small at first, but soon grew larger. Rebecca really started looking: She got books, went to the library, started reading health magazines. She found out about putting vitamin E on it, which helped more than anything. It looked better, stopped getting larger. Unfortunately, it didn't get much smaller. It's been this size for nearly a year."

"I've been putting on the E, swallowing 400 international units of vitamin E, taking 1,000 milligrams of vitamin C, some B complex, not eating sugar, and still this ulcer. That's why I'm here."

"Any zinc?"

"Oh, yes, zinc, 30 milligrams daily. We read about that, too. But it hasn't helped in the six months I've been taking it. Does it usually take longer?"

"Zinc usually starts to work in a month to six weeks, if it's going to help."

"Must be the wrong thing. I haven't gotten those white spots on my nails that go with zinc deficiency." Mr. Lehrman looked at me over his glasses. "I've been doing some reading, you see."

"White spots usually indicate zinc is needed," I said, "but they're not found every time. I've frequently seen zinc insufficiency in people with no spots on the nails."

"So if they're present, it means zinc is needed. But if they're not there, you still can't be sure?"

"Right."

# Prostate Problems

"Rebecca was suspicious of that. I'll tell her she was right again. I've been having prostate gland symptoms lately—difficulty getting urination started, getting up at night a lot more often. She told me she'd read zinc was supposed to help that, also."

"Zinc and essential fatty acids, usually." I made a note. "Have you been having any trouble with your digestion?"

"Not a bit. Why do you ask?"

"No problem with gas, bloating in the abdomen, constipation, diarrhea?"

"No."

"Bowels move every day?"

"Yes."

"Food doesn't sit in your stomach like it's not digesting?"

"No."

I made several further notes. "No particular symptoms, but we should check on your digestion anyway. Your wife's right: Zinc is indicated to help diabetic leg ulcers, as well as prostate problems. When there are two seemingly unrelated symptoms that usually are helped by the same nutrient, it makes it even more likely that the nutrient's needed. So if it doesn't work for you as for most people, it's wisest to make sure it's being absorbed before giving up."

"So what do I do?"

"I'd like you to get a mineral analysis on a hair specimen, to see what the zinc level is and for future comparison. Also, a gastric analysis to check acid levels and a blood test for pancreatic enzymes. In testing people with diabetes, I've found both these digestive functions are low quite frequently."

"That might cause me not to absorb zinc?"

"And many other nutrients."

Three weeks later Mr. Lehrman's tests were completed. He'd come in to go over them.

## Zinc Level Low

"Your mineral analysis definitely shows low zinc," I started.

"You're going to tell me it's like white spots . . . it doesn't have to be low to be needed."

"Right, but what made you think that?"

"Rebecca read it. She also read that cases like this better be advised by a doctor who knows nutritional therapy."

"It helps, especially for avoiding trouble. There are other reasons, too. For example, your copper level on your hair test is also low. If you took too much zinc with low copper, it might possibly lead to copper-deficiency anemia, cholesterol problems, or even abnormal heartbeats, called PVCs, although that's rare."

"Sounds dangerous. Why don't I take them both, together?"

"That's one alternative, but remember zinc and copper are in some ways 'antagonists.' I've observed that if taken together, frequently neither works."

"They push each other out?"

"Don't know for sure: not enough data. They might compete for absorption. It seems to help to take them at different times."

"So everyone who needs zinc should take copper, as long as it's taken at a different time?"

"Good grief, no. Most people have enough copper, some have way too much. It's just necessary to keep possible zinc/copper problems in mind when zinc is needed, and check for them."

## Pancreatic Enzyme Deficit

"However, I'm getting off the subject of your leg ulcer. Your stomach acid test was normal, but your pancreatic enzymes tested very low."

"That will keep me from absorbing zinc?"

"Yes, I've observed that over and over, particularly in children with eczema. There's something in pancreatic enzymes that's necessary for zinc. I don't know what it is, but when zinc is needed and pancreatic enzymes are low, zinc doesn't work well, even in fairly large doses."

"Is that the only thing that might keep zinc from being absorbed?"

"No. Some people with low stomach acid don't absorb zinc well until acid's supplied. I'm sure there are other factors, too, that haven't been found."

I wrote out a note for Mr. Lehrman, asking him to get pancreatin tablets, if possible the 1,300 or 1,400 milligram strength, to be used after meals, two or three at a time. I also wrote

down 50 milligrams of zinc three times daily; one gram of vitamin
C three times daily; 400 international units of vitamin E; 30,000
international units of vitamin A; 1,200 units of vitamin D; and one
tablespoon of linseed oil daily.

He looked at the note. "I understand the pancreatic
enzymes," he said. "Also the zinc, vitamin C to help healing, and
vitamin E. It obviously helped. But you lost me after that. And
what about copper?"

"If we had to use just a bare minimum to help the ulcer, I'd
say pancreatin, zinc, vitamins C and E, in your case. The other
items are most likely not to be absorbed when pancreatic enzymes
are low. Don't forget your prostate symptoms: The essential fatty
acids in the oil are important for solving those, along with zinc.

"I'd rather you didn't start any copper right now. Although
it's low on the test, it's not an extreme shortage. I'd like to give the
zinc a clear shot to help. We'll monitor your blood count and
cholesterol to make sure it's OK. Any problem, the copper can be
started.

"About diet: That's most important. Except for the pancreatin, a digestive aid, the other things are supplemental. Although
they're very important now, over the long run they're secondary
to a good overall diet program. I'd like you to follow the high-fiber
approach documented at the University of Kentucky by Dr.
Anderson." I gave him an order blank to send for Dr. Anderson's
guidebook. "Some people have even been able to discontinue
insulin over time by following this program."

"If that's so, I should be able to get off these pills. I hope so."

The first thing Mr. Lehrman noted was a considerable
decrease in intestinal gas, a problem he never realized he had. He
experimented by leaving out the digestive enzymes, finding they
really made a difference. "I guess I was so used to being gassy I
thought it was normal," he observed.

Slowly his ulcer healed. Nothing changed for six weeks; then
we both could see signs of improvement. It took a little over ten
months to fill in; at that point, he cut down the zinc supplement,
adding a little copper at a different time of day.

His prostate symptoms faded away over six months. Eighteen

months after starting his pancreatin, his supplements, Dr. Anderson's high-fiber approach to diabetes, and a serious exercise program, he was able to eliminate his prescription anti-diabetes pills.

# More to Zinc Research
# Than You Think

Several investigators have shown that zinc supplementation is effective in healing chronic leg ulcers. Research has also shown that serum zinc levels are lowered in individuals with leg ulcerations. It would seem logical to conclude that zinc is a useful treatment for leg ulcers, especially in persons whose serum zinc levels are low. Yet two out of three double-blind, placebo-controlled tests—the ultimate in scientific validation—failed to reach that conclusion. In another surprising twist, the consensus of opinion among zinc researchers is still that zinc is useful in the treatment of chronic leg ulcers. Puzzled? Read on . . .

A closer examination of the design of these scientific studies discloses faults common to many single nutrient studies, and provides clues to explain why most zinc and leg ulcer researchers believe that zinc is still effective.

The test which demonstrated positive results included both before and after measurements of serum zinc. That measurement established beforehand which persons with leg ulcers were low in zinc and which were normal. It also established which individuals actually absorbed the zinc they took.

The response assessment was divided into two groups: those with initially low zinc, and those without. As might be predicted, zinc was shown significantly more effective than a fake pill in the low-zinc group, but not effective in the normal-zinc-to-start-with group. Zinc was thereby established as effective in a subgroup of individuals with leg ulcers, namely those low in zinc.

In contrast, the two double-blind trials of zinc and leg ulcers that reported negative results didn't bother to include before and after measurements of zinc. Neither group of experiments had any way of knowing which individuals were more in need of zinc, or who absorbed the zinc, or who didn't. All individuals with leg ulcers were lumped into one group in both experiments. In both cases the zinc group did have greater healing, but the difference was not large enough to be statistically significant. Furthermore, in these two experiments, there was no way to know whether the zinc was absorbed or not.

Far too much research on nutrient effects that has been reported as "negative" has had the same defects as the negative double-blind zinc studies. If before-and-after blood, urine, and other tissue levels are not performed, there's no way to tell if experimental group individuals are low in the nutrient (sometimes this is important, sometimes not). The nutrient may not have been absorbed in the first place and, as you've read, if a nutrient isn't absorbed, it can't do much in the body. And absorption of a nutrient is no guarantee that it will penetrate to where it's needed, or be metabolized properly.

All nutrient research needs to be evaluated from these perspectives. Careful examination for all these factors—need, absorption, distribution, metabolism (as well as others)—must be made before accepting any report as valid.

Zinc is a particularly tricky nutrient. I have proof, both clinical and laboratory based, that zinc can be taken in a high dose, with a high-blood-zinc level achieved and a high-urinary-zinc output maintained, without effective penetration of tissue (in these cases, skin in need of healing) and hair. Changing the form in which zinc is given can result in better penetration of tissue, better healing, yet with only a fraction of the zinc dose and much lower blood levels.

At present, I'm involved with individual case work at the John Bastyr College in Seattle, comparing various forms of zinc, and a formal double-blind crossover study of various forms of zinc. Results will be published.

# Diabetics Have Low Stomach Acidity

Studies from the 1930s and 1940s reached the same conclusion: Diabetics are much more likely to have lowered gastric acidity. Thirty-two percent was the "average incidence" figure summarized by Elliot P. Joslin, M.D., of the Joslin Clinic in Boston, in 1946. That relationship has been confirmed and the percentage found higher in a recent investigation of insulin-dependent diabetics. Decreased acid secretion was also found characteristic of insulin-dependent diabetics by a group from the University of Texas Southwestern Medical School in 1978. Although I haven't been able to find recent data concerning acid secretion by the stomachs of noninsulin-dependent diabetics, work in our laboratory (using radiotelemetry) demonstrates the correlation more than half the time.

Also in the 1970s, two groups of investigators reported that the digestive function of the pancreas (enzyme production) is less in diabetics than in individuals without diabetes. As mentioned in Mr. Lehrman's case, normal pancreatic enzyme function appears critical to zinc absorption. I've encountered numerous cases where zinc won't work without pancreatic enzyme supplementation.

Research by Gary Evans, Ph.D., a biochemist at Minnesota State College in Bemidji, Minnesota, appears to have discovered why. In a conversation we had, he explained that pancreatic enzymes contain picolinic acid (a metabolite of tryptophan), which binds to zinc, aiding its absorption and tissue penetration. Although Dr. Evans's work is disputed by other investigators, results at my office indicate he's probably right.

## REFERENCES

**Diabetes**

Goldberg, David M., ed. "The Pancreas." In *Clinical Biochemistry Reviews—Vol. 2.* John Wiley & Sons, 1981, p. 95.

Rabinowitch, I. M. "Achlorhydria and Its Clinical Significance in Diabetes Mellitus." *American Journal of Digestive Diseases,* vol. 16, no. 5, pp. 322–331.

Rabinowitch, I. M.; Fowler, A. F.; and Watson, B. A. "Gastric Acidity in Diabetes Mellitus." *Archives of Internal Medicine,* vol. 47, pp. 384–390.

Richardson, Charles T. et al. "Diabetics Have Reduced Acid Secretion and Delayed Digestion." *American Family Physician,* June, 1978, p. 143.

Shay, H.; Gershon-Cohen, J.; and Fels, S. S. "Glucose Tolerance in Anacidity." *American Journal of Digestive Diseases*, vol. 7, no. 5, pp. 4–8.

## Diet

Anderson, James W. *HCF Diets: Guidelines for Carbohydrate, Fiber Diets*. University of Kentucky College of Medicine, 1978.

Anderson, James W.; Ward, Kyleen; and Sieling, Beverly. *HCF Diets: A User's Guide to High-Carbohydrate, High-Fiber Diets*. University of Kentucky College of Medicine, 1978.

## Zinc

Dachowski, E. J.; Plummer, V. M.; and Greaves, M. W. "Venous Leg Ulceration: Skin and Serum Zinc Concentrations." *Acta Dermatovener (Stockholm)*, vol. 55, 1975, pp. 497–498.

Greaves, M. W., and Ive, F. A. "Double-blind Trial of Zinc Sulphate in the Treatment of Chronic Leg Ulceration." *British Journal of Dermatology*, vol. 87, no. 632, pp. 632–634.

Hallbook, T., and Lanner, E. "Serum-Zinc Healing of Venous Leg Ulcers." *Lancet*, October 14, 1972, pp. 780–781.

Norris, John R., and Reynolds, Robert E. "The Effect of Oral Zinc Sulfate Therapy on Decubitus Ulcers." *Journal of the American Geriatrics Society*, September, 1971, pp. 793–797.

**Delayed wound healing, poor night vision, a decreasing sense of taste and smell, and a slightly enlarged prostate coupled with heavy alcohol consumption all add up to a need for zinc. A change in diet brings a new lease on life for this 72-year-old man.**

# A CASE OF HEAVY DRINKING AND ZINC DEPLETION

# 28

"I can't taste nothing or smell nothing. My hearing's failing, and my eyesight's starting to go," Mr. Dooley declared. "I told Katy the good Lord's trying to tell me something; it's time to pack it in, get ready to go. But she wants me around a few years yet—kept nagging at me, so here I am. If you can cure an old man's complaints, I'll be surprised." He crossed his arms and sat back.

"I really can't cure anyone's complaints. The best I can do is make suggestions about what you can do to allow your body to heal itself. It's important to realize it's your own living system that has the capability to heal, or not."

"That living system is pretty near worn out, I expect, with time, neglect, and abuse here and there."

"As long as you're here, we can try. How long have you had those problems?"

"Well, I'm 72 now. Haven't been able to smell much of anything for better than ten years, before I retired. Taste's been worse all the time the last four or five years. I told Katy I been eating her cooking so long I can't taste it no more. So she put a triple dose of chili peppers in the recipe, and I barely noticed. Said that proved it was me. She's right; I can't taste nothing at my sister's or at restaurants, neither."

"Your hearing?"

"Getting deaf—like my father, his father. Still hear good enough so I don't need a hearing aid. Some of it's from noise on my job; couldn't hear the trains like I used to the last ten years or so."

"You worked railroads?"

"All my life. Yardman, switchman, repair gang. You name it, I did it."

"Good exercise."

"Too good. At least my back and muscles are in shape."

# Poor Night Vision

"What about your eyes?"

"Last two years, fading away. Evenings, can't see good at all—dusk settling in on my eyes. Nighttime, bright lights bother me. Have to let Katy drive—can't go on my own, no more. Want to shoot pool evenings, but she don't want to go."

"So you don't drive at all?"

Mr. Dooley smiled. "I drive on down before dark sometimes, then wait till late when there's not much traffic on the road. Not safe though. Katy fusses a lot, so I don't do it much."

"You've been to the eye doctor?"

"Sure, Katy got me to go. He said to keep on taking the vitamin A she'd been giving me, but it hasn't done no good."

"How much vitamin A were you taking?"

"The big ones, 25,000 international units each, three a day, for the last year. Should've worked by now, shouldn't it?"

"Yes, if it was going to."

"Isn't that too much?"

"Not for an adult, usually."

"Why hasn't it worked?"

"Probably there are other factors. Incidentally, do you have any problems with urination?"

"Not really. Have to get up at night more than before—two or three times, that's all."

"Have to wait before urination?"

"Not really. What's that got to do with my eyes?"

"Factors that affect one part of the body affect others. Some of the problems you mentioned can have a common thread running through. So I thought I'd asked about other areas that could be part of the pattern."

We went over Mr. Dooley's health history. He'd been healthy most of his life. He'd had an appendectomy 30 years before, but no other surgery. He had no allergies, took no medications. His father had become deaf and had "a little diabetes" when he was older. His mother had "worn-out arthritis."

## "Knocked Back a Few Beers"

Mr. Dooley had smoked cigars for 50 years and said he "wasn't going to stop now". He also still "knocked back a few beers." I thought I'd better ask a little more about that point.

"I've really cut back, Doc. Since I retired, Katy's been after me. Don't buy more than four six-packs a week. Cut out almost all the hard liquor." He smiled again, "I remember them days on the railroad—working hard, gone from home days on end. Had some good times, me and the boys. Never did drink on the job, I want to tell you. Get killed that way. Always my own time. Knocked off a fifth or two a week."

"How long did you do that?"

"That's nothing. Some I know drank a pint a night. Don't get me wrong, I wasn't any alcoholic. Always could stop any time I wanted. Never showed any liver damage on checkups—some of those doctors looked real hard for that. Would've stopped in a minute if there was."

"How long were you drinking a fifth or two a week?"

Mr. Dooley frowned. "Maybe 10 to 15 years. Slowed down on my own. That's what I meant by abusing the old body. Saw what it was doing to some of my friends. Think it has something to do with my problems now?"

"Could be."

"Drank myself blind, like they say?"

"You're not blind yet."

"Help to stop the beer?"

"Maybe. Slow down a lot, anyway."

"That got something to do with not tasting?"

"Not smelling, too, possibly. What do you eat every day, starting with breakfast?"

"Well, for breakfast, coffee and hotcakes. Put syrup on them. For lunch: soup, salad, coffee. Dinner: meat, potatoes, corn, peas, or beans, less desserts these days. Katy's been trying to get me to cut down on sugar."

## Scratches Heal Slowly

I asked Mr. Dooley to come to the examining room. Despite his beer drinking, he was on the thin and wiry side, still muscular as he said. He had slight prostate gland enlargement; there were several cuts and scratches that appeared not to be healing well.

"Don't heal so good no more, at all," Mr. Dooley said when I pointed that out. "Figure it's all part of wearing out. Used to heal right up when I was a young whippersnapper."

Given his symptoms and physical findings, I thought he presented enough of a pattern so I could make a recommendation.

"I'd like you to take some zinc supplementation." I wrote out a note—zinc, 50 milligrams, three times daily—and handed it to him.

"That all?"

"For now. Before I make any other recommendations, I want to see what your tests show."

"Haven't done any tests for zinc, have you?"

"Sometimes looking and listening is enough of a test. For example, when healing is poor, the first thing to try is a small quantity of zinc."

Mr. Dooley looked at the note. "No small quantity here, is it? Could it be dangerous?"

"I think you need more than a small quantity. Besides poor healing, you have a minor prostate problem. That needs zinc, too."

## Sense of Taste Affected

"Fine, but I came in about the eyes, ears, taster, and smeller. Isn't worth eating if I can't taste no more."

"That, too. In fact, the first thing to suspect with loss of the sense of taste is a zinc problem. Likewise for smell. Both of those senses frequently come back, although slowly, with zinc supplementation."

"Maybe there's some hope for the old body yet."

"Can't say for sure, but it sounds probable."

"It's asking a lot, but what about my hearing, my eyes?"

"I don't think the hearing fits the pattern. First, there's deafness in your family, and secondly, you probably have had some noise damage, as you mentioned, from the job.

"Your eyes may be a different story. Researchers have found that night blindness that doesn't get better as expected with vitamin A improves when zinc is added."

"I should keep on with the vitamin A?"

"For now."

"Why does zinc help with vitamin A?"

"It appears that the transport protein for vitamin A isn't manufactured or released from the liver without enough zinc. Also, some of the enzymes affecting vitamin A in the eye are zinc dependent."

## How Alcohol Harms

Mr. Dooley shook his head. "I'll probably be sorry I asked, but what's that got to do with drinking alcohol? You were after me pretty close on that one."

"If you hadn't asked, I was going to tell you: Alcohol depletes zinc in the body. Low zinc levels are common in alcoholics. Now

I'm not saying you're an alcoholic, but you have done some fairly heavy drinking in the past."

"Don't apologize. Tell it to me straight. Should I quit?"

"That has to be your decision. Alcohol in small quantities may not be harmful, but considering your symptoms . . ."

"Got the picture. If I hadn't been boozing I might not be in trouble now."

"In your case, possibly not. But I don't want to give you the idea that only heavy drinking causes zinc depletion and symptoms like yours. People have turned up with loss of taste or smell, poor healing, or decreased eyesight associated with low zinc, with practically no backgound of heavy alcohol intake."

"Sure, you're saying there's more than one road to zinc problems, but if alcohol was mine, I'd better think on it. Alcohol causes other vitamin problems, too, doesn't it?"

"Of course. B vitamins, magnesium . . ."

Mr. Dooley held up a hand. "Enough. I didn't tell you, but Katy, she's been after me about the booze. Told me years ago it'd cause problems. Always told her I could quit if I wanted. Looks like I'll have to prove it."

I marked a slip for Mr. Dooley's lab tests. Among other things, I asked him to have a blood count done, since long-term zinc treatment has occasionally caused copper-deficiency anemia. I knew his zinc treatment would probably be long term.

I also requested that he eliminate all refined sources of sugar and flour from his diet, and include as many fresh, raw vegetables, nuts, seeds, and other whole foods as possible. His response was that he'd try, but it was "hard to teach an old dog new tricks."

Mr. Dooley's slow-healing skin was the first notable change, starting to improve within a month. His taste and night-vision problems started to respond in three months and appeared normal in nine. In six months, he noticed that he was getting up less often during the night. His sense of smell recovery was slowest, showing substantial improvement by a year's time. Even after three years, staying normal in other ways, his sense of smell was "good, but not like when I was young."

Mr. Dooley's hearing loss appeared unaffected by nutritional therapy.

Blood counts at intervals remained normal.

The only other change reported by Mr. Dooley was that on his regular visits to play pool at the tavern, he drank only mineral water with lemon.

# A Strong Case for Zinc

It's only occasionally possible to identify a single nutrient as responsible for most of a person's health problems. In Mr. Dooley's case, however, the collection of symptoms and signs appeared obvious. Delayed wound healing, decreased night vision, decreasing senses of taste and smell, and a slightly enlarged prostate, when considered together, make a strong case for zinc. Put together with heavy alcohol consumption—a known zinc-depleting agent—an excellent guess regarding zinc could be made even before any testing was done.

Mr. Dooley probably had many other nutrient problems associated with relatively large quantities of alcohol consumed over many years. However, none was as immediately obvious. Somehow he'd escaped detectable liver damage. As mentioned, I did persuade him later on to use B vitamins, dolomite (for magnesium), as well as vitamins C, E, and a multiple vitamin and mineral. After years of excess alcohol intake, I felt these were a minimum for him.

Zinc doesn't remedy all problems with taste, nor cure all or even nearly all cases of night blindness. The latter is routinely improved with vitamin A; zinc only enters the equation when there isn't enough to allow vitamin A to do its job. Likewise, zinc only remedies taste defects associated with zinc deficiency.

One reviewer summed up the situation best when he wrote: "Depletion of zinc can lead to decreased taste acuity, but decreased taste acuity is not necessarily associated with depletion of zinc."

## REFERENCES

**Alcohol**

Shorey, RoseAnn L. "Effects of Ethanol on Nutrition." *Journal of Chemical Education*, August, 1979, pp. 532–533.

**Taste**

Catalanotto, Frank A. "The Trace Metal Zinc and Taste." *American Journal of Clinical Nutrition,* June, 1978, pp. 1098–1103.

Greger, J. L., and Geissler, A. H. "Effect of Zinc Supplementation on Taste Acuity of the Aged." *American Journal of Clinical Nutrition,* April, 1978, pp.633–637.

Henkin, Robert I. et al. "Idiopathic Hypogeusia with Dysgeusia, Hyposmia, and Dysosmia: A New Syndrome." *Journal of the American Medical Association,* July 26, 1971, pp. 434–440.

**Taste and Smell Dysfunction**

Henkin, Robert I. et al. "A Double Blind Study of the Effects of Zinc Sulfate on Taste and Smell Dysfunction." *American Journal of the Medical Sciences,* vol. 272, 1976, pp. 285–299.

"Ineffectiveness of Zinc in Treating Ordinary Taste and Smell Dysfunctions." *Nutrition Reviews,* September, 1979, pp. 283–285.

**Vision**

Leopold, Irving H. "Zinc Deficiency and Visual Impairment." *American Journal of Ophthalmology,* June, 1978, pp. 871–875.

Morrison, Stanley A. et al. "Reversal of Night Blindness in Cirrhotics by Zinc Sulfate." *American Journal of Clinical Nutrition,* April, 1977, p. 612.

Morrison, S. A. et al. "Zinc Deficiency: A Cause of Abnormal Dark Adaptation in Cirrhotics." *American Journal of Clinical Nutrition,* February, 1978, pp. 276–281.

**Vitamins**

Bonjour, J. P. "Vitamins and Alcoholism: II. Folate and Vitamin $B_{12}$." *International Journal of Vitamin and Nutrition Research,* vol. 50, no. 1, 1980, pp. 96–121.

———. "Vitamins and Alcoholism: IV. Thiamin." *International Journal of Vitamin and Nutrition Research,* vol. 50, no. 3, 1980, pp. 321–338.

Knowing and understanding more about the health history of grandparents, parents, brothers, sisters, aunts, uncles, close cousins, and children can help document and solve problems of long duration. One family's history is reviewed.

# PROBLEMS THAT RUN IN THE FAMILY 29

A family health history is an important part of any individual's health background. While it's true that each of us is biochemically unique and may develop a problem that no relative has, it's just as likely that what's wrong with you or me has made an appearance (or will in the future) elsewhere in the family. Even if symptoms aren't identical, the underlying disharmonies in body chemistry are very similar. The following discussion of several members of the same family is an important illustration of the relevance of family medical histories.

Virginia Onofrio came in with four typewritten sheets of paper. "I thought it would be helpful to write everything out," she said. "There's so much the matter I can't believe it all myself. Besides, I get all flustered and forget things." She handed me two single-spaced pages, keeping copies for herself.

I took them with slight apprehension. Sometimes written lists are so disorganized or lengthy that it's impossible to make much use of them. This one, however, was well organized and to the point, starting with her symptoms in order of importance, with approximate duration and other details. She briefly noted previous treatments. She also included a short but comprehensive family health history, a summary of her eating habits, and a paragraph about "lifestyle."

Ms. Onofrio was 39, divorced, supporting herself and one daughter. Her most immediate concern was a series of infections that had caused her to miss several weeks of work in the past year. She was concerned about holding her job.

She'd had sinus problems for nearly 20 years, but they were increasingly worse. She'd had three serious infections in the previous 12 months. She'd also had a case of boils, several sore throats, repetitions of the flu, pneumonia once, and a recurrent vaginal infection.

## Fatigue, Headaches, and More

But her symptoms only started with infections. Also listed were chronic fatigue, even following adequate sleep. Sometimes the fatigue worsened in the late afternoon, other times not. She had headaches frequently; these, she noted, were a lifelong problem. She also noted a bad temper, chronic gas pains, constipation, low back pain, sometimes pain into the left leg, menstrual cramps ("for years"), heartburn, indigestion, nervousness, depression ("wondering if I'm going crazy sometimes"), and the recent onset of slight high blood pressure. Lastly, her fingernails were starting to break, she'd been waking up a lot at night, and she felt "too full" after meals.

As I finished reading the problem list, I looked at Ms. Onofrio. "Considering all this, I'm glad you're still with us."

She smiled. "Still in there kicking. I'm not going to let my body get in my way. But I've recently decided I'm going about it wrong, fighting against my body rather than trying to work with it, listening to it to tell me there's something the matter. A book I read recently said illness is just a signal that your whole life needs reevaluation. I believe that. I'm here to find out what to do to treat my body better."

I asked a few more questions about her symptoms and

problems, then went back to the second page. It started with family history. Her mother, who had arthritis, chronic headaches, and back pain, had recently been told she had osteoporosis. She had also had a painful bout of shingles a few months before. Her father tended to "drink a little," had a bad temper, but had no disease. Her teenage daughter was very moody, and had had asthma as a small child. Two grandparents (one on each side) had high blood pressure; another had "old-age" diabetes. A great-grandfather had pernicious anemia.

Her diet history showed recent attempts at improvement, mixed in with what she termed "bad old habits." Listed were alfalfa sprouts, brewer's yeast, and whole grains, along with sugary desserts and coffee. "A whole raft" of vitamins and minerals was noted, along with the remark: "They haven't helped much!"

Having finished her information sheets, I asked a few more questions, then asked her to go to the examination room. Her exam showed an apparent need for zinc, vitamin A, and essential fatty acids, a yeast infection, and a need for spinal manipulation. As I finished, I told her so.

"Well, that's better than a recommendation for a psychiatrist," she replied. "I've gotten a lot of those lately, especially since I'm divorced and chronically sick. If I take those vitamins particularly, and see a chiropractor, will that take care of me?"

## Low Stomach Acidity

"It'll help a little. But it probably would be more effective if you took hydrochloric acid supplement with meals, possibly pancreatic enzymes, too. Also, taking better care of your blood sugar problem, starting with the elimination of refined sugar, appears wise. You need to eliminate all your food allergies, and probably use vitamin $B_{12}$ injections, as well as other supplements. I might be wrong, but I think that all will be necessary."

"Whoa! Can you tell all that by looking at me, or are my symptoms that clear?"

"As I said, I could be wrong. Especially with something potentially hazardous like hydrochloric acid supplements, we'll test to see if you need it. The other things will need verifying, also. But aside from your own problems, your family history forms an interesting pattern.

"Your daughter had asthma. Decades ago, a striking association between asthma and hypochlorhydria (low stomach acidity) was described. I've found myself that most women with osteoporosis, like your mother, are also likely to have the low acidity problem. Of course, one of the diagnostic criteria for pernicious anemia is total lack of stomach acid. It's treated with B$_{12}$ injections.

"There's quite an overlap between low stomach acidity and allergy. Of course, your daughter had asthma. Your mother has arthritis: You noted it wasn't rheumatoid type, but osteoarthritis. There's a frequent association of nonrheumatoid, nongouty arthritis with allergy.

"One grandparent has diabetes. Your father tends to drink too much, which is frequently associated with blood sugar problems, as is your teenage daughter's moodiness. Of course that could be allergy, too.

"Now, I'm not claiming to diagnose your whole family, but it's possible to construct a picture that includes them all and relate the family pattern to your problems. If we then add your symptoms . . ."

"I see what you mean. Let's get started."

Ten months later, Ms. Onofrio was back, but not for herself. This time she accompanied her mother, Helen Shelton.

"I had to come in myself," Mrs. Shelton said. "When Virginia told me that almost all her problems fit into a family pattern, I could scarcely believe it. She's been ill so much more than the rest of us. But I've seen how well she's done on her low blood sugar and no-allergy diet. I can even tell when she's been taking her B$_{12}$ like she's supposed to.

"She said you said I probably needed hydrochloric acid supplements with meals as she does, and that I might be allergic. I told her that's nonsense. I've hardly had any stomach problems except some gas, and no allergies I know about. But I promised to come in if she improved . . . so here I am. Do you really think allergy testing might help my arthritis?"

"Which joints bother you?"

Mrs. Shelton held out her hands. "It's mostly here," she said. "But my knees do hurt on and off, and occasionally an ankle swells."

The middle joints of her fingers were most affected; the majority were thicker than usual; two were tender to touch. Three end joints were affected, also. "You've had tests for rheumatoid arthritis and gout?"

"Oh, yes, they tell me it's old-age-type arthritis—osteoarthritis. I'm supposed to take aspirin if it hurts. That's how I found out about my osteoporosis . . . they were taking x-rays of my joints and back because it hurts sometimes, too."

"Which side of the family has pernicious anemia?"

"That was my grandfather."

"By testing, I've found many women who have osteoporosis also have hypochlorhydria, the lack of stomach acid. An early edition of a major pharmacology textbook noted that gastric acidity was important for calcium assimilation. Your daughter has this problem, and probably your granddaughte. when she was younger. Of course, a lack of stomach acid is characteristic of pernicious anemia. So even with no symptoms, your chances are high."

## Allergy Often a Factor

"Allergy isn't always involved in osteoarthritis, but it frequently is. Your daughter's very allergic to foods; that was one of the principal causes of all her infections."

"And she forgot to mention her two uncles, my brothers, who both have hay fever. Of course she'd have no way of knowing they were both allergic to milk as infants. I remember, we had a goat."

"So it's possible, although not for certain, that you have hidden allergies, too. At least, it's worth checking."

"Also, I have headaches. I've been just amazed that Virginia's worst ones are caused by eggs, when she slips and eats one."

We went over the rest of Mrs. Shelton's history, as well as a checkup and tests. Although there were other minor findings, her principal problems turned out to be low stomach acidity and food allergies, as predicted by her family history and her own symptoms. Her arthritis came under much better control. Subsequent tests showed much better calcium assimilation.

Seven months after Mrs. Shelton's visit, she and her daughter both arrived, with Mr. Shelton and Susan Onofrio, Virginia's daughter. Each of the latter two were scheduled for a checkup.

"They've dragged us both in, kicking and screaming," Mr. Shelton declared. His granddaughter giggled. "These two have got us both diagnosed, based on them and the rest of the family. They've been watching us closely for symptoms, of course.

"I'm supposed to have blood sugar problems and so is Susan, because we both get cranky when we don't eat. Virginia here has hypoglycemia and my mother had diabetes. Also, I nip a bit more than Helen would like."

"Now, Father, you know it's more than that," Virginia said. She turned to me. "You said many children with asthma had low stomach acidity. Shouldn't we test Susan for that, considering my problem and Mother's?"

"Most children's stomachs normalize again as they mature. Unless she still has asthma, she's probably OK. But it frequently is helpful to check for hidden allergy, especially considering the family history. Allergies in children often don't go away, they just go 'underground.'"

We went through our usual procedures with Mr. Shelton and Susan. Although Susan didn't have a stomach acid problem, both she and her grandfather had reactive hypoglycemia. Susan had several food allergies. Mrs. Shelton and Virginia both agreed that when Susan and her grandfather cooperated with their program, they "behaved better" and felt better.

Certainly, not all families have health problems that fit together as neatly as this. Not everyone knows their family health history. But Virginia Onofrio and her family are an excellent example of the possible importance of a good family medical history in determining what an individual's own health problems might be.

While not everyone has an opportunity to know their family medical history, it's surprising how many individuals with health problems of long duration haven't made an effort to document theirs. Sometimes family health history isn't related to one's own problem, but it can on occasion be invaluable. A "health pedigree" going back a century or more isn't necessary, but knowledge of the health history of grandparents, parents, brothers, sisters, aunts, uncles, close cousins, and children is definitely a good idea.

An extreme case of fatigue along with irritability, headaches, sleep difficulty, and occasional gas problems leads to the discovery of multiple food allergies. Avoiding the allergenic foods clears up the problems.

# 30 A CASE OF FATIGUE AND FOOD ALLERGY

Mr. Jackson looked tired. His eyes were very slightly reddened; there were lines and slight darkening beneath them. He rubbed his forehead occasionally, as if to wipe away fatigue. "Eleanor thought some vitamins would pick me up," he said, gesturing toward his wife, who had come in with him. "She says I'm too tired all the time. I tell her that I'm not getting younger, and I put in a lot of hours, but she still thinks there's something the matter, so here I am." He smiled, crossed his arms, and sat back.

"Now, Daniel, you admitted yourself that a lot of the time you don't feel right," she chided. "You've been to doctors three times in the past five years, on your own. So you know things aren't just right."

"But they all told me I was in good health. Just relax, get more sleep, take a little more time off. Even the last psychiatrist I saw didn't think there was that much the matter with me."

"So fatigue is your only problem, then?"

"Mainly, yes. It's quite bad."

"There's a few other things, too. Daniel, tell the doctor. You

get headaches, and you get real grouchy and irritable sometimes."
She turned to me. "Daniel's basically very good-natured. But
sometimes I can't believe how his temper changes. When we were
first married 20 years ago, it hardly ever happened. The last 5
years, it's been more and more. I don't think it's me."

Mr. Jackson smiled. "I keep telling you it isn't you, honey. It's
just when I get so tired, everything seems to bother me. Used to be
a good night's sleep would take care of it, but I don't sleep so well
anymore."

## Wakes Often during Night

"Do you get to sleep easily?"

"It varies. Mostly I do, but some nights not. I wake up a lot.
And sometimes can't get back to sleep. The psychiatrist said
sometimes that's a sign of hidden depression, even though I didn't
seem depressed. He tried me on an antidepressant drug. I quit
after a month. It made me feel all weird in the head, kind of
hopped up. Tried another one, that didn't help, either."

"Did it help the tiredness?"

"Not really. I felt tired as ever but like something was
pushing me at the same time. Not good at all."

"Not sleeping certainly can be a symptom of depression, but
it can be a symptom of other things, too. Many people who have
hypoglycemia don't sleep well. It seems that in the daytime
they're abnormally tired, but at night can't sleep. Waking up,
particularly at roughly the same time each night, is frequently a
hypoglycemic symptom. Of course, depression is often associated
with low blood sugar, so the two are often confused."

"That's one reason we're here," Mrs. Jackson said. "I've been
reading about low blood sugar and tiredness. Daniel's agreed to
take a blood sugar test if you think it's necessary."

"With symptoms of fatigue and waking up at night, hypoglycemia sounds like at least a possibility." I looked at my notes. "You
said something about headaches?"

"Yeah, I've been getting a few, but everybody does. I think
it's just tension. I'm an electrician, working at construction sites.

There's always a push on to get something done, or some problem or other. It's all part of the job. I think I just let it get to me sometimes."

## No Lunch—No Headache

"Do you get headaches especially when there's job pressure?"

"Sometimes. But that's a funny thing. Other times, when I'm working really hard—long hours, up early, home late, skipping meals—I don't get a headache. You'd think I would. I even feel better, not as tired."

"Daniel just thrives on his work," Mrs. Jackson said. "That's why I can't believe this tiredness is all in his head."

"How often do you get headaches?"

"From twice a week to every couple months. It's not a big thing. Aspirin takes them away, so I don't keep track."

"You don't get them if you don't eat all day?"

"Can't say I do. Like I said, when I work hard all day and don't stop, sometimes I feel fine."

"Have you been checked for high blood pressure?"

"Several times. That's in my family, but mine's always normal."

"I assume you've been checked for anemia?"

"Yes, that was one of the things done when I told the first doctor about this tiredness. He said that was fine."

"He was checked for that sickle-cell kind of anemia, too," Mrs. Jackson said. "No problem."

"You mentioned high blood pressure in your family. Who has that?"

"My mother."

"Any other health problems in your family?"

"Mother has asthma, too. Daddy's fine, won't go near a doctor. One of my sisters has a trace of diabetes, but she's way overweight. Let's see. Grandmother died of a stroke; all the other grandparents are alive, in their nineties. That's all I can think of."

"You forgot Uncle George."

"Oh, yes, he died of cancer."

"And one of our daughters has a little hay fever every summer, but it's not bad," Mrs. Jackson added.

"Anyone in the family have a thyroid problem?"

"No."

"Do you smoke?"

"No"

"Drink alcohol?"

"Beer on weekends, when I'm watching the games on TV, but not during the week."

"Coffee, tea, cocoa, chocolate?"

"I gave up everything with caffeine in it to see if it would help me sleep. Didn't work. So I drink some coffee every once in a while. But not in the evenings."

"Does it give you a lift from tiredness?"

"Not really. I know it makes Eleanor all shaky if she drinks too much, but I don't feel a thing."

## A Problem with Gas

I reviewed my notes again. "Tiredness the main problem, irritable more often lately, headaches in no particular pattern, don't sleep well, waking up a lot. Can you think of any other symptoms?"

"Well," Mr. Jackson looked embarrassed. "Sometimes I get all gassed up. It can be a problem."

"Does your stomach bloat right after you eat?"

"No, hardly ever that."

"Two to three hours after meals?"

"Sometimes—but it's odd—sometimes I don't get very gassy at all for days or weeks, then it'll come on for a while."

"Have you noticed any foods particularly cause gas?"

"Well, beans, but then that happens to everybody. And milk, but nobody in my family can handle milk—it gives us diarrhea or gas. Never have liked it, anyway."

"Do you use anything with milk in it?"

"We've just cut it out," Mrs. Jackson said. "I know lactose

intolerance is common in black people, so we don't use it at all. Doesn't seem to be Daniel's problem. I can't figure it out, either."

"Do you get constipated, or have diarrhea?"

"No constipation. Sometimes loose bowels with the gas, but sometimes not."

"No blood with bowel movements?"

"No."

"Have you tried anything else for this fatigue?"

## Diet Change Didn't Help

"We changed our diets. Eleanor, tell him."

"I was looking for anything that would help, so five years ago, we cut out all refined sugar, stopped eating white bread, cut down on canned food as much as possible, started eating as many fresh raw vegetables we could."

"It didn't help?"

Mrs. Jackson looked dejected. "If anything, Daniel seemed a little worse."

"The kids did a lot better, especially our boys. They got less nervous. Only Alice, she's the one with hay fever, didn't behave better. But four out of five isn't bad. So we stuck with it, for them especially. I thought I'd best check with a doctor, though, if I was eating better and feeling worse. Then they all tell me I'm fine. One even said all that health food is probably making me sick, but I know that's not right because I was tired out before then."

"We tried vitamins, too," Mrs. Jackson said. "I gave him lots of B vitamins for energy. It always made me feel fine, but Daniel said he was worse, so we quit." She looked frustrated.

Mr. Jackson took a deep breath before he spoke. "You know, Eleanor's right. I blamed her for me being here, because I've been told so often I'm healthy that I argue with myself about whether it's all in my head. But I'm worried, even though I don't let on a lot. When I say tired, I don't mean just a little. I get so bone-tired and weary sometimes it's hard to keep going. I can't think straight. On my job that's not good. That'll go on for weeks, then it's gone for a while. If it was anything serious, it'd be all the time, wouldn't it? So I don't think it's serious, but I don't feel good a lot of the time. Do you think any vitamins would help, if we found the right ones? After all, I'm 42. I probably could use a little help in that department."

"I'd like to check you over first. I know you've been checked before, but sometimes things look different from a nutritional-biochemical angle. Also, we'd best run some tests."

"Which tests?"

"Well, a glucose tolerance test, as Mrs. Jackson suggested. There is diabetes in your family. A mineral test for trace element deficiency, or heavy-metal excess. Tests for nutrient assimilation. Good diets that don't help are frequently not being fully assimilated. General biochemical screening, since this is the first time you've been here. But especially food allergy tests."

## Clues Point to Allergy

"Allergy? I'm not allergic to anything. Never have been. Didn't even break out with poison ivy like the rest of the family when I was growing up. I don't get hay fever or sinus trouble. I can breathe just fine."

"Allergy doesn't cause just hay fever, asthma, sinus problems or skin problems. Actually, allergies can cause any symptom you can think of, sometimes. Everything considered, I think food allergy is a likely possibility. It is a major and common cause of fatigue. Anemia, hypothyroidism, hypoglycemia, vitamin and mineral problems are all common reasons for tiredness, but food allergy is equally common.

"Also, your mother has asthma, and your daughter has hay fever. Whenever there's obvious allergy in the family, hidden allergy is more likely a cause of mysterious symptoms in other family members.

"Lastly, remember you mentioned you actually felt a little worse when you switched from a refined food diet to more unprocessed, whole foods? And only your daughter with hay fever didn't do better behaviorally? That is another clue for food allergy. Highly refined and processed foods have much of the nutrition removed, and aren't good for us. But all that refining and processing also removes some of the allergenic properties, so some people who are quite allergic do feel worse eating whole, raw foods that they're allergic to."

"What a choice," Mrs. Jackson said. "Eating junk food, being poorly nourished, but feeling better—or eating whole, nutritious food, and feeling worse. Sounds like an advertisement for the junk food industry."

"Not really, because you're quite right about the low-grade malnutrition. And sometimes it gets worse than low grade. No, the solution is eating whole, nutritious foods you're not allergic to, and feeling well. But we may be getting a little ahead of things. Let's do the checkup and tests and see."

Mr. Jackson subsequently proved quite allergic to almost precisely 50 percent of the food he'd been eating, and mildly allergic to another 20 percent. After the initial shock wore off, he became acquainted with many new foods, being careful to test for new allergies. He eliminated the bad allergens, and ate the mild ones on a rotation plan so they wouldn't bother him much. One of his worst allergens turned out to be brewer's yeast, which explained his problem with the type of B vitamins Mrs. Jackson had given him. He found he had to be very careful to pick out vitamin and mineral supplements with nothing in them he might be allergic to.

His blood sugar test did show mild hypoglycemia, in his case probably secondary to his food allergies. His other tests indicated a degree of poor absorption, but this condition improved after he strictly eliminated his food allergens.

As might be expected, his fatigue, sleeping difficulty, irritability, headaches, and gas problem were all traced to food allergy and only reappeared in varying combinations when he slipped a little on his allergy-free diet.

## Allergies Do Run in Families

If you're not feeling as well as you'd like and can't discover why, look first for the same types of problems other family members have had. We share more biochemical traits with relatives than nonrelatives and we're much more likely to share biochemical disorders with them, too.

The tendency to allergies is definitely one that runs in families. Food allergies are extremely common. If you still have any doubts, please read the books by Marshall Mandell, M.D., William Philpott, M.D., James C. Breneman, M.D., and Theron Randolph, M.D. (listed in the Recommended Reading List). Since, at present, medical practice mostly ignores food allergy or denies its existence, I'm forced by circumstances to probe for food allergy with more than half of the people who come in. As awareness of food allergy, food sensitivity, and chemical and environmental sensitivity spreads in the medical profession, many more people will find explanations for their symptoms.

Food allergy is one of the most common causes of fatigue in both adults and children. In an excellent review of the problem in children, Dr. Randolph notes that it was first described in print in 1898 by an educator who called it "abnormal fatigue" and clearly described many symptoms now recognized as allergic in origin.

Whenever possible, avoidance of allergenic foods is the best treatment. When it isn't possible, then desensitization to food allergens is second best. As is the case with inhalant allergy desensitization, it doesn't always work, and some methods and procedures appear to be more effective than others. At present, I refer individuals who wish to be desensitized to one of my colleagues specializing in the branch of allergy termed clinical ecology.

There are vitamins which alleviate allergic symptoms to a degree. None of them singly or in combination cure allergic disease, but they can make symptoms much more tolerable. These include vitamin C, which I usually recommend with appropriate precautions at body tolerance levels. Pantothenate and vitamin $B_6$ are helpful individually; the entire B complex, derived from a nonallergenic source, should also be used. Essential fatty acids, especially those found in primrose oil, have been shown by David Horrobin, M.D., to favorably alter parameters of "allergic bio-chemistry." (Remember to take vitamin E whenever essential fatty acids are used.) And Stephen Levine, Ph.D., a sufferer from chemical allergies himself, has found the mineral selenium to be especially helpful against symptoms of chemical allergy.

Many food supplement companies will now disclose the source of all the ingredients in their various products. Allergic individuals should avoid products by companies who don't offer full disclosure, or risk symptoms from that source. Hypoallergenic supplements, both multiple and individual nutrient, are beginning to appear more frequently in health-food stores. Whenever allergy permits, it's best to stay with nonallergenic natural sources, using synthetics only when necessary.

How can you tell if food allergy might be the cause of your undiagnosed symptoms? Aside from statistical probability being great, there are a few physical signs to remember. The most common are:

- Dark circles under the eyes (in nonpregnant, nonhormonally treated individuals)
- Puffiness under the eyes
- Several horizontal creases in the lower lid
- Chronic nasal and sinus stuffiness (Of course, this usually indicates environmental allergy, too. But most people who are allergic to environments have food allergies, too.)
- Chronically swollen glands with no cause found, especially in children
- Chronic noncyclic fluid retention, again with no other cause found.

Don't forget family history. It's one of your more important clues to what may be the matter. If someone else in your family is allergic, you may be also.

## REFERENCES

**Allergic Fatigue**
    Randolph, Theron G. "Fatigue and Weakness of Allergic Origin (Allergic Toxemia) to Be Differentiated from Nervous Fatigue or Neurasthenia." *Annals of Allergy,* November–December, 1945, pp. 418–428.

Rowe, Albert H. "Allergic Fatigue and Toxemia." *Annals of Allergy*, January–February, 1959, pp. 9–18.

**Allergies and Behavior Disorders**
Fowler, William M. et al. "Electroencephalographic Patterns in Children with Allergic, Convulsive and Behavior Disorders." *Annals of Allergy*, January 20, 1962, pp. 1–14.

Randolph, Theron G. "Allergy as a Causative Factor of Fatigue, Irritability and Behavior Problems of Children." *Journal of Pediatrics*, November, 1947, pp. 560–572.

Speer, Frederic. "Allergic Tension-Fatigue in Children." *Annals of Allergy*, March–April, 1951, pp. 168–171.

Weinberg, Eugene G., and Tuchinda, Kontri. "Allergic Tension-Fatigue Syndrome." *Annals of Allergy*, April, 1973, pp. 209–211.

**Allergy Therapy**
Horrobin, David. *Clinical Uses of Essential Fatty Acids*. Eden Press, 1983.

Philpott, William H., and Kalita, Dwight K. *Brain Allergies: The Psychonutrient Connection*. Keats Publishing, 1980.

Randolph, Theron G., and Moss, Ralph W. *An Alternative Approach to Allergies*. Lippincott & Crowell, 1980.

**Food Allergies**
Breneman, J. C. *Basics of Food Allergy*. Charles C Thomas, 1978.

Gerrard, John W. *Food Allergy: New Perspectives*. Charles C Thomas, 1980.

Mandell, Marshall, and Scanlon, Lynne Waller. *Dr. Mandell's 5-Day Allergy Relief System*. Thomas Y. Crowell, 1979.

Easily cracked, chipped, peeling, and breaking fingernails are a key symptom in nutritional medicine. In this case, breaking fingernails was only the tip of the iceberg.

# 31 A CASE OF BREAKING FINGERNAILS

"Really, I hate to bother you about such a minor problem, but it's been going on for so long. A few other things were bugging me, too, so I finally decided to come in. Besides, it's about time for a checkup, Pap smear, and all that." Poised nervously in her chair, arms crossed, Mrs. Cole looked worried, defensive.

"If you're trying to stay healthy, it's just as well to come in when a problem's minor, before it gets bad. Sometimes people come in with no health problems, just to check on blood pressure, cholesterol, mineral levels . . . to monitor if diet and exercise programs are working as planned."

"I know that, but this is a minor problem that's just going to stay minor. I mean it won't ever be a major disease or anything."

"Why don't you tell me what it is?"

"All right, but I hope you don't think I'm foolish. My husband thought it was a laugh, and an expensive one, too. I told him I worked and saved my own money, so I'd come in if I wanted to." She paused for a moment. "Oh yes, I didn't say yet . . . it's my fingernails. They're cracking, breaking, splitting, weak. Every time one starts to grow decently, it breaks off. I haven't been able to grow good nails for years. It's a little thing, but it really bothers me." Having spoken her concern, she relaxed a little and sat back.

"How long have your nails been like this?"

"This bad, at least ten years. I'm 49 now. I don't expect to be a beauty queen, but I try to keep myself up. No matter what I do, my nails just break. Even before they got bad, though, I had trouble with them."

"What have you tried?"

"All the usual things. Protein, gelatin, calcium, multiple vitamins. None of it works. When I was younger, if I took a lot of calcium or ate a little extra protein it helped, but not anymore. I apply external hardener, which helps a little, and I use those artificial nails, but those aren't a real answer.

"You know, what I've gotten worried about these last few years is, if my body can't grow good fingernails, maybe there's something the matter in general with its ability to grow and repair other tissues. Tissues I can't see, or won't feel until things get bad. That's probably an unnecessary worry—it's only fingernails—but I might as well mention it."

## Hair Starting to Thin

"That's not as unlikely as you think. Have you also had any problems with your hair?"

"I do seem to be losing more than I should. I'm not going bald or anything, but my hairdresser says my hair's thinning out and doesn't look as good as it should."

"You're not taking estrogen hormones, birth-control pills, or any other medications?"

"No. Do they make hair fall out?"

"In a few people who seem especially sensitive."

"Well, I'm not taking any hormones or birth-control pills. We've had our family; my husband's had a vasectomy."

"How about skin problems?"

"Maybe a little dry, but that's all."

"Any other symptoms you can think of?"

"One other main thing: I'm tired, all the time. That's been going on for years, too. I've been checked for anemia and thyroid problems, but the results are normal. I keep on pushing, getting things done. I'm not going to let something like fatigue stand in my way, so even my husband doesn't believe me when I tell him I'm tired all the time. I go to bed tired, wake up tired, and I'm tired all the way in between."

"Have you been checked for hypoglycemia, low blood sugar?"

"No, but I decided to get rid of all the sugar and refined foods in my diet 10 or 12 years ago, when I was taking another shot at growing fingernails. I did feel a little better overall, prevented a few headaches, improved my digestion, but I stayed just as tired and my fingernails kept right on splitting."

"You still don't eat sugar or refined food?"

"Maybe once every few months, when we're out. Otherwise, I developed the habit of reading labels on everything, making sure my diet is as whole and natural as possible. My reading convinced me that's the best thing to do. Now if it could just work on my fingernails . . ."

"You're right, even if it doesn't help your nails to avoid sugar, it's still best. By the way, no digestive symptoms now?"

## Constipation and Gas

"Nothing like before. I still get a little gassy, burp a little, and occasionally I'm a little constipated, but I'm sure it's nothing out of the ordinary. Before I eliminated sugar and white flour, I was constipated all the time—a regular air balloon."

"You don't bloat in the stomach?"

"Maybe after an especially big meal, not otherwise."

"As far as you know, do you have any allergies?"

"No."

"Never had—even when you were growing up—any hay fever, eczema, asthma, hives?"

"No."

"Recurrent infections?"

"No."

"Any allergies in your family?"

"No. Why so many questions about allergies? I know a lot of things can be caused by allergy, but you're not thinking of allergic fingernails, are you?"

I laughed. "No, I'm not, though I've learned to look for allergy much more often than I used to, particularly when a problem is stubbornly puzzling. What I was thinking of was your fatigue. Chronic fatigue is frequently associated with allergy."

Mrs. Cole thought for a moment. "No, there's just no one in my family I can think of who's had allergies. Actually, my family health history isn't terribly helpful. Both my parents are quite well, except my father has a little high blood pressure. It's controlled with medicine. I have no brothers or sisters. My children are OK. One set of grandparents was killed in an auto accident; the other two are in their eighties and quite well."

We went over Mrs. Cole's past medical history for other symptoms, but aside from her stated complaints of bad fingernails, thinning hair, slightly dry skin, occasional constipation and gas, there wasn't much else.

Her examination was mostly normal, too. Her fingernails were indeed in poor condition: chipped, cracked in two or three places, none very long. Her hair appeared a little thin, although not badly so. Her skin was slightly dry, particularly the lower legs, but once again, not pronounced. She had two misaligned vertebrae. Otherwise, physically, everything seemed normal.

"Well, I guess I didn't expect you to find much," Mrs. Cole said. "I knew about that back problem, but I didn't mention it because my chiropractor takes care of it, and besides it isn't hurting right now. Anyway, what's next?"

"Routine screening: blood tests, urinalysis and an analysis of minerals on a hair specimen."

"Just routine analysis?" She looked disappointed.

"Hold on there. I think the chances are good we'll get an indication of the problem from those tests, especially the mineral analysis."

"You've run into this kind of problem before?"

"Yes. Frequently, fingernails like yours are, as you thought, an indicator of other problems."

# Mineral Levels Low

Mrs. Cole returned a month later. We looked at her mineral analysis first, as it gave the best clues. Calcium, magnesium, iron, manganese, zinc, chromium, and nickel were all below the lower limit of normal.

"I read a little about this," she said. "When that many minerals are low, it might mean I'm not absorbing them?"

"That's right. Usually the absorption defect that goes with terrible fingernails is hypochlorhydria, lack of sufficient stomach acid production."

"Really? Does that happen often?"

"Often enough that when I hear about poor quality fingernails, I make sure to check for stomach acid problems."

"How do you do that?"

"It could be done by stomach pumping, but our lab uses a test called gastric analysis by radiotelemetry."

"Why didn't we just do that to start with? It's been a month since I was in."

"I know, but you didn't have very pronounced symptoms suggesting hypochlorhydria or lack of stomach acidity, so I thought it might be best to see what your mineral analysis report might be."

"What do you mean by 'pronounced symptoms'?"

"For low acidity, there's usually bloating in the stomach after meals, burping during or after meals, a feeling that some foods are just sitting in the stomach not digesting, and constipation. However, quite a number of people with only minor problems in these areas have insufficient stomach acid. Occasionally low stomach acidity exists with no symptoms at all."

"I guess my symptoms are in the minor category. Should I get some hydrochloric acid capsules?"

"Not yet. I'd rather you had the test. Remember, the acidity problem is only one of the possible causes of a mineral pattern like yours, although I think it's the most likely."

# Blood Test Results

Mrs. Cole looked at her blood test results. They were mostly normal, although her pancreatic enzyme determinations were low, another reason for poor assimilation of nutrients and a frequent accompaniment to low stomach acidity. Her attention was drawn to another test result.

"It says here my calcium is normal in the blood test. How can that be if my hair test is low?"

"That's not a surprise. Let's use osteoporosis for an example. You've heard of that?"

"Isn't that what happens when there's calcium lost from bones and they break easily?"

"Exactly. I've seen x-rays showing severe demineralization of bones, obviously marked calcium loss, and yet the blood calcium is normal."

"Why's that?"

"Remember, the levels of calcium and some other minerals in the blood are regulated very carefully by the body, because so many vital functions—such as muscle contraction and heartbeat—depend on them. So if there's too little, more is taken from bone and tissue storage. If there's too much, the excess is stored in the tissues or excreted. High or low levels of calcium and certain other minerals in the blood are quite unusual, and not necessarily indicative of levels elsewhere in the body."

"The hair test is?"

"It comes closer. It isn't perfect either. More needs to be known about interpreting it, but it's still very useful."

"I see. So should I have my stomach acid checked? What vitamins and minerals should I take?"

"It'd probably be just as well to wait until after the stomach acid test before taking any appreciable quantities of minerals. Probably not that much would be absorbed anyway if you have an acidity problem."

# Stomach Acid Low

Mrs. Cole checked back after her stomach acid test. As expected it showed a poor acid secretory response to a standard challenge. I asked her to start with 5 grains of betaine hydrochloride per meal and build up slowly towards 45 grains per meal. At this recommendation, she looked surprised, and took a bottle from her purse.

"I bought these just to see. I even took one a few days ago; didn't feel anything. They're five grains. The bottle says one or two with meals. Forty-five grains is . . . that's nine tablets with every meal. Isn't that too much?"

"Not at all . . . in fact, that's the same as the average adult dose of liquid hydrochloric acid solution, which is one teaspoon (five milliliters) of the 10 percent strength."

"Wouldn't that be easier? One teaspoon instead of nine capsules?"

"Not necessarily. The one teaspoon has to be dissolved in 8 to 12 ounces of water, and sipped through a glass straw so it doesn't destroy tooth enamel."

"Good grief. Either 8 to 12 ounces of water with acid, sipped through a glass straw, or nine of these tablets per meal, just for fixing my fingernails! Maybe they aren't so bad after all."

"Remember, your fingernails and thinning hair are probably a distant early warning of other, more serious problems. I can't tell you what might happen first, but something's bound to go wrong sooner than it should if your levels of all those minerals stay low. Besides that, if you haven't enough stomach acid, proteins probably won't be digested properly. Some of the stores locally have ten-grain hydrochloric acid capsules. Perhaps you should look for those."

"It would be easier, only four to five per meal. Actually, I was just kidding. I realize I could run into health trouble worse than just poor fingernails if I'm not absorbing nutrients. Still, that is a lot of hydrochloric acid. Are there any precautions?"

"Don't take it with aspirin or any 'anti-inflammatory' drugs.

Don't take it if it makes your stomach hurt. When in doubt it's wisest not to take any, and to call in.

"One other thing: In some cases the liquid is easier to tolerate and works more effectively than tablets. But I'd have to write you a prescription."

"I'll check back here if I need it. But how will we know?"

"By how you do, and if your mineral analysis shows a good change or not. Also remember you should follow each meal with pancreatin because your enzyme tests were low."

"How about a combined hydrochloric acid-pancreatic enzyme tablet?"

"Those are hardly ever strong enough. Remember, even the ten-grain hydrochloric acid capsules are needed four or five at a time."

"Will all this help my fatigue?"

"Probably. If your assimilation is poor, you're likely to be fatigued. However, the nurse will show you how to give yourself vitamin $B_{12}$ injections. Those help tiredness in nearly all cases of hypochlorhydria."

"Good grief. Acid capsules, enzyme pills, vitamin $B_{12}$ injections, and a whole list of minerals and vitamins. All this over one set of fingernails! If I don't prevent a few other problems, too, I'll be surprised."

I wrote out a list of minerals for Mrs. Cole, along with a few basic vitamins. She decided to try the large dose hydrochloric acid capsules first, instead of the prescription liquid.

Her fingernails started to show noticeable improvement in two to three months. After six to nine months she showed me "long, hard, uncracked, unchipped" nails. Her hair quit thinning; her hairdresser said it was looking much better. Her fatigue left, although she's needed periodic vitamin $B_{12}$ injections to fully maintain her energy levels.

Just as important, her mineral levels showed substantial improvement, probably an indication of better digestion and overall nutrient assimilation. Although neither of us could guess with certainty what health problems she's avoiding, I'd say her chances of continued better health are much improved with better nutrient assimilation.

## Breaking Fingernails: A Key Symptom in Nutritional Medicine

Probably because she'd been following a good diet and getting enough exercise for over a decade, Mrs. Cole's digestion and absorption problems hadn't led to more than fatigue, thinning hair, and easily broken fingernails. Others less aware of good health habits aren't as fortunate: Poor quality fingernails are usually only one of a whole collection of symptoms caused by suboptimal diet and poor digestion and absorption in a large majority of people.

Easily cracked, chipped, peeling, and breaking fingernails are a key symptom in nutritional medicine. More than 90 percent of the people with poor fingernails tested in our laboratory don't have enough stomach acid. Textbooks of medicine list fingernail trouble as a possible symptom of weak thyroid (hypothyroidism). Remember the overlap between low stomach acidity and various diseases? Low stomach acidity and hypothyroidism are two of the most closely correlated problems. Not surprisingly, thinning hair and fatigue are two other symptoms of hypothyroid conditions, also.

Supplementing hydrochloric acid and pepsin won't correct hypothyroidism. Occasionally, supplementing thyroid will correct a minor weakness in stomach acid production, but this isn't usual. Since a deficiency of stomach acid production is frequently associated with an *overactive* thyroid, too, it appears probable that there's another unknown cause (or causes) for both.

As noted in "Good Digestion: Why We Can't Take It for Granted," I recommend powdered encapsulated preparations of betaine hydrochloride with pepsin or glutamic acid hydrochloride with pepsin, and usually don't recommend the tablet forms at all anymore. Unfortunately, almost all capsules are made from just one or two types of animal gelatin, which on rare occasion is a problem for allergic individuals. Hopefully a greater diversity of materials for capsules may appear in the stores if there's enough need.

The key items for fingernail improvement appear to be protein and calcium, neither of which is well digested or absorbed by individuals with hypochlorhydria. Other nutrients are important, too, as fingernails are made of more than just calcium and protein. In practice, however, these make the biggest difference.

Recently, improvement in fingernail quality through the use of essential fatty acids, specifically those found in primrose oil, has been reported. I've not yet had very many occasions to recommend primrose oil specifically for fingernail improvement, since digestive correction, calcium, and protein usually suffice (and primrose oil is expensive), but the few times it's been tried it appears to have been helpful.

I don't know why toenails don't seem to cause the same problem fingernails do. Perhaps we don't notice them as much, or perhaps long elegant toenails aren't as desirable, but whatever the reason, very few people complain of easily broken, cracked, or peeling toenails.

## REFERENCES

**Evening Primrose Oil**

Campbell, A. C. "Treatment of Brittle Nails with Evening Primrose Oil." Paper presented at Efamol Symposium, 1981.

Horrobin, David. *Clinical Uses of Essential Fatty Acids.* Eden Press, 1983.

Allergies to a number of common foods like milk, coffee, and even lettuce, as well as uncontrolled blood sugar are two high-powered causes of this 40-year-old woman's chronic problem of fluid retention. A diet eliminating refined sugar and highly allergenic foods, supplemented with potassium, completely reverses the discomfort she suffered since childhood.

# 32 A CASE OF CHRONIC FLUID RETENTION

"I'm fortyish, and a little overweight," Betty Arens said with a smile. "I can't do much about the age, but I could do something about the weight more effectively if it weren't for water retention. One doctor called it 'chronic idiopathic edema.' I thought it'd finally been figured out the first time I saw that diagnosis, but I found out 'idiopathic' means roughly the same as 'cause unknown.' "

"No other health problems?"

"None I'm aware of. I've only been in the hospital for babies. If I had anything serious wrong, I'm sure it would have been found by now. I've been to doctors on and off to see what I could get done about fluid. Tests were negative: What worked best was just taking 'water pills.' Diuretics. One doctor told me I'd probably need them on and off the rest of my life. But I don't feel good when I take them: Nothing specific, I just feel a little 'off.' I read about diuretics causing potassium, magnesium, and other nutrient losses, so I decided taking them wasn't a good idea. Oh, I still keep a few around for when I really get bad, but only very occasionally."

"What do you mean by really bad?"

"Ten pounds or more. When my shoes won't fit, my rings get too tight, and my clothes are tight all over. Even then I put up with it unless I have to go out socially or travel."

Considering Mrs. Arens's age, and that she'd been checked before, I decided that problems such as heart failure, kidney disease, liver disorders, diabetes mellitus, and other "serious illness" would be very unlikely.

"How long has fluid retention been a problem for you?"

"Ever since I can remember. Probably all my life, but I first recall noticing it when I was a teenager, and becoming concerned with my appearance."

"How much does your weight fluctuate?"

"Anywhere from 4 to about 15 pounds. That's about how much water comes off quickly, in just a few days, with diuretics. It can't be all fat if it comes off that fast."

"Worse before menstrual periods?"

"Sometimes, but not every time. It's certainly not the main problem. Before you mention it, I did try $B_6$, up to 200 milligrams, three times a day. It keeps down the 'extra' premenstrual weight, and perhaps a pound at most of what I call my 'regular' fluid, but that's all."

## Troubled by Salty Food

"Have you noticed anything else that makes it worse?"

"If I eat a lot of salty food. I learned that a long time ago. We don't even have a saltshaker now."

"Nothing else?"

"No, it just comes on its own, it seems."

"Besides diuretics, have you ever found anything else that would make fluid go away, even temporarily?"

"If I put myself on a no-carbohydrate-at-all diet, the water just drains away after a week or two. Then some comes back, but not as much as my 'regular' amount. If I persist, and I have, twice, for three or four months, I lose a significant amount of fat. But I still have some persistent 'water,' and I just can't stay on an all-protein-and-fat diet the rest of my life. Among other things, from what I read, that wouldn't be healthy."

"What sort of foods do you eat now?"

"I still stay more with proteins, as that helps with easier 'fat control.' Let's see: beef, eggs, fish, cheese, milk. Vegetables are mostly the nonstarchy ones: lettuce, tomato, carrots, pepper, celery, bok choy, that sort of thing. Only one slice of bread a day, rice, potatoes, beans occasionally. No soft drinks, mostly coffee or tea."

"What about snacks?"

"I try to keep those down, but I do eat crackers and ice cream."

"Does much of your food come in cans, boxes, or bottles?"

"Quite a bit."

"Do you read all the labels to exclude salt and sugar?"

"I'm careful about salt. The only thing I ever add sugar to is coffee, but if there's some in packaged food I let it go."

"Do you take any vitamins?"

"C, E, B complex, and two potassium tablets, 99 milligrams each, I think."

"Tell me about your family health history."

"My father died in an accident when I was young. His mother, as well as my oldest brother, have high blood pressure. My mother's well, except she had her gallbladder out a few years back. She has a little arthritis. Her father had maturity-onset diabetes. No cancer in the family. Two of my children have hay fever, but so does my husband. That's all I can think of."

## Puffy under the Eyes

After a few more questions, we went to the examination room for a general checkup. She definitely had a lot of fluid: Her fingers, backs of hands, and ankles up to midcalf were puffy. She had puffiness under the eyes, along with a minor bluish discoloration.

"I've always had that, to one degree or another. When I was a kid, it was so bad sometimes I thought I looked like a raccoon, with big blue-black circles under my eyes. It's been better since I was a teenager, except during my pregnancies."

There were no other obvious physical abnormalities. "I'd like you to have basic screening blood tests done, in case there are any problems, as well as for preventive reasons. Also, please have a mineral analysis, a six-hour glucose tolerance test, and a test for allergies to foods."

"I'm sure I don't have diabetes," Mrs. Arens said. "I know my children have allergies, but that's all from my husband's side of the family."

"It may be from your side of the family, too. Dr. James Breneman has demonstrated that at least a substantial number of people with gallbladder difficulty are food allergic. You said your mother had her gallbladder out?"

"Well, I'm not sure what it has to do with fluid retention, but if you think so, OK."

"I don't think you have diabetes, either. The glucose tolerance test is to see if you have hypoglycemia (low blood sugar) or simply abnormal sugar tolerance."

The allergy tests and mineral tests had to be sent away for analysis, but she had the glucose tolerance and other tests the next day. The only abnormality was a mild problem with hypoglycemia.

## Cutting Back on Sugar

She was asked to completely eliminate any form of refined sugar from her diet. This included sucrose, maltose, lactose, dextrose, corn syrup, corn sweetener, fructose, dextrin, and, just to be sure, anything she was suspicious about. She was also asked to continue her vitamins B, C, and E, but to add a larger amount of potassium (one gram). She was not asked to adopt any particular "hypoglycemia diet," as I preferred to wait until her allergy tests returned.

About a month later, she was back.

"You look like you have a little less fluid today," I remarked. "Or is it just a 'random good day' today?"

"No, there's progress . . . maybe one-third, up to one-half. Three to six pounds of fluid off, on the average. But definitely not all of it.

"You know, I never realized how much refined sugar was in everything until I had to get rid of it. Seems like it's on every label I read. But what I don't understand is how eliminating refined sugar helps get rid of retained fluid. Or was it the extra potassium?"

"Probably both. Refined carbohydrate, especially sugar, and sometimes just carbohydrate excess, is a common cause of fluid retention, especially in people who have a family history of diabetes. Even though you don't have diabetes yourself, your glucose tolerance test showed a degree of sugar intolerance. Also, animal experiments show that sugar promotes excess sodium retention.

"Research indicates the same amount of sodium that wouldn't 'bother' someone else may be a liability to hypertensives and many of their relatives, due to genetic factors."

"So sodium isn't 'bad' for everyone?"

"In great excess, anything is. For some an average amount is 'neutral,' and for a few, extra sodium may be helpful. Obviously, in your case, low sodium is wisest. The extra potassium counteracts sodium to a degree. I'm sure it's part of what's helped you a little so far."

## Allergic to Several Foods

"However, your main problem appears to be allergy. Your test shows definite problems with wheat, rice, tomato, cow's milk, apples, coffee, lettuce, pork, Cheddar cheese, and oranges."

Mrs. Arens looked dazed. "Would you repeat that?"

I did so, and then observed, as gently as possible, that

probably wasn't her entire allergy list, as we'd tested only 20 items.

Collecting her thoughts, she asked the most common follow-up question. "Are you sure about that test? I just don't have allergic symptoms."

"Edema is one of the most common symptoms of allergy. Dark circles under your eyes are another. In fact, many pediatric allergists call them 'allergic shiners.'

"As for the accuracy of the test, I've evaluated that extensively. It's not perfect, but works very well in practice. As far as I'm concerned, the only thing better is extensive evaluation by a clinical ecologist."

It took several weeks to get organized, particularly as further allergy testing was required. Mrs. Arens slowly put together an allergy-free, sugar-free, high-potassium and otherwise well-balanced diet . . . as she reported, "no small job."

On this program, all of her chronic fluid retention disappeared. She found that allergens were even worse than salt or refined sugar, even though all three caused trouble. She also found, like many allergic people, that she could now control her overall weight (not just the fluid) with only a moderate degree of calorie counting.

## Allergies—a Frequent Cause of Fluid Retention

A recent medical textbook describes "idiopathic" edemas as a problem affecting predominantly women between ages 25 and 40. It occasionally varies with the menstrual cycle, but not as clearly as so-called premenstrual edema. Idiopathic means cause unknown. Therapeutic measures have included elastic stockings, drugs similar to adrenalin, diuretics, and low-sodium diets. Success has been variable.

It's been my experience that chronic idiopathic edema is frequently caused by food allergy. Discovery and strict elimination of all food allergens often eliminates the problem.

Salt restriction is usually also necessary, since individuals with edema frequently report being "sodium sensitive." I recommend total elimination of refined sugar and refined carbohydrate for anyone's good health, but refined sugar has also been found to promote sodium absorption. However, despite the often beneficial effects of salt restriction and refined carbohydrate elimination in cases of idiopathic edema, food allergy is definitely the most important factor.

Exactly how allergy leads to edema isn't known. My guess (and it's only a guess, not proven) is that it represents a mild to moderate degree of "kidney allergy." It's known that some cases of nephrosis (extreme edema and failure of kidney function) can be caused by food allergy, particularly in children. Cow's milk is one food implicated. Again, it's just a guess, but it's possible that cases of idiopathic edema found due to food allergy could be allergic nephrosis in a milder form.

Even if my guess about reasons is wrong, results remain the same. When other causes of edema are excluded—and it's labeled idiopathic—food allergy is frequently the cause, and elimination of allergy the cure.

# REFERENCES

**Allergy and Gallbladder Disease**
Breneman, J. C. "Food Allergy as a Cause of Gallbladder Disease." In *Basics of Food Allergy*. Charles C Thomas, 1978, pp. 67–69.

**Allergy and Kidney Disease**
Cairns, Stephen A.; London, Alison; and Mallick, Netar P. "Circulating Immune Complexes Following Food Delayed Clearance in Idiopathic Glomerulonephritis." *Journal of Clinical and Laboratory Immunology*, vol. 6, 1981, pp. 121–126.

Freed, D. L. J. et al. "Antibodies Against Foods in Renal and Mental Disease." *Clinical Allergy*, vol. 9, 1979, pp. 421–424.

Pirotzky, E. et al. "Basophil Sensitisation in Idiopathic Nephrotic Syndrome." *Lancet*, February 13, 1982, pp. 358–361.

Richards, Warren; Olson, David; and Church, Joseph A. "Improvement of Idiopathic Nephrotic Syndrome Following Allergy Therapy." *Annals of Allergy*, November, 1977, pp. 332–333.

Sandberg, D. H. et al. "Severe Steroid-Responsive Nephrosis Associated With Hypersensitivity." *Lancet*, February 19, 1977, pp. 388–390.

**Blood Pressure and Sodium and Sucrose**
Srinivasan, S. R. et al. "Effects of Dietary Sodium and Sucrose on the Induction of Hypertension in Spider Monkeys." *American Journal of Clinical Nutrition*, March, 1980, pp. 561–569.

**General**
Wintrobe, Maxwell M. et al. *Harrison's Principles of Internal Medicine*. McGraw-Hill, 1974, pp. 176–182.

**Sodium**
Maffly, Ray H. "Disorders of Water, Sodium and Potassium." In Section 10: Nephrology, *Scientific American Medicine*. Scientific American, p. 15.

**The real cause of gallbladder problems may be as simple as their solution. A woman with a ten-year-long history of suffering from the misery of gallbladder pain finds renewed health once she eliminates the foods that are the cause of her problem.**

# 33  A CASE OF GALLBLADDER PAIN AND ALLERGY

"I don't want to have my gallbladder removed! I've never had *any* surgery—except my tonsils out when I was six years old and too little to fight back. I don't want any more done. Besides, my older sister had her gallbladder out, and she's still having gallbladder attacks. Her doctor says there's nothing more to do because her gallbladder's been removed already. So why should I have surgery if it might hurt afterward anyway? I just don't want surgery!"

Susan Vlasuk's report from the radiologist showed one and possibly two stones present in her gallbladder. I'd just read it over with her and she let me know just how she felt about her problem. We'd had the x-rays done, partly at my insistence, to make sure of what her problem was. There really wasn't much doubt: Her symptoms had been fairly typical, and worsening for the last two years.

Starting about ten years ago, she'd noticed "indigestion" after some meals; her "stomach didn't feel right"—maybe a little nauseated—but as it didn't happen very often, she ignored it.

Three to four years later, the symptoms became worse. She started to have more pain, which sometimes was in the stomach, but increasingly seemed to shift to "under my ribs, on the right side."

About this time, her older sister had gallbladder surgery, so she'd become suspicious that her symptoms meant a gallbladder problem. After some reading, she cut down on eating fats, which "helped a little, but didn't get rid of the problem entirely."

Still, she didn't go to a doctor, "because all they could do is take out my gallbladder, and I don't want that." But two years ago, the symptoms became much worse. Her first major attack came in the middle of the night, after an especially big meal. She woke up with intense pain under the ribs on her right side. Her husband drove her to the emergency room, where the diagnosis of cholecystitis (gallbladder inflammation) was made. She was seen by the emergency room doctor and a surgeon, given injections of a strong painkiller, intravenous fluids, held a few hours until the pain started to subside, and sent home.

## Symptoms Worsen

Since that attack, she'd had several more, but only went back to the emergency room once. Her regular doctor had urged her to have x-rays taken and to see a surgeon, as he was convinced it was gallbladder trouble. But she'd resisted. "I thought if the attacks weren't too often, I could just get through. Also, my sister was still having pains after her operation."

Unfortunately, her symptoms increased and intensified. During the months prior to visiting my office, she reported that nearly every day she had a small degree of discomfort or pain in the gallbladder area. Several times each month, she had to take painkillers for two or three days. Four to five days each month, she was in bed with pain. She eliminated all fats, oils, and spices from her daily diet, even though she had previously cut them down considerably.

But that didn't seem to help, either. So she made an appointment "to see if maybe proper diet, vitamins, minerals could give me some help. My doctor said he didn't think so, but why not try, it couldn't hurt. But he said I'd be back to have my gallbladder out, anyway."

At her first visit, I'd upset Mrs. Vlasuk a little by insisting we get x-rays done. She explained she didn't like x-ray exposure, and "that just sounds like the other doctors." I replied that while I agreed her symptoms were unlikely to be anything but gallbladder problems, I wanted to be as certain as possible before recommending any treatment. Also, if I couldn't help her, she'd have to have x-rays before surgery, anyway. She reluctantly agreed.

"So, now what?" she asked, settling down from her initial outburst. "You haven't really said. Isn't there any kind of diet program I can try?"

"Yes, there is. But of course we can't be sure it will work. Sometimes it doesn't."

"Does it dissolve gallstones?"

"I don't think so. But sometimes it relieves all the pain quite well."

"What diet plan is it?"

# The Elimination Diet Approach

"First, I want you to follow Dr. Breneman's elimination diet for people with gallbladder problems. Frequently, that's sufficient to start. If not, I'll want you to try a five-day fast with only distilled water."

"Elimination diet? That sounds like allergy. I've got gallbladder problems! And who's Dr. Breneman?"

"That's exactly right . . . it is an 'allergy-elimination' program. Dr. Breneman's the doctor who discovered and has proven that in many cases gallbladder problems are brought on or aggravated by food allergies."

"That sounds a little far out. I never heard of being allergic in your gallbladder. Are you sure about this Dr. Breneman?"

"Positive. The idea might sound far out, but Dr. Breneman isn't. He's a former member of the board of regents of the American College of Allergists, and past chairman of their Food

Allergy Committee. He kept track of a group of gallbladder patients, all of whom had had stones, and some who'd had their gallbladders removed but still had pain. As long as they didn't eat anything they were allergic to, they had no pain in all that time."

"Did their gallstones go away?"

"I don't know. But what's most important is that the pain disappeared, and in those who still had their gallbladders, no surgery was required."

"Sounds good. Lead me to the diet!"

"Remember, it isn't guaranteed to work. Sometimes it doesn't. But if the initial elimination program isn't helpful, or only partially, then I usually recommend proceeding to a five-day fast. That's because once in a while a person will be allergic to some food on the elimination program. However, Dr. Breneman picked out 'low allergy-risk foods,' so if it's going to work, it usually does on just the elimination program without fasting."

"I hope so. I suppose I'd lose weight fasting, but I'd rather not."

"The list of foods to use is a short one. Please don't eat anything at all not on this list."

"For how long?"

"One week. Usually, if it works, symptoms disappear in three to five days."

"Then what?"

"Then you start adding in foods, one at a time, and we see what your gallbladder tells you. But let's worry about that later, if the elimination program works."

"Then I'd have to fast?"

"I'd recommend trying it. But that doesn't always work either . . . let's see what happens."

## Narrow Choice of Foods for Test

I gave her a list of the foods advised by Dr. Breneman for the elimination trial: beef, rye, soy, rice, cherry, peach, apricot, beet, and spinach. I reminded her to eat or drink nothing else, except water.

One week later, Mrs. Vlasuk was back. She was obviously elated, and pain free. "It worked!" she said. "I had my last pain three days ago! I could just hug that Dr. Breneman. I don't have to have surgery!"

"Hold on. We've only got part of the proof, and it's only been a week. It could be coincidence, too. The hard part is finding out what you're allergic to, because that can bring on the pains again."

"Couldn't I have skin tests, or that new blood test I've heard about? That way I could just eliminate what the test said."

"Skin tests for food allergy really aren't reliable, and while I've seen good clinical results from blood testing, it's not 100 percent perfect either. Remember, the blood test is still new, and relatively expensive. Since you've been able to put up with the pains until now, why not let your body do the rest for you? After all, that's the ultimate test."

Mrs. Vlasuk thought for a minute. "It's been so nice to be pain free for the last three days. I'm sure this is going to work . . . I just feel better all over." She thought again. "You're probably right . . . I should just try the foods on myself. But is it OK if I just stay on this elimination program for a while longer, maybe two or three weeks, before trying other foods again?"

"That makes sense. Then if you change your mind, you could try the blood tests first."

"So what foods do I try? How do I do it?"

I gave her a list of foods taken from Dr. Breneman's article. (See accompanying box.) "Start with the 'high-risk' foods at the top of the list, and work down. If you don't get any reaction, try each one several times before going on to a new food, just in case it takes some time to bring on a reaction. Keep a diary, so you'll remember. Also, notice the large percentages for 'other foods' that aren't specified on the list, and medications. Anything you eat or drink you might be allergic to, so test everything.

"Also, for general good health, it's wise not to eat any refined sugars or refined foods. Even though they might not be allergens for your gallbladder, they cause other health problems. Why not

# Allergy and the Gallbladder

| Food Sensitivity | Percentage of Patients Affected | Food Sensitivity | Percentage of Patients Affected |
|---|---|---|---|
| Egg | 93 | Apple | 8.7 |
| Pork | 64 | Tomato | 8.7 |
| Onion | 52 | Cabbage | 5.8 |
| Fowl | 34.8 | Peas | 5.8 |
| Milk | 24.7 | Peanut | 4.3 |
| Coffee | 21.7 | Spices | 4.3 |
| Orange | 19 | Fish | 2.9 |
| Beans | 14.5 | Rye | 1.5 |
| Corn | 14.5 | Medications | 20.3 |
| Nuts | 14.5 | Other | 42.0 |

SOURCE: Adapted from J. C. Breneman, *Basics of Food Allergy*, 1978. Courtesy of Charles C Thomas, Springfield, Illinois.

get off to a fresh start on a good food program while you're doing this?"

"I've been meaning to do that, anyway. From what I read, I know I should," she replied. Looking at the list, she exclaimed: "Eggs? Onions, fowl, milk? Those are at the top; eggs are 93 percent! No wonder I have trouble. Well, I'll give it a try. Looks like it could take weeks or months to get through everything. But it's worth it, if I can stop these pains and avoid surgery."

Mrs. Vlasuk subsequently found that the foods which provoked her gallbladder were egg, chicken, coffee, peanuts, onions, carrots, and wheat. It's been two years since her last gallbladder attack; her sister, who tried allergy elimination, too, is also pain free. While two years isn't long, Dr. Breneman's original group of patients had gone ten years pain free at the time of his report. I'm reasonably certain that Mrs. Vlasuk will, too.

# The Real Cause
# of Gallbladder Attacks

There's not much more to say about gallbladder disease that wasn't said already in the chapter "Food Sensitivity: Often the Hidden Reason for Persistent Problems." The success of the program created by James C. Breneman, M.D., makes somewhat irrelevant the many and costly studies on dissolution of gallstones with chenodeoxycholic acid—a hot topic in medicine for the past decade or more. If gallstones aren't the real cause of gallbladder attacks, then dissolving them may be an exercise in futility.

Some practitioners of natural medicine advocate a gallbladder flush, using lemon juice, oil, and other substances to persuade the gallbladder to squeeze out its stones through the bile ducts into the intestine and pass them through the bowels. Although that procedure appears to be often successful, it has hazards. If a stone should happen to get stuck in the bile duct, it could precipitate a quick visit to surgery for its removal. The same theoretical hazard exists with gallstone dissolution: A larger stone, too big to pass easily into the bile ducts, could do so as it got smaller, and (again theoretically) get stuck.

Given these theoretical hazards, I don't presently recommend either gallbladder flushes or gallstone dissolution. Putting an end to gallbladder attacks by allergy elimination instead appears to be the best method.

## REFERENCES

**Allergy**
Breneman, J. C. "Allergy Elimination Diet as the Most Effective Gallbladder Diet." *Annals of Allergy*, February, 1968, pp. 83–87.
————. *Basics of Food Allergy.* Charles C Thomas, 1978.

A man suffers severe headaches for ten years without learning their cause. Tests reveal hypoglycemia and allergies to milk products and eggs, among others. A week after altering his diet to eliminate the allergenic foods, his headaches disappear entirely.

# 34 A CASE OF FREQUENT HEADACHES

Sam Roberti came in holding his forehead with his left palm. Distractedly, he looked around for a chair and sat down. Before I could say anything he rubbed his forehead hard, asking: "Do you mind if I take a couple aspirin or something for this headache? I know I'm not supposed to eat before having my checkup and blood tests, but I can tell this is going to be a migraine if I don't take something soon."

I got up to get some water. "That's OK: We can certainly reschedule any tests that medicine would interfere with. Do you have medication with you, or shall I give you something?"

"Well, if it's OK, I have these." He pulled out a small vial from his pocket. "This feels like one of my migraines. If I take them soon enough, they usually cut the pain down to a dull roar. I'm only supposed to take so many per week or my fingers fall off, or something like that."

"Sounds like some sort of ergot preparation." I brought the water; Mr. Roberti swallowed his medicine, rubbed his forehead, and sat down again.

"Thanks. I was afraid you natural-medicine people wouldn't want me to take drugs."

"That's a common misunderstanding. Drugs have their place when absolutely necessary or when nothing else safer works. We do try to find effective natural alternatives as often as possible, though . . . I assume you came in about headaches?"

"Yeah, that's mostly it. Otherwise, I feel pretty good. More tired than I think I should be, but that's probably job pressure."

"How long have headaches been a problem?"

"Twenty years, at least . . . since I got out of college. I'm 43 now and the last ten years have really been bad. Most weeks, I have three or four headaches. Little ones, big ones. I take pain medications all the time."

"You've been told they're migraine?"

"Some of them, definitely. Those are the ones I can tell are coming. They hurt just the left side of my head. Sometimes they last a couple of days. My vision sometimes blurs; occasionally I throw up. It's confusing: Some headaches hurt all over my head instead of just half like a migraine's supposed to. Migraine medicine doesn't work on those."

"What does?"

"Different things. Aspirin, Tylenol, Darvon, codeine, Talwin . . . I've tried nearly everything. Sometimes just a couple cups of coffee helps."

"What sort of tests have you had done?"

"All kinds. I've been to the university, the Mayo Clinic, to a pain clinic, to see several neurologists. Every couple of years for the last ten, I've taken another shot at it. This year my wife, Barbara, talked me into coming here. She thinks vitamins might help, or something like that."

"So you've had x-rays?"

"X-rays, brain scans, brain-wave tests, all sorts of body and urine tests . . . at least they say I don't have a brain tumor."

## Tried Special Diet

"Have you noticed any pattern in your headaches?"

"Yes, I have them all the time! Seriously though, for a while, my wife thought she noticed I was getting more of them in the late afternoon than other times. She thought I got more cranky and irritable at those times, too. I told her, 'Who wouldn't after the days I put in at work,' but I went along. After all, nothing else helped. She got rid of all the sugar, put me on one of those high-protein, low blood sugar diets with whole grains instead of white flour—a health-food diet.''

"What happened?"

"It seemed to help for about a week, but it must have been psychological, because after that I had the worst headaches I'd had in a while. We got rid of the late afternoon ones all right: I had them morning, afternoon, and evening instead, mostly the migraine kind. After three weeks, I gave up, went back to junk food."

"What kinds of food had you eaten more of on the low blood sugar diet?"

"Mostly proteins: more eggs, a little more beef, considerable cheese for snacks—I never have been much of a cheese eater— whole wheat, but not a great deal, since it was a low carbohydrate diet."

"Your late-afternoon headaches went away?"

"I guess so. But I had more headaches overall than before."

"Do you sleep well?"

"Not really. That's another reason I'm tired. I wake up at three or four A.M. and have a hard time getting back to sleep."

"Do you wake up at three or four with a headache?"

"Not always. Maybe every 10 days, two weeks or so. Mostly I just wake up."

"What happens if you don't eat for six or eight hours during the day? Do you get a headache?"

"Frequently, but not always. Helps if I drink coffee, sometimes."

"Do you put sugar in your coffee?"

"Half teaspoon."

"Do you lose your temper easier than you did a few years ago, or get annoyed when there isn't any serious reason?"

Mr. Roberti looked embarrassed. "That's what Barbara says. She's probably right. But I know what you're driving at, the low blood sugar thing. I've tried it, like I told you. It didn't work.

Besides that, some of the doctors I've mentioned it to say there's no such thing as low blood sugar, anyway."

"I don't want to get into that debate at present, except to agree that it is a controversial subject. In my experience, as well as that of most nutrition-oriented physicians, low blood sugar, or hypoglycemia, is found to be one of the most frequent causes of headaches. It does sound like that's part of your problem."

"Why didn't I get any relief then?"

"Low blood sugar is in itself a symptom, the result of disruption of the blood sugar control system. Sometimes it's symptomatic of a sugar-filled, refined diet. Often it's more complicated. Sometimes it has to do with nutrient malabsorption, emotional stress, weak adrenals, food allergy, hormonal problems, lack of exercise, and, I'm sure, other things. Often the causes are multiple."

"So you're saying you think at least some of my headaches are a symptom of hypoglycemia, which might be also a symptom of something else?"

"Possibly."

"What else, then?"

## Allergies Suspected

"Didn't you say you'd gotten worse headaches when you changed your diet, not only going off sugar but altering your food pattern?"

"Yes, but it was all stuff I'd eaten before."

"More of some things, though."

"Sure."

"Does anyone in your family have hay fever or chronic sinus problems?"

"My son has hay fever. So did my mother. How did you know?"

"Didn't. Just thought it possible. Besides hypoglycemia, another common cause of headaches—migraine and other types— is food allergy. So I thought I'd ask about allergy in your family."

"My mother says I had a milk allergy when I was very small, but I grew out of it. I don't have any allergy symptoms now, that I know of."

"Sometimes allergies seem to go away as we grow. Other times they just change symptoms."

"You think my headaches might be allergic?"

"Allergic and hypoglycemic. Those are two very common causes. You've had nearly everything else checked. Why not see if that's it?"

"Sounds too simple. Why didn't anyone tell me that before?"

"Can't say exactly, but you wouldn't see a podiatrist to remove your tonsils, would you?"

"I see what you mean. So what do I do?"

"To nail it down, I think you should have a glucose tolerance test, and tests for food allergies."

"What sort of allergy testing?"

"There are various systems . . . fasting, pulse testing, cytotoxic testing, elimination diets, kinesiology. The one I use most frequently at present is the radioallergosorbent, or RAST test."

"What about skin testing?"

"The commonly used type, scratch testing, isn't accurate. There's another type used by physicians specializing in clinical ecology, which is quite accurate. Clinical ecologists also use sublingual testing. However, it takes specialized training in clinical ecology, which I don't have."

"Well, let's do the type you use now. I've heard of fasting—my wife was telling me—and I don't have time for it."

"Incidentally, it makes a difference where RAST testing is done, too. Different labs get quite different results."

I marked a slip for Mr. Roberti's tests. As I gave it to him, I asked him if he'd been to see an osteopath or chiropractor.

"Did that a few years back," he replied. "Couple of my friends got their headaches cleared up that way. But the osteopath said I didn't have any spinal problem."

I made a note. After his examination was over, he left for the laboratory.

Four weeks later, he was back about his test results. "Well, what's the news?" he said as he sat down.

"Your wife was right. Your six-hour glucose tolerance test did show reactive hypoglycemia—low blood sugar. However, that's not all. You definitely have allergies."

"Which ones?"

# Allergic to Cheese

"Cheddar cheese and milk are the worst. Eggs also are bad. Unfortunately, so are wheat, coffee, corn, and oranges."

"Good grief. No wonder I felt worse when I went on that high-protein diet. I ate a lot of cheese, which I usually don't, plus more eggs and whole-wheat bread. Funny about coffee though. Sometimes it helps my headaches."

"People with hypoglycemia notice that often. Also, some doctors point out that a dose of an allergen will sometimes clear up symptoms caused by its withdrawal. It's like an addiction."

"You mean you can get addicted to something you're allergic to?"

"Clinical ecologists say that's definitely so. Again, it's a controversial point, but I've seen the evidence."

"I do feel worse if I don't get my coffee . . . wait a minute. Does that mean I'll have withdrawal symptoms if I quit all these allergenic foods?"

"Possibly. Also, people often have withdrawal symptoms when they eliminate refined sugar, refined flour, any other sources of caffeine, as well as coffee."

"That's what I should do then? Eliminate all allergy-causing foods, refined sugar, refined flour, coffee, tea, and anything else with caffeine?"

"Looks that way."

"Maybe I better take a few days off work to go through withdrawal."

"Not everyone has withdrawal symptoms. Some don't have any. But if you do, it helps to use extra vitamin C, five to ten grams a day, or more, temporarily, and extra B complex vitamins."

"That's for the withdrawal period?"

"Yes."

"What about later on?"

"Let's discuss that after you fix up your diet. You may not need as many vitamins after you get rid of the allergenic and refined foods."

"Seems reasonable." After some discussion about books concerning hypoglycemia and food allergy, Mr. Roberti left the office.

He subsequently reported that after a withdrawal period of nearly a week, his headaches, the migraine type as well as the nonmigraines, cleared up entirely. Since then he's suffered migraines only when he eats foods he's allergic to.

## Tension Is *Not* the Number One Cause of Headaches

Emanuel Cheraskin, M.D., Ph.D., once told me that "a headache isn't caused by aspirin deficiency." A headache isn't due to a deficiency of stronger pain relievers, either. There's always an underlying cause, yet few of those in orthodox medicine look for one.

In my experience, tension is not the number one cause of a headache. Actually, there are three main causes, which are spinal problems (best treated by a skilled osteopath or chiropractor), allergy or food sensitivities, and blood sugar difficulties. If all these causes are properly searched for and treated when found, the number of headaches truly due to tension becomes very small.

Certainly, brain tumors and other serious problems cause headaches, too. However, the percentage is extremely low. Before wasting considerable time and money on sophisticated medical diagnostic techniques such as CAT scans, EEGs, and the like, I always look for the more common causes first.

Migraines are among the most devastating of all headaches. Many appear to be due to food sensitivity, including allergy, an identification which has been made in dozens of publications since the 1920s. Despite the success of food allergy elimination reported by many authors, it's resolutely ignored by almost all physicians, except allergists. Even among allergists, agreement on foods as a principal cause of migraine is variable, in large part depending on the accuracy of the test system used to uncover food allergy. The subgroup of allergists called clinical ecologists appear to have the greatest success with migraine treatment. They are concerned with tracking down the cause or causes of the migraine whether it be from food, water, air, or environmental chemicals.

For doctors not trained in clinical ecology, RAST testing can show with great success which cases are due to food allergy, and identify the individual food culprits with a high degree of accuracy. (Care must be taken to use an accurate variety of the RAST test, however.) Nearly all individuals I've worked with who suffer from migraines have had some type of food allergy involvement.

A publication in the *Annals of Allergy* further confirms allergies as a cause of migraine. According to Ernst Thonnard-Neumann, M.D., and Leonard M. Neckers, Ph.D., levels of blood cells involved in the allergic response are significantly different in migraine sufferers. The same investigators reported that substantial relief from migraine can be obtained with low doses of heparin, a natural substance in the body that prevents blood clots. In individuals responding to heparin, migraine relief coincided with changes in the number of cells involved in the allergic response.

Nonallergic food and chemical sensitivity due to a deficient intestinal enzyme has been identified. One form of the enzyme phenolsulfotransferase, which breaks down both natural and synthetic food chemicals containing phenols, has been found at lower than normal amounts in the intestines of migraine sufferers by Vivette Glover, Ph.D., of Bernhard Baron Memorial Research Laboratories and Queen Charlotte's Hospital for Women, London. It's been suspected for years (and confirmed in the case of phenylethylamine, a chemical naturally present in chocolate) that foods containing chemicals comprised partly of phenyl groups may contribute to migraine. This research reported in *Family Practice News* appears to have uncovered one of the reasons.

Some headaches diagnosed as migraine can be relieved by removal of refined sugar, processed foods, and by adding more frequent small meals, and other hypoglycemia treatment. Some argue that any headaches relieved in this manner are not "true migraines," but some other kind. Exact definitions are important in medicine, but to the headache sufferer diagnosed with migraine, relief is more important than what the headache is called. As I've observed many migraine headaches (diagnosed by competent neurologists) partly or completely relieved with hypoglycemia diagnosis and treatment, I think hypoglycemia should be looked for in all headache sufferers, including those said to have migraine.

# REFERENCES

**Allergy**

Balyeat, Ray M., and Brittain, Fannie Lou. "Allergic Migraine: Based on the Study of Fifty-five Cases." *American Journal of Medical Science*, vol. 180, 1930, pp. 212–221.

Catterall, William E. *Allergy as the Cause of Migraine—A Literature Review*. William E. Catterall, 1979.

Grant, Ellen C. G. "Food Allergies and Migraine." *Lancet*, May 5, 1979, pp. 966–968.

Heymann, Harry. "Migraine and Food Allergy: A Survey of 20 Cases." *South African Medical Journal*, November, 1952, pp. 949–950.

Messer, William. "Headache and Allergy." *Annals of Allergy*, October, 1960, pp. 1117–1125.

Monroe, Jean et al. "Food Allergy in Migraine." *Lancet*, July 5, 1980, pp. 1–4.

Randolph, Theron G. "Allergic Headache: An Unusual Case of Milk Sensitivity." *Journal of the American Medical Association*, October 14, 1944, pp. 430–432.

Sandler, M. "A Phenylethylamine Oxidising Defect in Migraine." *Nature*, July 26, 1974, pp. 335–337.

Shapiro, Richard S., and Eisenberg, Ben C. "Allergic Headache." *Annals of Allergy*, March, 1965, pp. 123–125.

Sheldon, John M., and Randolph, Theron G. "Allergy in Migraine-like Headaches." *American Journal of Medical Science*, vol. 190, 1935, pp. 232–235.

Unger, Albert H. "Allergy and Headaches." *Annals of Allergy*, September–October, 1955, pp. 523–532.

Unger, Albert H., and Unger, Leon. "Migraine Is An Allergic Disease." *Journal of Allergy*, vol. 23, 1952, pp. 429–440.

Unger, Leon, and Cristol, Joel L. "Allergic Migraine." *Annals of Allergy*, March, 1970, pp. 106–108.

Wilson, C. W. M. et al. "The Clinical Features of Migraine as a Manifestation of Allergic Disease." *Postgraduate Medical Journal*, September, 1980, pp. 617–621.

### Headache

Caviness, Verne S., and O'Brien, Patrick. "Current Concepts: Headache." *New England Journal of Medicine*, February 21, 1980, pp. 446–450.

"Lack of Digestive Enzyme May Cause Dietary Migraine." *Family Practice News*, September 1–14, 1982, p. 26.

Skultety, F. Miles. "Headache—Part I." *The Female Patient*, vol. 5, 1980, pp. 22–24.

### Immunity

Thonnard-Neumann, Ernst, and Neckers, Leonard M. "Immunity in Migraine: The Effect of Heparin." *Annals of Allergy*, November, 1981, pp. 328–332.

———. "T-Lymphocytes in Migraine." *Annals of Allergy*, November, 1981, pp. 325–327.

### RAST Test

Adkinson, N. Franklin. "Cost, Quality Control, Clinical Threshold Still Problems of RAST." *Family Practice News*, April 15–30, 1982, p. 49.

### Sucrose

Dexter, James D.; Roberts, John; and Byer, John A. "The Five Hour Glucose Tolerance Test and Effect of Low Sucrose Diet in Migraine." *Headache*, May, 1978, pp. 91–94.

> Three years ago, a man begins having PVCs—premature ventricular contractions. He runs 20 miles a week, eats a good diet (no caffeine, little beef or eggs, a variety of vegetables and whole grains, and little milk or cheese), and takes vitamin supplements, yet his condition remains the same. Though most tests come out negative, a mineral analysis shows an imbalance in his copper and zinc levels. By adjusting those minerals, the PVCs are completely eliminated.

# A CASE OF IRREGULAR HEARTBEAT 35

Mr. Harold Herter looked fit. Although dressed in slacks and a casual shirt, his running shoes hinted at one reason for his "in-shape" appearance. I thought perhaps he was here for a "staying-healthy" visit and checkup, but he had a bothersome symptom.

"It's my heartbeat," he said, pointing to his chest. "One cardiologist says it probably isn't dangerous, and that I shouldn't worry about it. The other cardiologist agrees it probably isn't going to kill me, but he thinks I ought to take medication anyway, particularly since it's getting worse, not better. I did a little reading. It's confusing. But with my family history, I'm still worried. I'd like to see if these isn't something I can do about it with diet or vitamins."

"What sort of problem is it?"

"One cardiologist called it 'PVCs'—premature ventricular contractions; the other said ventricular premature beats. The book I was reading said those were the same thing."

"That's so. Have you had any other problems, like chest pain?"

"No, never. The last few years, I've been watching my diet, running regularly. I'm up to 20 miles a week, and never have a twinge."

"Do you have more irregular beats when you run?"

"About the same, maybe a little less."

## A Fluttery Feeling

"Tell me how it feels."

"Like I said, no pain. I get a fluttery feeling in my chest. Sometimes just once, sometimes repeatedly for several hours. Also, occasionally there's a . . . well, the closest I can describe it is a large thump. Really a surprise when it happens."

"How long have you had the PVCs?"

"About three years. They're more frequent recently, which is why I went to the cardiologist. My father died of heart trouble when he was only 66, and my grandfather, Mother's father, took digitalis for a heartbeat problem before he died of a heart attack. You can see why I'm worried."

"In addition to running, you're watching your diet?"

"Yes. I cut out all the caffeine, coffee, tea, chocolate, and colas, because I heard caffeine could aggravate heartbeat problems. I eat very little pork or beef anymore, butter and eggs only occasionally. You might know, the last two years my cholesterol reading has gotten higher! The last time, I had one of those high-density cholesterol tests done, and it wasn't so good. It's frustrating, because I'm running, watching my diet, taking my vitamins, and I'm getting more PVCs and worse cholesterol tests. I'm beginning to think maybe heart trouble is just inevitable in my family."

"Don't give up yet. There may be some other things to do, or not do. Is there still any sugar in your diet?"

Mr. Herter looked embarrassed. "Yes, although we don't have a sugar bowl in the house anymore. I do have an occasional weakness for sweets. And we don't read labels as carefully as we should on packaged foods. Just the other day I noticed the salt container . . . we use that very lightly . . . said it also contained dextrose. That's a form of sugar, isn't it?"

"Yes."

"There is diabetes in my family, too. But the books I looked at didn't say anything about diabetes or sugar and PVCs."

"That's true. Most of the books don't say so, but sometimes hypoglycemia (low blood sugar) is associated with a variety of heartbeat irregularities, including PVCs. I think you'd best check for that, especially since there's diabetes in your family."

"Six-hour glucose tolerance test?"

"That's the one."

"My daughter had it a few years back. She was having weak spells, passing out. They told her it was negative, but she cut out all the sugar, and the spells went away. She's been after me about cutting out sugar ever since. I don't have fainting spells, though, or get weak."

"Hypoglycemia doesn't always produce the same symptoms. The range of symptoms is incredibly diverse. We'd better check, anyway."

"That's fine. I wasn't arguing."

We reviewed the rest of Mr. Herter's diet. Except for not eliminating refined sugar and artificial food chemicals, he'd done well. He ate a variety of vegetables, both raw and cooked, mostly steamed. Beans, nuts, seeds, and whole grains were all included. Animal protein was comprised mostly of fish and chicken, with beef or eggs occasionally. He ate cheese and drank milk from time to time. Several years before, he'd switched to distilled water, to avoid chlorine, fluoride, and asbestos, all known to be in his city's water.

## Prostate Problems

Most of his health history was negative. He had had hay fever as a teenager and in his twenties, however, and lately a touch of prostate difficulty. I thought I'd better ask more about these problems.

"You have hay fever anymore?"

"Not really. Haven't had much trouble for over 30 years now. I do get a little nasal stuffiness every once in a while, but that's all."

"Any other allergy symptoms?"

"Such as?"

"Nearly any symptom can be allergy related, even heartbeat irregularity. That's why I'm asking. But what I meant were common symptoms, like hives, eczema, or sinusitis."

"None of those. Except for prostate symptoms and occasional colds, I'd been well for years, until these PVCs showed up."

"Any allergies in your family?"

"Well, yes, my daughter, the one who seems to be sugar sensitive, she still has allergy troubles—eczema. She could have gotten that from my wife's side, though. They have lots of asthma and allergy."

"Even so, I'd recommend some allergy screening."

"OK, if it's possibly involved in causing irregular heartbeats."

"You mentioned prostate symptoms?"

"Those are gone now. That's another problem my father had. Needed surgery, he got so bad. I think I have my problem taken care of, though."

"What symptoms did you have?"

"When I was 55, I started having to get up to urinate more often at night. I tried to ignore it, but during the next year I couldn't anymore. I had to wait to urinate. The force of the stream was definitely decreased; there was more dribbling. Not only that, the doctor told me there was definitely enlargement.

"I did some reading on prostate trouble. First I tried pumpkin seeds. Then I found an article that talked about zinc and essential fatty acids from vegetable oil. I took 50 milligrams of zinc, and 1½ tablespoons of linseed oil daily, and six months later, no more prostate symptoms, and none since. I've continued to make sure my prostate stays normal. I also take digestive enzymes to make sure the zinc and oil are absorbed properly."

"Sounds like you do a lot of reading."

"Have to. Don't want to let these problems just sneak up on me. I realize I have to take an active part in staying healthy. That's why I'm bothered that I can't get these PVCs to go away, with all I'm doing."

"I can understand that. What other vitamins do you take?"

"Vitamin E, 400 international units, both for general health and to prevent any possible side effects from taking the vegetable oil for essential fatty acids. Vitamin C, one gram twice daily. B complex for stress, a multiple vitamin, and lecithin. I added that two years ago when my cholesterol went up, but it hasn't helped."

Mr. Herter's examination was normal except for his PVCs, which "cooperated" by showing up at the rate of approximately one every two minutes. He had no spinal problems that might contribute to heartbeat abnormality. Even his prostate examination was normal: no enlargement. Apparently it had receded, along with his symptoms.

As we'd discussed, I asked him to have a six-hour glucose tolerance test done to check for hypoglycemia. Also, I recommended allergy screening tests, a mineral analysis of a hair specimen, and routine "blood chemistry" screening, which included cholesterol and high-density cholesterol (HDL) measurements.

# Blood Sugar Normal

When Mr. Herter returned, he mentioned his glucose tolerance test right away. "In a way, I'm disappointed," he said. "The nurse said my test was normal. She said you don't recommend eating refined sugar anyway, just on general health grounds, but there was nothing else special to do. I was certain that was the cause of my problem, with diabetes in my family."

I looked at his test record. "I've seen low blood sugar elimination clear up many benign heartbeat irregularities, but in your case there really isn't any low blood sugar problem to eliminate."

"I got rid of the sugar anyway, as the nurse said. I'd been meaning to all along. But you're right, I still have the PVCs. So what about any allergies?"

"There's a minor one reported for Cheddar cheese, and another minor one for beef. That's all."

"Not enough to cause my problem?"

"Probably not, although even minor allergies can do strange things sometimes."

Mr. Herter looked disappointed. "So you don't know what's causing the PVCs then?"

"Not yet. There is a configuration of evidence in your case, however, that points to a possible explanation. And even in cases where the cause is uncertain, treatment with minerals—magnesium, manganese, copper, and others—can sometimes be helpful."

"What other evidence is there in my case?"

"To start, you're slightly anemic. Not bad, just a little, but still anemic."

"That's odd, the doctor last year said I was close to being anemic. He didn't recommend iron—he was sure it would correct itself. It's worse now?"

"Looks that way. Second, your cholesterol is still a little high, 293, and the HDL is too low at 41."

Mr. Herter pulled out a slip of paper. "I brought in the numbers from last year. Cholesterol 288, HDL 44. This year's a little worse. But what's that got to do with PVCs?"

## Low Copper Level

"Putting that together with the copper and zinc levels on your mineral analysis, it suggests strongly that too much zinc and/or too little copper may be the problem."

"Is my zinc level high?"

"No, it's low-normal. But your copper level is very low. It's probable zinc wouldn't cause trouble if your copper levels were better."

"Too much zinc and too little copper can cause PVCs?"

"Yes, and cholesterol abnormalities, besides. There's quite a bit of work by Dr. Klevay on the zinc/cholesterol problem. Zinc and PVC difficulty so far has only been described in three cases, by Dr. Spencer, an alert clinician who wrote a letter to the editor of the *American Journal of Clinical Nutrition* about it. Since that time, I've seen a few other cases. Yours appears to be one of them.

"Also, excess zinc and too little copper can lead to anemia."

Mr. Herter looked thoughtful. "It all fits. I started taking zinc for my prostate four years ago. Started getting PVCs three years ago, cholesterol got a little higher two years ago, almost anemic last year, anemic this year. And I drink distilled water. I understand a lot of copper comes from water pipes."

"That's so. But considering what else comes from water pipes, it's frequently better to get copper elsewhere."

"My prostate symptoms have done so well. You even said the size is back to normal. I don't want to stop zinc. Can I take zinc and copper both?"

"Yes, although the amount of zinc should be cut back temporarily until the copper starts to work. As you can see on your mineral test, you do need zinc. The levels are only low-normal. If you stopped it and took only copper, the copper would probably in time lead to the opposite problem—too little zinc."

"My prostate symptoms could return?"

"Possibly, or perhaps another low-zinc difficulty."

# A Matter of Balance

"So it's not really that zinc is bad or good, or copper either. It's a matter of balancing the two properly."

"Exactly, in your case and most others. Too much zinc with too little copper, you get anemia, PVCs, cholesterol abnormalities. Too little zinc, you get prostate problems. Enough of both, you should be OK."

Mr. Herter took 30 milligrams of zinc and 5 milligrams of copper daily for six months. He took them at different times of day, as (theoretically) they might "compete" for absorption.

His PVCs disappeared in a month. His anemia was gone in three months, reverting to a normal blood count. By six months, his cholesterol was 233, with HDL 47, a much better cholesterol/

HDL ratio. Also in six months, his hair mineral analysis was nearly normal for copper. His zinc level, however, had dropped slightly.

After another readjustment of dosage, he's settled on 50 milligrams of zinc and 3 milligrams of copper daily. His prostate symptoms and PVCs have both stayed away; his blood count and cholesterol are rechecked regularly, and remain normal.

## No Therapy Is Risk Free for Everyone

As a general rule, vitamins, minerals, and other natural therapies are much safer than drugs. Side effects produced by nutrients are frequently beneficial; nearly all drug side effects are harmful.

Despite a greater degree of safety, no type of therapy (vitamin, mineral, and other natural therapies included) is totally risk free for everyone. As more research is done on nutrient therapy, it's almost certain other hazards will be uncovered.

Ordinarily, overdoing zinc leads to copper-deficiency anemia and lower levels of HDL cholesterol, rather than irregular heart-beat. Carl Pfeiffer, M.D., Ph.D., a pioneering researcher in nutritional biochemistry, reported a case in which an average 2,300 milligrams of zinc was taken daily. The individual had extremely low levels of copper, undetectable copper transport protein, a low white blood cell count, slightly low blood proteins (albumin and globulin), and very high levels of an enzyme, alkaline phosphatase. (She had also taken extra vitamin C, which may have protected against some adverse effects.) No effects on the heart were reported.

Stopping excess zinc intake and starting copper treatment successfully reversed all abnormalities in one to four weeks. This case represents "most zinc taken" as far as is known.

Sometimes side effects can be put to good use. Wilson's disease is a metabolic disorder in which large excesses of copper accumulate in the body. Symptoms can be severe. Three groups of investigators have reported that zinc, taken orally, can prevent the accumulation of copper in the body, and rid the body of already accumulated excess. Symptoms of the disease improve; many of them disappear. Although zinc treatment requires monitoring, one individual was reported to have taken it for 14 years, with great improvement in Wilson's disease and no serious side effects. The investigators, overlooking zinc's identity as a mineral, stated that "zinc sulfate can be regarded as a relatively nontoxic drug." It also appears that zinc treatment may be preferable to the standard drug therapy for this disease.

# REFERENCES

**Copper**

Allen, Kenneth G. D., and Klevay, Leslie M. "Hyperlipoproteinemia in Rats Due to Copper Deficiency." *Nutrition Reports International*, August, 1980, pp. 295–299.

**Copper/Zinc Ratio**

Klevay, Leslie M. "Coronary Heart Disease: the Zinc/Copper Hypothesis." *American Journal of Clinical Nutrition*, July, 1975, pp. 764–774.

Murthy, Lalitha, and Petering, Harold G. "Effect of Dietary Zinc and Copper Interrelationships on Blood Parameters of the Rat." *Journal of Agricultural and Food Chemistry*, July–August, 1976, pp. 808–811.

Porter, K. G. et al. "Anemia and Low Serum Copper During Zinc Therapy." *Lancet*, October 8, 1977, p. 774.

Spencer, Jack C. "Direct Relationship Between the Body's Copper/Zinc Ratio, Ventricular Premature Beats and Sudden Coronary Death." *American Journal of Clinical Nutrition*, June, 1979, pp. 1184–1185.

**Zinc**

Hoogenrood, T. U.; Koevoet, R.; and de Ruyter Korver, E. G. W. M. "Oral Zinc Sulphate as Long-Term Treatment in Wilson's Disease (Hepatolenticular Degeneration)." *European Neurology*, vol. 18, no. 3, 1979, pp. 205–211.

Hoogenrood, T. U. et al. "Oral Zinc in Wilson's Disease." *Lancet*, December 9, 1978, p. 1262.

Hooper, Philip L. et al. "Zinc Lowers High-Density Lipoprotein Cholesterol Levels." *Journal of the American Medical Association*, October 24/31, 1980, pp. 1060–1061.

Pfeiffer, Carl C.; Papaioannon, Rhoda; and Sohler, Arthur. "Effect of Chronic Zinc Intoxication on Copper Levels, Blood Formation and Polyamines." *Journal of Orthomolecular Psychiatry*, vol. 9, no. 2, 1980, pp. 79–89.

A man suffering for years from heartburn uncontrolled by antacids finds relief by avoiding nicotine, caffeine, and fatty foods. These dietary changes plus supplements of choline and lecithin tightened the lower esophageal sphincter muscle, which had malfunctioned and caused his problem.

# A CASE OF HEARTBURN 36

"I'm tired of swallowing antacids all the time. I've bought hundreds of pounds the last few years. That can't be good. Besides, my wife's been nagging me to eat differently since she started reading about nutrition. So here I am."

Morris Goldberg was at the office for his first visit. He spoke with energy and great intensity.

"How often do you take antacids?"

"Every day. I get burning pain that starts here, and goes up my chest. Sometimes practically to my throat." He indicated his stomach, sweeping his hand upward through the middle of his chest. "Typical heartburn, goes with the job, but nobody can give me a reason other than that. Stress, pressure is what I'm told."

"What sort of work do you do?"

"I own a small company. It's doing OK, considering, but keeping it that way is two full-time jobs, at least."

"How about when you're on vacation?"

"What's a vacation? Seriously, it might be a little better when we're away, but I had one of my worst attacks in Hawaii last year.

Even went to the hospital, my wife was worried it was a heart attack. It wasn't—just the same thing, worse."

"Is it worse after you eat, or when your stomach's empty?"

"Either one. I can't figure that out."

"Does the pain wake you up at night?"

"Sometimes, nights in a row. Other times, not for weeks."

"Ever have blood in your bowel movements, or black ones, like tar?"

"No, no, I know what you're thinking, like digested blood from an ulcer. It's not an ulcer. I've had upper GI x-rays twice, all clean. No ulcer. Not even one of those what-do-you-call-them hernia things."

"Hiatus hernia?"

"That's it. The one from the stomach into the esophagus that lets the acid come back up, right? They were sure I had that, but I don't."

"When were you x-rayed last?"

"A couple years ago. I take a shot at this thing every two or three years. Don't have time more often."

# Personal Habits Questioned

"Do you smoke?"

"Yeah, cigars, three to six a day."

"Drink coffee?"

"Three, four cups a day. One doctor told me coffee probably made it worse, so I cut down from 10, 12 cups."

"Do you eat any refined sugar?"

"Some, but I don't make a habit of it. You're starting to sound like my wife. 'Morris,' she says, 'Morris, if you'd just stop smoking, drinking coffee, and eating sugar, I'm sure you'd feel so much better.' So, maybe she's right, but I want some proof before I stop everything I like."

"Do you get any constipation or diarrhea?"

"Not really. Maybe a little constipation every once in a while, but nothing to speak of."

I asked Mr. Goldberg other general questions about his health and his diet. He had few other symptoms: sometimes slight headaches if he didn't eat, waking up at night and not getting back to sleep. He ate too few fresh vegetables, and still consumed refined sugar and flour.

His physical examination was fairly normal. A little out of shape, but no obvious disease. As we finished, I advised him of this.

"So you're going to tell me it's stress—I'll have to put up with it until I retire or sell out? Or is it the cigars and sugar?"

"Let's look for some proof first, as you said. I'd recommend we do tests for stomach acid and blood sugar, as well as routine screening tests."

"I understand the routine screening; my wife told me this checkup is for preventive reasons, too. She wants to be sure I get my cholesterol checked. But why check the blood sugar or stomach acid? Isn't it obvious I have too much? I've had two x-rays already."

"You could have too much stomach acid, or a normal amount, or even too little. In fact, sometimes too little stomach acid goes with heartburn symptoms. I'll admit, your symptoms sound like too much acid, but I'd like to know for sure.

"The only other symptoms you mentioned, headaches when you don't eat and waking up at night frequently, are characteristic of poor blood sugar control, hypoglycemia."

"Doesn't everyone get headaches if they don't eat?"

"Definitely not. People with good blood sugar control can go all day without eating, with no headache."

"That so? OK, let's check. That's what I'm here for."

## Some Improvement Reported

Several weeks later, Mr. Goldberg was back. His tests had shown a mild reactive hypoglycemia (low blood sugar), and an overproduction of stomach acid. Screening tests disclosed low blood levels of pancreatic enzymes and a few trace element deficiencies.

As he'd had his glucose tolerance test for hypoglycemia just a week after his checkup, his wife had already bought books on hypoglycemia and removed all the refined sugar from his diet at home. He'd kept on the program when eating out, and had stopped drinking coffee as advised.

"So I'm sleeping better at night," he said. "But I'm still getting headaches if I don't eat, and my heartburn isn't much better, only a little. What's that got to do with heartburn, anyway? I came in here about acid stomach pain up into my chest and taking antacids. You tell me I've got a little hypoglycemia, not to eat sugar or coffee, but I'm still taking antacids. Only my wife's happy; she's been telling me about coffee and sugar for years."

"You're right, that's not the whole picture, but it is related. Remember your radiotelemetry test showed a little too much stomach acid? Well, in the long run, reducing overproduction of stomach acid will be helpful, even if you don't have an ulcer. Sure, the main thing is keeping the acid in the right place, your stomach, instead of up in your esophagus. But less of it would be helpful, too.

"It's fairly well known that caffeine stimulates stomach acid production. Not just caffeine in coffee, but in chocolate, black tea, and cocoa. But hypoglycemia stimulates stomach acid production, too. So cutting out caffeine and controlling hypoglycemia should be helpful in the long run."

# Pressure You Need

"Now, about keeping the acid where it belongs: Have you ever heard of something called the lower esophageal sphincter?"

"No, what's that?"

"Unfortunately, it's a slightly misleading term. Sphincter means a ring of muscle, like a valve, and there actually isn't a well-defined ring of muscle separating the esophagus from the stomach. But there is a high pressure zone normally present at the lower esophagus that prevents regurgitation of stomach contents. That keeps most of us from having chronic heartburn. I think you have a malfunction of this zone, allowing the acid to come back up. In your case, too much acid makes it worse."

"That sounds like one of those hiatus hernia things that lets stomach acid through."

"No, in fact it's possible to have a hiatus hernia and no heartburn if the lower esophageal sphincter pressure is normal. It's also possible to have no hiatus hernia and heartburn if the pressure is too low. I think that's your problem."

"So what I need is higher pressure at the lower esophageal sphincter? That'll keep the acid in the right place—my stomach not my esophagus—and I won't have heartburn, if I follow this. So what do I do"?

"Well, one thing is to stop smoking."

"Smoking? That, too? Rachel will be so happy. I can hear it now, 'I told you so, Morris.' Why smoking? I knew maybe smoking causes cancer, but heartburn?"

"Remember that proof you asked about? Well, researchers have measured lower esophageal pressure before and after smoking. Smoking decreases the pressure, allowing the stomach contents to escape back into the esophagus."

"So why doesn't everyone who smokes have bad heartburn?"

"Some have stronger esophageal sphincters than others. By the way, nicotine in tobacco isn't the only thing these researchers found to lower the pressure. Caffeine and fatty meals do, also. There are certainly unknown factors, too, that will lower it."

Three months later, Mr. Goldberg reported his heartburn was much better. "The hardest part was stopping smoking. But as long as I don't smoke or drink coffee or go off my diet, I only have to take antacids maybe twice a week.

"By the way, you didn't say sugar lowers the esophageal pressure, but when I eat it, I get more burning."

"I don't know about sugar for sure. I can't find any reports of tests. But I hear that frequently."

# Choline and Lecithin
# May Relieve Heartburn

While removing tobacco and coffee, both of which relax the lower esophageal sphincter and allow acid reflux, is very important, there are also two food supplements available which can promote tightening of the sphincter and aid in reflux prevention.

The first of these is choline. One of the many important functions of choline in the body is to serve as part of the acetylcholine molecule, a major nerve-transmitter substance. Choline research is very popular at present in psychiatry and neurology, since it's been observed that extra choline can stimulate the formation of more acetylcholine in the body, and possibly influence the course of nervous system ailments. In my own practice I've found it useful, along with pantothenate, thiamine, and manganese, for individuals with myasthenia gravis—a disease of progressive muscle weakness caused by a loss of receptors for acetylcholine on muscle membrane. Presumably by increasing the supply of acetylcholine, choline can aid in this disease, although definitely not as a cure.

Donald Castell, M.D., who's published considerable practical research on the function of the lower esophageal sphincter, found that a synthetic drug which mimics the function of acetylcholine would increase lower esophageal sphincter pressure, decreasing acid reflux and the symptoms of heartburn. Taking the cue from Dr. Castell's work, and following the more conservative approach of nutritional biochemistry, I've tried choline and found that it also works. I've concluded this, however, more from the reduction of symptoms than from measurements of sphincter pressure, as I don't have the equipment for the latter.

Sometimes choline is effective all by itself, in amounts from one gram daily to one gram four times a day. Sometimes it has to be accompanied by extra thiamine, pantothenate, and manganese.

Lecithin is the other supplement that's frequently effective. Studies have shown that lecithin acts like time-release choline, producing much longer sustained blood levels of choline. (Remember, choline is one of the components of which lecithin is made.)

There appears to be a group of chronic heartburn sufferers with lower esophageal sphincter incompetence. The sphincter zone just doesn't work right, even if no known inhibitors of it (such as tobacco or coffee) are being used. These individuals have the problem without (as far as is known) causing it themselves.

# REFERENCES

**Antacids**
Castell, Donald O., and Levine, Stephen M. "Lower Esophageal Sphincter Response to Gastric Alkalinization: A New Mechanism for Treatment of Heartburn with Antacids." *Annals of Internal Medicine*, February, 1971, pp. 223–227.

**Choline**
Hirsch, Madelyn J.; Growdon, John H.; and Wurtman, Richard J. "Relations Between Dietary Choline or Lecithin Intake, Serum Choline Levels, and Various Metabolic Indices." *Metabolism*, August, 1978, pp. 953–960.

**Diet**
Castell, Donald O. "Diet and the Lower Esophageal Sphincter." *American Journal of Clinical Nutrition*, November, 1975, pp. 1296-1298.

**Heartburn**
Castell, Donald O. "Heartburn: A Modern Look at an Ancient Problem." *Medical Opinion*, July, 1971, pp. 20–25.

**Hiatus Hernia**
Cohen, Sidney, and Harris, Lauren. "Does Hiatus Hernia Affect Competence of the Gastroesophageal Sphincter?" *New England Journal of Medicine*, May 13, 1971, pp. 1053–1056.

**Smoking**
Dennish, George W., and Castell, Donald O. "Inhibitory Effect of Smoking on the Lower Esophageal Sphincter." *New England Journal of Medicine*, May 20, 1971, pp. 1136–1137.

A man suffering from an embarrassing case of herpes between his upper lip and nose eliminates chocolate and peanuts and finds relief after years of suffering. Adding supplements of the amino acid lysine helps keep his attacks under control.

# 37 A CASE OF HERPES SIMPLEX (COLD SORES AND FEVER BLISTERS)

George Herbert knew exactly what his problem was. Everyone else could see it, too. He had a large, angry red sore between his upper lip and nose.

"I just can't go to work like this, " he remarked. "Would you buy a car from a salesman who looked like me? People cross the room to avoid me. I've gotten used to missing work from two to three weeks when I feel it coming on. The boss is understanding, but I'm going to have to look for another line of work, away from people, if this keeps up. I've lost too much income over the last four to five years, with several weeks layoff each year."

"I assume you've tried various treatments before?"

"Sure. I've been to two or three dermatologists, and up to the university. They all tell me the same thing: It's herpes simplex infection, and there isn't any treatment that'll kill it. I've had dyes put on it, with light shined on the dye. Lots of ointments. None of that helped at all. What seems to help the most is putting vitamin E on it, and taking lots of vitamin C, ten grams a day or more. I figured that might help because it's a virus, and vitamin C is supposed to help against viruses. But even that only helps it feel a little better. It still looks just as bad, and lasts as long. Still, since the vitamins did a little bit better than anything else, I thought I'd come over here to see if there was anything else in the vitamin line to do."

"Let's have a look at it." I got up, and motioned for Mr. Herbert to come into the examination room.

"Excuse me, this will be a little warm." I pulled the light closer, and shined it on the sore for a better look. It was roughly circular, and between the size of a quarter and a half-dollar. There were numerous tiny blisters, about the size of a pinhead or a little larger, all clumped together, appearing to be set on a base of red, angry-looking skin. The blisters appeared to be filled with clear-to-yellowish fluid.

"Looks like a herpes sore, all right," I said, turning the light off.

"I know you have to look for yourself, but I told you that. It always comes back in the same place, too, like herpes is supposed to. I guess I'm just lucky it doesn't spread. It's contagious, so I can't just put a bandage over it and go to work. I'm told that wouldn't stop the spread that much."

"Probably not. Has your wife caught it?"

"She's had herpes on and off since she was a girl, but not near as bad."

"Come on back to my office, please."

Mr. Herbert and I went back to the adjacent room and sat down.

# A Taste for Chocolate

"Tell me what you eat every day."

"Regular meals: meat, potatoes . . . "

"Please start with breakfast, and mention as many items as you can think of that you might have at each meal."

"Well, for breakfast, I have eggs, ham, or some kind of cereal, toast, jam. My wife gets sugar-free cereals, and jam with honey, but I'm afraid I do drink cocoa quite frequently. Really like the stuff.

"I usually take sandwiches to work for lunch. Whole-wheat bread, usually peanut butter or tuna fish. Usually hot chocolate or coffee to drink. Sometimes, though, I get a salad and cottage cheese.

"Dinners vary a lot. Usually beef, chicken, or fish. Always potatoes and vegetables. I really like peas, beans, corn. Salad with that. Sometimes we have spaghetti or casseroles."

"Do you drink soft drinks?"

"No. I really do avoid sugar most all the time. My only vice is chocolates. I eat more chocolate and peanut bars than I should."

"Several a week?"

Mr. Herbert looked embarrassed. "Yeah, I guess so. But I avoid all the other sugar. My other snacks are mostly nuts like almonds, walnuts, cashews, or pumpkin or sesame seeds. My wife says those are really nutritious: She keeps track of those sorts of things better than I do. She says I'm doing lots better than I used to on my diet, and actually I feel better, too. I take the vitamins she gives me every day."

"Which ones are those"?

"Let me think . . . C, E, A, and D. I don't know the rest. I really do feel better than when I used to eat more junk food. If it weren't for this darn herpes. I actually think it may be worse, since I've changed my diet over."

"Unfortunately, you may be eating your way into recurrent herpes attacks, even though your are doing better on your diet."

Mr. Herbert looked surprised. "Really? Don't tell me I have to give up chocolate. It's the only sugar-containing food I still eat. Sugar doesn't cause herpes, does it? Besides, I'm eating lots less sugar than I ever did."

"No, it's not the sugar in this case, although as you know sugar of the refined sort isn't good for anyone. But the chocolate may be part of the problem."

Mr. Herbert looked disgruntled. "There goes my last food vice. But if it'll help get rid of this . . ." He pointed to his upper lip. "What makes you think I'm eating my way into herpes attacks?"

# Two Key Amino Acids

"Let me explain. Do you know what amino acids are?"

"Sort of."

"They're the subunits that proteins are made of. Proteins are amino acids linked together in long, complex chains. Proteins are mostly digested into smaller amino acid subunits, absorbed, and rearranged into our own body proteins.

"The two amino acids that appear to be important in herpes infections are lysine and arginine. Scientists reported that arginine induces the growth and reproduction of the herpes simplex virus, while lysine inhibits the virus. What's important is the ratio of arginine to lysine. The higher the arginine to lysine ration, the more herpes virus is likely to grow. Conversely, if lysine is high with respect to arginine, the growth is inhibited."

"So, if my food has a high arginine to lysine ratio, I'm more likely to set off herpes?"

"Exactly. Scientists have shown this in virus cultures, and are starting to prove that the same thing happens in people who have herpes virus in their tissues."

"The next thing you're going to tell me is that chocolate has more arginine than lysine"?

"I'm afraid so. The arginine to lysine ratio in chocolate is approximately two to one. But that's not all: Peanuts are about three to one. Most cereal grains, nuts, and seeds have more arginine than lysine."

"What things that I eat have relatively more lysine?"

"Meat, potatoes, milk ... do you take any brewer's yeast? That's almost two to one in favor of lysine."

"My wife's been trying to get that in me. Looks like I'll start ... but nuts, seeds, and whole grains are very good nutrition, aren't they? And I really like them."

"Hold on. I didn't say those should be eliminated; perhaps cut back just a little. But not eliminated. In your case, the worst offenders are chocolate and peanuts. I know you like cocoa and chocolate. But besides the arginine and lysine problem, there's caffeine, too, and, of course, chocolate usually comes with sugar.

Perhaps you could continue with nuts, grains, and seeds if you eliminated chocolate and peanuts, which have a really bad ratio.

"Also, there are lysine supplements available that investigators report help people with recurrent infections. Tablets of up to 500 milligrams are sold in most nutrition stores."

## Keeps Virus Suppressed

At this, Mr. Herbert brightened considerably. "So I could take those every day, keep my arginine to lysine ratio adjusted, and keep this infection away. I'm not clear on that though. Does this kill the virus?"

"Unfortunately not. It just stops its growth and reproduction. You could think of it as a birth-control pill for herpes virus."

He laughed. "Does it work as birth control for any other viruses? How about the common cold?"

"As far as I'm aware, that's not been tried. In fact, it apparently has only been tried on encephalitis virus in mice, which it appears to inhibit, also. Progress is slow."

"Could it be harmful?"

"I don't think so, especially not in the doses required to keep the virus suppressed. Also, there's a congenital error of amino acid metabolism rarely found, called 'hyperlysinemia.' People with this problem have excess lysine in their bloodstreams at all times; it's reported to be harmless."

"So what do I do?"

"First, I advise that you stop eating chocolate or peanuts. Secondly, get some lysine tablets. Since you have an active infection, start with 1,200 milligrams daily. That is reported to take the pain away promptly. Keep this dose up until the sore is gone, then cut down to 300 to 600 milligrams daily. You'll have to experiment on your own to find the smallest amount to keep the virus suppressed. One other thing. Take it in between meals with no other protein. Theoretically, it should absorb better if it doesn't have to compete with other amino acids. Probably, a little carbohydrate with it would be helpful."

# A High Success Rate

"Think it'll work?"

"Can't say for sure, but the report I mentioned before looks encouraging. In 45 herpes patients followed for two months to three years, the treatment only failed in 2 of them. Just as important, the biochemical research underlying it looks solid."

"Forty-three of 45? Not bad odds. Thanks a lot. But I'm going to miss my morning cocoa."

Mr. Herbert's herpes infection took six days to suppress, instead of lasting the usual two to three weeks. He reported that when he felt new sores coming on (which happened much less frequently as long as he took 500 milligrams of lysine daily), he raised his dose to 1,250 milligrams daily, and "the attack goes away before it ever starts."

# Lysine Is a Safe Treatment for Herpes

Lysine appears to be safe for self-treatment, especially short term. In experiments unrelated to herpes infection, 14 individuals took 40 grams (40,000 milligrams) daily for three to five days with no reported toxicity. Another person took 20 grams a day intermittently for five months. There's a congenital condition, hyperlysinemia, in which circulating blood lysine remains at high levels throughout life. Obviously, adjusting food eaten to attain a favorable lysine to arginine ratio (without compromising diet quality otherwise) is the preferred option. If diet alone is insufficient to control herpes, however, lysine supplements appear to be a safe alternative.

In 1979, N. Milman and associates reported a scientific study of the effects of 1,000 milligrams of lysine in recurrent herpes of the lip. Their study was "placebo-controlled, double-blind crossover." (That type of study is designed to eliminate psychological effects, and to test both the active ingredient and the placebo [fake pill] in the same individual. Scientifically speaking, it's considered very accurate.) The results were partially positive, but distinctly less overwhelming than the original studies. When analyzed, they illustrate the old principle of biochemical individuality.

Even though the number of recurrences for those taking 1,000 milligrams of lysine daily was only slightly less than while taking the placebo (91 versus 104), the number of people who had no recurrences at all while taking lysine was significantly greater than while using the fake pill (14 versus 4). Apparently lysine works well for some individuals, and not others.

How can you tell if it would work for you (assuming the misfortune that you need it)? There's no way to tell in advance. Experience at this time appears to be the only way to find out.

Why didn't lysine work as well in the Danish study as in the first trial? Aside from the distinct possibility that it isn't really as effective as first thought, there are other possible explanations.

The American investigators advised their study group to avoid nuts, seeds, and chocolate, in addition to taking lysine. That eliminated substantial amounts of arginine from the diet, in effect producing a more favorable lysine to arginine ratio before adding in the effects of supplemental lysine. Although it can't be stated for certain, individuals in the American study probably had a substantially better lysine to arginine ratio, since the Danish researchers recommended no dietary alteration. The key to the effect isn't the total amount of lysine taken, but rather the amino acid ratio.

Neither set of researchers reported whether they requested any particular timing of lysine dosage. Since amino acids often compete with other amino acids of similar type for absorption, taking any therapeutic amino acid at the wrong time could theoretically impair its effectiveness. That may not be relevant with these lysine studies, but there's no way to tell.

Since it appears safe, I've sometimes recommended (when lesser amounts aren't effective) that individuals use as much as two to three grams of lysine daily in two separate doses, on a relatively empty stomach (no protein), to prevent recurrences, and up to six grams a day (if necessary) for a few days to more quickly beat down early eruptions. Most of the time, the higher doses are effective when the lower ones aren't.

A study presented at a herpes virus workshop asked 1,543

individuals with cold sores and canker sores, as well as herpes, to fill out questionnaires about lysine's effectiveness. Eighty-four percent of those returning the questionnaire said lysine either prevented recurrence or decreased the frequency of the type of sore each suffered from.

Healing took place in 6 to 15 days without lysine, according to 90 percent of those returning the survey, compared to healing in only 5 days or less for 83 percent with lysine. That type of study can be criticized, however, since those for whom the treatment works may be more motivated to return questionnaires than those for whom it doesn't. The placebo (fake pill) effect isn't screened out.

In my experience, lysine has been quite effective for the prevention and treatment of herpes, especially when the dosage is varied as needed. There are a few for whom it doesn't work, but they appear to be a minority.

Another possible breakthrough in the natural treatment of herpes infection has been reported by Gordon Skinner, M.D., of the University of Birmingham in Birmingham, England. Using a specially prepared ointment containing lithium, zinc, and vitamin E, 17 of 21 individuals with genital herpes reported a decrease in discomfort, and 12 of 18 reported a decrease in the duration of healing, compared to the other treatments they were receiving.

Even more significantly, seven out of ten individuals reported a distinct lessening of symptoms in a second scientifically controlled study. Six out of ten individuals has less virus discharge from oozing sores, which could be important in controlling transmission of the virus. Although the study group was very small, these early results seem most promising. The ointment appears safe, and larger-scale experiments are planned for the future.

# REFERENCES

## Amino Acids

Griffith, Richard S; Norins, Arthur L.; and Kagan, Christopher. "A Multicentered Study of Lysine Therapy in Herpes Simplex Infection." *Dermatologica*, vol. 156, 1978, pp. 257–267.

Kagan, C. "Lysine Therapy for Herpes Simplex." *Lancet,* January 26, 1974, p. 137.

Milman, N.; Scheibel, J.; and Jessen, O. "Lysine Prophylaxis in Recurrent Herpes Simplex Labialis: A Double-blind, Controlled Crossover Study." *Acta Dermatovener (Stockholm),* vol. 60, no. 2, 1980, pp. 85–87.

Pearson, Harold E.; Lagerborg, Dorothy L.; and Winzler, Richard J. "Effects of Certain Amino Acids and Related Compounds on Propagation of Mouse Encephalomyelitis Virus." *Proceedings of the Society for Experimental Biology and Medicine,* vol. 79, 1952, pp. 409–411.

Tankersley, Robert W., Jr. "Amino Acid Requirements of Herpes Simplex Virus in Human Cells." *Journal of Bacteriology,* March, 1964, pp. 609–613.

Van Gelderen, H. H., and Teijema, H. L. "Hyperlysinaemia: Harmless Inborn Error of Metabolism?" *Archives of Disease in Childhood,* vol. 48, 1973, pp. 892–895.

Walsh, David E.; Griffith, Richard S.; and Behforooz, Ali. "Subjective Response to Lysine in the Therapy of Herpes Simplex (An Epidemiological Survey)." Paper presented at the International Workshop for Herpes Virus Research, August 1, 1983.

## Vitamin E

Fink, Merton, and Fink, Judith. "Treatment of Herpes Simplex by Alphatocopherol (Vitamin E)." *British Dental Journal* vol. 148, no. 11–1, 1980, p. 246.

## Zinc

Tennican, Patrick et al. "Topical Zinc in the Treatment of Mice Infected Intravaginally with Herpes Genitalis Virus." *Proceedings of the Society for Experimental Biology and Medicine,* vol. 164, 1980, pp. 593–597.

Wahba, Asher. "Topical Application of Zinc Solutions: A New Treatment for Herpes Simplex Infections of the Skin?" *Acta Dermatovener (Stockholm),* vol. 60, no. 2, 1980, pp. 175–177.

**A hyperactive nine-year-old boy's irritable and sometimes uncontrollable behavior was stabilized only by drugs. His concerned and emotionally torn parents put him on the Feingold diet, eliminated refined sugar, added vitamins C and B complex, and some short-term perception therapy. Within days his behavior improved dramatically and eliminated his need for drugs—a relatively simple solution to a long-standing problem.**

# A CASE OF HYPERACTIVITY 38

Many children at one stage or another sorely try their parents with their abundance of energy. And that is perfectly natural. But when we say a child is "hyperactive," we mean something rather different. Hyperactive children are not only extremely active, but they are so disruptive, particularly in elementary school classrooms, that both teachers and parents are willing to try almost anything to control their behavior.

Probably the most frequently used means of behavioral control has been two drugs, Dexedrine and Ritalin. While the improvement is frequently dramatic, the potential side effects for the children have been disturbing to parents and to physicians who treat hyperactive children. In several communities, the subject of "drugging small children" has become a highly emotional controversy, especially when it has become known that these drugs (frequently called "speed") are two of the most widely abused.

It has become increasingly apparent to me that hyperactivity, like many other health problems, arises from violation—whether intentional or not—of one of the laws of nature. Simply stated, this "natural law" is that a living being adapted to a specific environment will probably be harmed by a significant environmental change. And a radical change in diet is one of the most serious environmental changes. For some of us, this change—from traditional natural foods to processed foods—is as challenging as if the very air we breathe had changed its composition.

I believe the following case and discussion will make the meaning of this more clear, as well as provide information on natural approaches to the treatment of hyperactivity.

In May, 1976, David and his mother returned for follow-up on David's hyperactivity. David's mother's report was a very good one—he no longer had a problem with hyperactivity.

She specifically listed a number of behavioral changes. David's personality had become entirely different. He was no longer always grumpy and irritable. He had stopped a type of "rocking" behavior he had always done before. He was much better able to cope with a variety of situations.

She also noted that David's violent temper was gone. Certainly, he still got angry, but there were no longer frequent violent explosions for no apparent reason. Also, he was able to sit still for much longer periods of time.

David had always been reluctant to join any activities, even though it seemed he wanted to. Now, he'd become involved in athletics, and joined the Cub Scouts.

David mentioned that even his grades in school had improved. He'd had average reports before, but during the past year he'd gotten one A and all the rest Bs. David's mother noted that his memory had improved, and he could concentrate better.

Both David and his mother were very pleased with how he was doing, as was I. But I couldn't take much of the credit, since David's parents had gone most of the way toward getting him improved before consulting with me. I'd only helped with some of the final "touches," and perhaps provided some needed encouragment.

David had only been in to the office a few times, and I'd not gotten to know him very well. He was now nine, and I'd met him for the first time when he was eight. So, at this point, I asked David's mother if she would write me a background letter, covering his earlier years and the difficulties she and his father had in dealing with his hyperactivity.

## Portrait of a Hyperactive Child

A few weeks later, this letter arrived. It provides such a good example of a "hyperactive" child's problems (and those of his parents) that with David's mother's permission, much of it is excerpted below.

"David started out as a very colicky baby. He hardly slept at all, never more than one or two hours at a time. . . .

"After he started walking, he was always into things. He never seemed to walk; it was always running. He got a rocking horse for his first birthday . . . he would rock first thing in the morning, whenever he was mad or hurt, and always right before bed. It seemed to pacify him to be rocking. . . .

"He seemed to have so much more energy and was more restless than other children his age. . . . He was very impulsive, and would always act and then think. . . .

"He would throw temper tantrums for no reason at all. It was like having a time bomb around, never knowing when it would go off. . . .

"David cried so easily just from being unhappy with himself . . . he couldn't understand why he acted the way he did when he knew it was wrong. He had no patience and was easily frustrated. . . .

"He had one year of preschool . . . he did fairly well because he was allowed to do what he wanted, and spent most of his time playing with blocks and big trucks. . . . He would never stick with any one thing for any length of time, and would never sit still to color or do puzzles or anything like that. . . .

"I was concerned when he started kindergarten, and discussed him with his teacher. She never required him to sit for any length of time, or do a lot of paperwork. . . .

"When he entered first grade he had three teachers . . . one refused to believe his was a learning problem and treated him as a discipline problem.

"David's small motor coordination was not good. . . . He wouldn't do his work because he was so frustrated, and she would keep him in at recess and make him sit at his desk. . . .

"David always rocked whenever he was sitting or standing and during this time his rocking increased. He would come home from school crying, not wanting to go back. He started twirling his hair from nerves and almost created a bald spot on one side. I called the doctor when he stopped eating for almost three days.

"He prescribed a small quantity of Ritalin. . . . It was unbelievable; David changed immediately. He was quiet, no rocking. We were able to get through to him . . . it was almost like having a new boy around. In school he was able to sit still and do the work. He was able to cope much better in school."

## Exhausted by Drug Therapy

Both his teachers and doctor agreed there had been a marked change, and advised he be continued on it. Despite the good result from Ritalin, David's parents were uneasy.

"He had trouble with math. . . . He had very little ability to retain information. His coordination was poor, so he shied away from games or group activity. . . .

"During gym or any school party, he would always stay off by himself and not participate. It was as if he was afraid to enjoy himself, afraid of failing."

Further, David's parents were becoming increasingly concerned about the side effects of Ritalin.

"His appetite was not very good . . . he complained of stomachaches frequently. At night he would be so mentally exhausted that when he would finally fall asleep, he would sleep very deeply. . . . He would be grinding his teeth, and his fists would be clenched tight . . . you could not wake him up for anything. We stopped giving him Ritalin on vacation days or weekends."

David's mother kept looking for other answers to his problem. She took him to the university for tests to determine specific problem areas. Once she had the results, she went over them with his next year's (second-grade) teachers. Unfortunately, there seemed to be no alternative to restarting the Ritalin when school started. That was, however, the last school year it would be needed.

## Trying the Feingold Diet

"In March, 1975, I was given an article . . . about a book by Dr. Ben Feingold . . . titled *Why Your Child Is Hyperactive*. At first we followed the book exactly. . . . We stopped Ritalin on April 18, 1975, and he never had any more. . . .

"David became much more relaxed and easier to get along with. After a while he became conscious of it himself and made comments that he didn't cry as much and didn't get in trouble as much. It was almost like an inner peace with him."

David's parents had observed firsthand the results of a return to a natural diet. For what Dr. Feingold prescribed, in brief, was a diet entirely free of artificial colors, flavors, and preservatives. Dr. Feingold's theory of the causation of hyperactivity, based on long clinical observation, was that much of it was due to "salicylate" sensitivity. As the majority of artificial colors, flavors, and preservatives are based on the salicylate molecule, they should all be avoided. Also, aspirin (chemically, acetylsalicylic acid) and anything with aspirin in it is to be avoided.

Finally, Dr. Feingold recommended the avoidance of many fruits and berries, as some of these contain natural salicylates.

In effect, the recommended diet removes all food intake from any chemical sources whatsoever.

In working with many hyperactive children, I have found that a chemical-free diet is always essential. However, avoidance of natural-salicylate fruits is sometimes important, but often is not. As David's mother observed:

"Eventually we added back the fruits one at a time, without any adverse effects."

About this time David and his mother both came to our offices for an initial consultation. I encouraged them to continue with David's diet program, and also recommended that we obtain a mineral analysis of a hair specimen.

When the analysis returned from the laboratory, it showed two results which occur very frequently in hyperactive children. One was a mineral pattern characteristic of persons with hypoglycemia (or low blood sugar). The second was an increased level of copper.

When David's mother telephoned about the results, I emphasized that all refined sugar and refined carbohydrates, such as white bread and puddings, should also be eliminated from David's diet. While we did not have "absolute" proof—such as a glucose tolerance test—that David was hypoglycemic, the mineral pattern was highly suspicious.

But, just as part of a natural-food diet, David's mother had already done most of this, anyway.

## Vitamins and Visual Therapy Added

In addition, I asked that David be given B complex vitamins, which are essential to proper sugar metabolism. Of these, vitamin $B_6$ also is thought to help remove excess copper. I recommended a daily quantity of ascorbic acid (vitamin C), well above the so-called Recommended Dietary Allowance, as this extra amount is important to optimum health.

These were the only diet and vitamin recommendations that appeared necessary, but, as David's mother pointed out, these seemingly simple instructions were difficult to follow. Putting together a no-sugar, no-artificial-chemical diet from the average supermarket is no easy job.

David's parents didn't stop with trying to help his body chemistry. Concerned about his poor condition, they looked around for further answers.

"We took him for an eye examination because we were concerned over his coordination and were looking elsewhere for answers. . . . An optometrist . . . specialized in the vision of children . . . and worked with children with perceptual and visual problems . . . they set up a training program. . . .

"He would go for one hour each week . . . and then . . . work at home . . . exercise to help distinguish left and right, to help eye tracking movement, to build his balance, coordination. . . .

"He learned to do jumping jacks. He had never been able to do them before and he was so proud when he could do them with the rest of his gym class, and not sit there and cry."

In addition to his hyperactivity, David had a problem that some hyperactive children seem to suffer from, often termed "metabolic dysperception." Apparently due to a disordered metabolism brought about by an unsuitable diet, sufferers from this problem do not perceive many things in their environment in precisely the same way as do persons with more normal metabolism, especially brain metabolism. In some children, such things as depth perception and spatial interrelationships seem altered. Alone or in combination with poor motor control, also brought about in part by abnormal metabolism, clumsiness can result.

While a return to normal metabolism—normal body chemistry—is basic to correction of this additional problem, retraining is frequently necessary. Particularly with a child like David, whose learning of motion and balance had apparently taken place under abnormal metabolic conditions, much basic learning had to be repeated under more normal conditions of metabolism.

The type of retraining that David took is available in many centers in the United States and elsewhere under the name "perceptual motor therapy" (as well as similar names). As David's mother reported:

"During the 13 weeks of training, he improved greatly. He was able to do so many more things, and he was beginning to think he was not so dumb after all. He started getting involved in group activities, started playing sports at school, joined Cub Scouts, and was able to learn and retain much more."

I should add here that not all hyperactive children need or

benefit from perceptual motor therapy. But unfortunately, many who would be benefited don't receive this retraining.

When David visited my office last, he had been on his no-chemical, no-sugar diet for over a year. His perceptual motor therapy had been completed the prior year. He continued to take his small quantities of vitamins.

I could detect no sign of hyperactive behavior. Quoting his mother once more:

"We have been so pleased with the results of all this. David is a much happier and calmer child and he is so much more aware of what all this has done for him. . . .

"He still had a little trouble doing a lot of seatwork, and handwriting is hard for him to adjust to, but he is now able to cope with these frustrations, and understand them. He is still impulsive, but he doesn't have the violent temper anymore."

Luckily, David's parents got to his problem at an early enough age. Unlike some children, especially older ones, who are frequently so attached to sugar-laden, chemically preserved foods that holding them to a natural diet is difficult, David was no problem this way.

"The diet made him feel so good that he has never eaten candy or anything he's not supposed to because he knows what it does to him. I have never had to worry about him 'cheating' on it."

# A Caution about "Progress"

Thus, a simple return to a natural diet was enough to "cure" David of his "disease," hyperactivity. But David never really had a disease to begin with. I'd like to add here an example of another hyperactivity cure, to further illustrate my original observation about health problems caused by violation of the laws of nature.

In a paper published in *Academic Therapy* by Drs. Ott, Mayron, Nation, and Mayron, the effect of types of light on hyperactive behavior is described. Very briefly summarized, this paper describes an experiment showing that hyperactive behavior could be made worse by fluorescent room lighting while a spectrum more like that of the sun improved the hyperactive behavior immediately.

And, just to be complete, it should be mentioned that allergy, malnutrition, lead toxicity, and radiation from television sets have all been found to cause hyperactive behavior.

How does this relate to the "law of nature" I mentioned at the beginning of this article? Let me state it once again: A living being adapted to a specific environment will probably be harmed by a significant environmental change.

David—like any of us—is a living being adapted to a very specific environment. That environment has, for hundreds of thousands of years, contained entirely natural foods, with no preservatives, flavorings, colorings, or refined sugar. The available light has been, for those same hundreds of thousands of years, only that from the sun, or that provided by fires of wood or the flames of candles. Only in the past 100 years or so have these new factors occurred in our environment—and the same can be said of lead exposure or television radiation. Of all the causes of hyperactivity, only allergy to natural substances has existed for any appreciable length of time in our environment.

Of course, none of us has been alive long enough to remember this entirely natural environment. But our bodies, inherited from many thousands of generations of ancestors, have much the same biochemistry, adapted to the same natural environment. So, any significant environmental change—such as chemicals in the diet, unnatural-spectrum lighting, lead exposure, television radiation— is more likely to be harmful to the health than beneficial.

For David, the harm was hyperactivity. This is only one of many health problems caused by deviation from a natural environment. Probably, many are yet unknown.

This is not an argument to dispense with the benefits of civilization. It is simply a caution—to be aware of our departure from natural ways, and particularly the effects of these largely unrecognized changes on health.

# Eliminating Problem Foods
# Is the First Step

Hyperactivity is a classic example of sensitivities caused by a wide variety of common substances: refined sugar, synthetic food chemicals, artificial light, inhalants—even to natural foods. While most hyperactive children are sensitive to more than one of these categories, no two children react to exactly the same things. That's one reason why experiments designed to prove or disprove whether one specific substance causes hyperactivity frequently aren't conclusive. Such experiments mistakenly focus on the categories capable of causing reactivity, rather than on the hyperactive children themselves.

While the Feingold (salicylate-free) program is helpful for many hyperactive children, I find it unusual that it relieves *all* symptoms. A large majority have to stop all refined sugar; a similar (and overlapping) majority have allergies. Parents of the typical hyperactive child have to eliminate all three—salicylates, refined sugar, and food allergens—and quickly discover the degree of importance each one carries.

Of course, I don't believe that refined sugar or artificial food chemicals should be eaten by anyone, hyperactive or not. But these supersensitive children show adverse effects immediately, while most of the rest of us take years longer, so the cause and effect aren't always as clear.

A smaller but still significant percentage of hyperactive children I've worked with have additional sensitivities to preservatives, artificial light, or inhalants. But these problems are almost always in addition to the more common dietary ones. They rarely exist on their own.

I'm amazed that some authorities are still making statements about hyperactivity such as "it appears now that diet plays at most a minor role." A pediatrician who works frequently with hyperactivity, William Crook, M.D., reports that 70 percent (128 of 182) of the parents of hyperactive children judged that their child's hyperactive behavior was definitely related to specific foods. Sugar was the worst, followed by food additives (especially red food color). The parents of 101 children (55 percent of the 182) reported a good to excellent response after eliminating the allergic food.

As Dr. Crook says: "Is it not reasonable to give all hyperactive children the benefit of a carefully designed and executed elimination diet, rather than putting them immediately on medication or continuing to argue about the relationship of diet to hyperactivity?" A trial of chemical, sugar, and allergen elimination is beneficial for health in any case; if hyperactivity improves coincidentally, nothing is lost. If such a program doesn't work, more radical means can still be used. If an elimination diet program proves useful, then attention to ensuring adequate quantities of all nutrients is the only further step required.

## REFERENCES

### Allergy

Hughes, E. C. et al. "Case Report: A Chemically Defined Diet in Diagnosis and Management of Food Sensitivity in Minimal Brain Dysfunction." *Annals of Allergy,* March, 1979, pp. 174–176.

Kittler, Fred J., and Baldwin, Deane G. "The Role of Allergic Factors in the Child with Minimal Brain Dysfunction." *Annals of Allergy,* May, 1970, pp. 203–206.

O'Shea, J. A., and Porter, S. F. "Double-Blind Study Reconfirms Link Between Allergens and Some Hyperkinetics." *Journal of Learning Disabilities,* vol. 14, no. 4, 1981, pp. 189–191.

Rapp, Doris J. "Food Allergy Treatment for Hyperkinesis." *Journal of Learning Disabilities,* vol. 12, no. 9, 1979, pp. 608–616.

Tryphonas, H., and Trites, Ronald. "Food Allergy in Children with Hyperactivity, Learning Disabilities and/or Minimal Brain Dysfunction." *Annals of Allergy,* January, 1979, pp. 22–27.

### Behavior

Adler, Sol. "Behavior Management: A Nutritional Approach to the Behaviorally Disordered and Learning Disabled Child." *Journal of Learning Disabilities,* vol. 11, no. 10, 1978, pp. 49–56.

Schauss, Alexander G. "Behavior Problems and Biochemicals." *Science News*, April 18, 1981, p. 247.

**Drugs**
Bressler, R.; Bogdonoff, M. D.; and Subak-Sharpe, G. J., eds. *The Physician's Drug Manual—Prescription and Nonprescription Drugs*. Doubleday, 1981.
Long, James W. *The Essential Guide to Prescription Drugs*. Harper & Row, 1982.

**Feingold Diet**
Brenner, Arnold. "A Study of the Efficacy of the Feingold Diet on Hyperkinetic Children." *Clinical Pediatrics*, vol. 16, no. 7, 1977, pp. 652–656.
Crook, William G. "Many Pediatricians See a Relationship Between Diet, Hyperactivity." *Pediatric News*, July, 1979, p. 3.
Feingold, Ben F. *Why Your Child Is Hyperactive*. Random House, 1975.
Feingold, Ben F., and Feingold, Helene S. *The Feingold Cookbook for Hyperactive Children*. Random House, 1979.
Salzman, Louis K. "Allergy Testing, Psychological Assessment and Dietary Treatment of the Hyperactive Child." *Medical Journal of Australia*, August, 1976, pp. 248–251.

**Hyperactivity**
Langstreth, L., and Dowd, J. "Glucose Tolerance and Hyperkinesis." *Food and Cosmetics Toxicology*, April, 1978, pp. 129–133.
Rapp, Doris J. "Does Diet Affect Hyperactivity?" *Journal of Learning Disabilities*, vol. 11, no. 6, 1978, pp. 383–389.
Wunderlich, Ray C. "Treatment of the Hyperactive Child." *Academic Therapy*, Summer, 1973, pp. 375–390.

**Lighting**
Mayron, Lewis W. et al. "Light, Radiation, and Academic Behavior." *Academic Therapy*, Fall, 1974, pp. 33–47.

A six-year-long pregnancy attempt leads this desperate couple to seek medical help. The husband's sperm count doubles in only six weeks after supplementing his diet with the amino acid, arginine. Pregnancy is not far behind.

# A CASE OF INFERTILITY 39

Arnold and Amanda Shenkin came in together. The appointment was for Mr. Shenkin. Perhaps accordingly, he appeared somewhat nervous, while Mrs. Shenkin was more relaxed. As soon as they were seated, she came straight to the point of their visit.

"We've been trying to get me pregnant for nearly six years," she said. "No luck. I'm not approaching menopause yet—I'm 31—but we're getting concerned. You see, we'd postponed starting a family until I was 25. We'd both worked a few years, and saved our money so we could afford it. Of course, we never thought I wouldn't get pregnant right away, or we might have started sooner."

"You've been to see a doctor before, haven't you? What have you found out?"

Mr. Shenkin shifted his feet and looked a little more embarrassed. "We've found out it's probably me," he said.

"Let me tell the doctor what all we've been through, in order," Mrs. Shenkin said. "I'm sure he wants to know what has and hasn't been done.

"Let's see . . . it's been six years. The first two, we just stopped using any form of birth control, and waited for me to miss a period."

"Excuse me for interrupting, but what form of birth control? Pills?"

"No, I only took those for one year, just after we were married. I was 20 at the time, stopped when I was 21. They made me just a little queasy. I hadn't read about taking $B_6$ and other B vitamins with birth-control pills. Then I read that sometimes it's harder to get pregnant if you've been taking the Pill, so I decided to stop."

"You'd been off the Pill for four years before trying to get pregnant?"

"Yes. I used a diaphragm. One of the doctors said four years is plenty for the Pill to 'wear off.' "

"Usually."

"So, where was I? Oh yes . . . after two years of no luck, I went to see my gynecologist. He referred me to a colleague, a fertility expert. The next two years I went through all sorts of tests and procedures."

"Can you remember which ones?"

"I certainly can. I had my tubes checked to make sure they were open. I had several cervical mucus tests, complete hormone checks, tests for sperm antibodies. I took my temperature for the whole two years to make sure I was ovulating. I even had that 'Band-Aid' surgery, laparoscopy I think it's called, so they could look around inside. Absolutely everything was working perfect."

"Did you take any fertility drugs?"

"No. It was suggested but not pushed because my tests were OK. Besides, why take drugs if I was ovulating normally?"

## Tried Better Diet

I turned to Mr. Shenkin. "You had a sperm count done at that time?"

"No, I'm a little ashamed to say I didn't. Maybe a little bit of the old male ego thing, I suppose. But also, after two years of seeing doctors, Amanda was starting to get interested in this nutrition thing, so I . . . we . . . decided to see where that would go."

"Since I'd had all kinds of tests with no results, I started to do some reading on my own. One of my friends, whom I used to call a health nut, started giving me books and magazine articles. I was doubtful at first—"

"I was really skeptical, too," Mr. Shenkin broke in. "All our friends were having children despite eating what the books called junk food. I figured if it made that much of a difference, there should hardly be any babies born at all."

"Skeptical isn't the word for it, Arnie. Hostile is more like it. Remember the first time I refused to go to the fast-food place for hamburger and cola? But he came around slowly, particularly after he saw what happened to me. I hadn't been sick—in fact, all the doctors told me I was perfectly healthy—but I hadn't been feeling the best either. After three months on a whole-food-no-junk program, I was really surprised."

"She'd been coming home from work really tired every night. She seemed to need nine hours sleep every night, and was really cranky for about a week before menstrual periods," Mr. Shenkin said. "We never did much on weekends, because we were mostly resting up from the previous week."

"All that changed," Mrs. Shenkin said. "I needed only seven-and-a-half hours of sleep; my premenstrual time was lots easier. But what really made him notice was when we went on a bicycle and camping trip."

"She was still going strong and I was worn out. So I switched over to her health-food diet, and I must say I've been feeling better the last year or so, too."

"I even got him to take a few vitamins."

"Before you get to that, tell me what you did with your diets."

"Nothing really far out. We still go to regular grocery stores.

We stopped buying anything with refined sugar or refined flour in it. We eliminated all artificial colors, flavors, and preservatives, except on rare occasions.

"On the positive side, we eat more raw vegetables, fruits, nuts, seeds. We cut back on animal protein, though we still eat some. We eat more fish. We have a copy of *The Supermarket Handbook* by the Goldbecks and follow that."

"Sounds good. No allergies in your families?"

"No. From what I've read, we're lucky.

"Now, what about vitamins?"

"Nothing unusual. A good mega-multiple with 25,000 international units vitamin A, approximately 50 of each B vitamin, and so on. Extra vitamins C and E. A multiple mineral. That's all.

"I'm glad we did all that," Mr. Shenkin said. "I really do feel better, even though I 'cheat' a little every few weeks and buy a hamburger. But, the problem is, Amanda's still not pregnant."

"So, a few months back, I went back to the fertility doctor. He checked me over again, looked at the tests I had done before, looked at the temperature records I'd been keeping again, and told me I was fine. He suggested once more that Arnie get a sperm count."

"So I did. There really wasn't anything else to do," Mr. Shenkin said. "Amanda had been through everything, we'd changed our diets entirely, and still nothing." He reached into his shirt pocket. "Here's the report. What surprises me is that with all the 'good health' things we've done the test is still bad."

"Unfortunately, you don't know how bad it might have been a few years back before you made these changes. It could have been the same, possibly worse. There've been reports of declining sperm counts in apparently healthy young men the last few years; probably diet has something to do with it. Let me look at this report for a few seconds."

The laboratory reported approximately 25 million sperm per milliliter, with less than 50 percent motile (moving). Like many labs, they noted "normal" as more than 50 million per milliliter, with more than 50 percent motile.

"This is moderately bad, but not severe," I observed. "Under 20 million is cited as a severe problem."

"What can I do about it?"

"I think we should go ahead with your medical history, do a checkup, and at least routine screening tests. After that, I'll have a recommendation."

Two weeks later, the Shenkins were back.

"You certainly have no 'diseases,'" I said. "A few vitamin and mineral insufficiencies, but actually better than average." I wrote out a brief list. "Please add these to your present program."

Mrs. Shenkin looked at the list, disappointed. "We were really hoping . . ."

"That's not all," I said. "Besides that list, there is a more specific treatment, reported in the *Journal of Urology* as well as elsewhere, that's improved the sperm count and motility in a majority of cases like yours.

"Actually, it's just as well you've been through your diet and vitamin changes before finding out what the specific problem might be," I said. "It's always wisest, and undoubtedly better for the babies, if parents put themselves on the best possible diet and take their vitamins and minerals, before even trying to get pregnant. Would you rather get pregnant now, or back when you were eating substantial quantities of junk foods?" I asked Mrs. Shenkin.

"Now, of course," she replied.

## Arginine Recommended

"So maybe this has all been for the best. Enough editorials, and on to specific treatment. Please take four grams of L-arginine a day," I told Mr. Shenkin. "If you have trouble finding it, here are some addresses and telephone numbers."

"What's L-arginine?"

"An amino acid. The journal article report I mentioned stated that of 178 men with mild to severe problems with sperm count and motility, 111 had marked improvement, and another 21 had a moderate improvement after taking this amount of arginine. Forty-six, or 25 percent, had no improvement."

"That's 75 percent improved. Not bad," Mr. Shenkin observed.

"There is one theoretical hazard, though. Increasing the amino acid lysine and decreasing arginine in the diet has been reported to suppress the growth of the herpes virus. It's possible that doing the opposite by increasing arginine could stimulate its growth."

"I've never had herpes. Arginine won't make me catch it, will it?"

"No. And this is only a theoretical hazard. The *Journal of Urology* article didn't report any side effects. I haven't seen any, although I haven't used the treatment often."

"I won't worry. Any other side effects?"

"None known. Arginine is a natural amino acid component of protein, remember."

"We'll try it. If it improves sperm counts, and that's the problem . . ."

"Maybe I'll get pregnant, finally," Mrs. Shenkin finished.

"Remember, the report didn't guarantee pregnancy," I said. "Just a 75 percent chance of improved sperm count. Incidentally, please get another one done in six weeks."

Six weeks later, the lab reported a 100 percent improved laboratory test. Shortly thereafter, Amanda Shenkin called in to let us know she was pregnant.

# Is Arginine An Effective Fertility Promoter?

In a follow-up investigation of arginine and fertility, another research group stated; "Arginine was no more effective than the placebo in improving fertility or the semen quality of infertile men with severe oligozoospermia." This paper, reporting on "double-blind, placebo-controlled" research, would seem to contradict the report by A. Schacter and associates. Instead, it demonstrates the necessity of close reading of scientific data before reaching definite conclusions, a point so ably made by Linus Pauling, Ph.D., in his reviews of "negative" vitamin C studies.

In a follow-up study, Pryor and associates investigated the effects of arginine on men having a total motile (live) sperm count of less than 10 million per ejaculate. Schacter's group included 93 men with less than 20 million sperm per milliliter, and 85 with between 20 and 50 million per milliliter. Dr. Pryor's group didn't state any number of milliliters, so estimate of total sperm count isn't possible for comparison with Schacter's group. However, it's clear that Schacter's group had a large number of men with a much milder impairment of sperm production.

In Schacter's group, results in terms of increased sperm production were worse in the more severely impaired group. Only 11 of 93 (12 percent) had an increase of 100 percent or more in sperm count, compared to 31 of 85 (36 percent) in the "mild" group. In Dr. Pryor's group, all severely impaired, 13 of 64 (20 percent) had an increase of 100 percent or more in sperm count, a result actually better than Schacter's positive study.

Dr. Pryor's yardstick of success was an improvement in conception rates, comparing arginine to a placebo (fake pill). His group found no difference in the more severely impaired men. Schacter's yardstick was both improved sperm count and conceptions. His group reports a total of 28 conceptions, but doesn't say whether they were attributable to the "mildly impaired" or "severely impaired" men. (All of Schacter's group had had infertility for at least a year, and usually considerably longer.)

The only conclusion to be drawn from these two investigations is not that arginine does or doesn't work for infertility due to a diminished sperm count, but that it may be effective in cases of mild to moderate severity, with a sperm count of between 20 and 50 million per milliliter.

# REFERENCES

**Arginine**

Pryor, J. P. et al. "Controlled Clinical Trial of Arginine for Infertile Men with Oligozoospermia." *British Journal of Urology,* vol. 50, 1978, pp. 47–50.

Schacter, A.; Goldman, J. A.; and Zukerman, Z. "Treatment of Oligospermia with the Amino Acid Arginine." *Journal of Urology,* September, 1973, pp. 311–313.

**Nutrition**

Goldbeck, Nikki, and Goldbeck, David. *The Supermarket Handbook.* Harper & Row, 1973.

**An unusual case of itching suggests a possible blood sugar problem. A high-protein, low-carbohydrate diet along with no refined sugar or junk foods, and a mineral regimen, completely eliminates the problem.**

# A CASE OF ITCHING 40

Anita Carson came into my office scratching her arm. As she sat down, she rolled up her sleeve and said, "I might as well show you. See?" She extended her arm. "Nothing there, besides my arm, is there?"

I agreed that all I could see was her arm, which appeared normal upon quick observation.

"Then why does it itch? Not just my arm, but my legs, the other arm, sometimes my back. I've gone crazy trying to figure it out."

"How long has this itching been going on?"

"Really bad for two, three months now. But actually it started about two years ago, a little. At first I got occasional itching on this arm, and sometimes my ankles. It lasted a few hours, and went away. I'd only get it a few days a month. About six, seven months ago my back started to itch, and larger areas on my lower legs and right arm as well as the left. Now it's to the point where something's itching on and off all day, and at night. Lately it's been particularly bad at night."

"Does your skin ever break out, or have you seen anything on your skin?"

"No, that's why I showed you my arm. Everything always looks normal. I've spent hours looking for bug bites or bugs, and never found any. We don't have animals, but I searched our whole bedroom, and checked the kids more than once in case they picked up something at school. Couldn't find anything."

"No bumps or hives?"

"Never. The only thing abnormal is a little bleeding if I scratch too hard."

"Have you ever been allergic to anything?"

"Not as far as I know. There's no allergy in my family either, as far as I know. No hay fever, sinus, asthma, or anything like that. But I did try changing laundry and dishwashing detergents, wearing only cotton underwear, using cotton sheets. Didn't help."

## Looking for Clues

"What illnesses are in your family?"

"Well . . . my father had a heart attack when he was 56, but he's fine now. My grandmother, his mother, had diabetes when she was older. Grandfather died of cancer. Mother's got a little high blood pressure. My Aunt Dorothy had cancer. Mother said she itched a lot before her cancer was found. Of course, she was almost 70 . . . I couldn't have a cancer, could I?"

"That's always a consideration in cases of persistent itching, but it's quite far down the list. How old are you now?"

"Forty-three."

"Have you noticed any swelling anywhere, any lumps or bumps?"

"No. I've checked since Mother told me about Aunt Dorothy, but I want you to make sure. It could be internal cancer, too, couldn't it?"

"If it is cancer at all, yes. But that's still only a remote possibility. Have you noticed any other symptoms or malfunctions besides itching?"

"I've been a lot more tired lately, but I keep waking up at night itching and not getting back to sleep. Sometimes I wake up with no itching. Maybe I'm just worried."

"No pains anywhere?"

"No."

"Noticed any gray or light-colored bowel movements, or brownish urine?"

"No. What would that be from?"

"Liver problems. Those frequently are a cause of considerable itching."

"Nothing like that, and I haven't turned yellow, either. Isn't that supposed to happen with liver conditions?"

"Yes, some of them. Ever have any kidney problems?"

"No."

"Do you still have refined **sugar** or white flour in what you eat?"

"Mother said you'd ask that. I've been trying to cut down, but sugar's in everything."

"Drink soft drinks?"

"Sometimes."

"How about chemical colors, preservatives, flavors?"

"I haven't tried to eliminate them, if that's what you mean."

## Physical Exam Is Negative

I asked other questions about what she ate, her general health background, then asked Mrs. Carson to go to the exam room. A check on her skin surface showed, as she said, no rashes, hives, or any other changes, except a little dryness. She had no swollen glands, no breast lumps, no physically detectable signs of cancer. I told her so as the examination finished, and suggested some lab tests.

"I'd like you to go to the lab to have blood and urine tests done, to see if anything can be turned up."

"What kind of tests?"

"Liver function tests, kidney function, cholesterol, triglyceride, blood sugar, another screening test for diabetes called Hemoglobin A1c, red and white blood cell counts . . ."

"How about one of those hair mineral tests?"

"Yes, for general mineral status evaluation, but it probably won't tell us much about the itching."

"That's OK, I'd still like to know what minerals I need."

"Also, tests for food allergy. Since you don't have much allergic background, we'll only do a few for the most common foods, just to see."

"Sounds reasonable, especially if I can get rid of this itching. Is there anything I can try in the meantime, while I'm waiting for these tests?"

"Try eliminating all the artificial flavors, colors, and preservatives from your diet. Sometimes that will get rid of itching."

"That's quite a job."

"I know, but all of those synthetics don't belong in our bodies anyway. Getting rid of them is a good idea even if it doesn't help itching."

"OK. I've been meaning to do that anyway—I've just been postponing it." She gathered her things and left for the lab.

A few weeks later she was back about the results. "I ought to tell you first that I haven't had any synthetic anything for three weeks; it might have helped a little, but not much. I'm still itching in various places every day. What did my tests show?"

"According to the RAST allergy tests, you don't have any significant levels of antibodies for wheat, milk, eggs, corn, oranges, chocolate, peanuts, tomatoes, or beef. Chances are you're not significantly food allergic.

"Your liver function tests were all normal. You didn't appear to have any liver problems, and I think this confirms it. Likewise, your kidney function tests, blood count, cholesterol, and other screening tests were normal."

"So we didn't find anything?" She reached over to scratch her leg. "There's got to be something. I'm still itching."

"Well, there's a suspicious pattern on your mineral analysis;

your screening tests for blood sugar were suspicious, but not conclusive. Your triglycerides were a little high."

"Do high triglycerides make you itch?"

# A Suspicious Pattern

"No, but they do fit a pattern. High triglycerides are frequently found with blood sugar problems. There's not been any study done, or published proof, but after looking at thousands of mineral tests, I've found that when one looks like yours, with slightly high zinc, moderately high calcium and magnesium, and low potassium, manganese, and chromium, it frequently is associated with blood sugar problems, such as hypoglycemia or mild diabetes."

"Oh. But didn't you do a blood sugar test?"

"Yes, it was normal, but toward the high end. It's 98, with normal being 60 to 110."

"How could I have diabetes with normal blood sugar?"

"Remember, that's just the fasting blood sugar, not a glucose tolerance test. Since the mineral pattern's suspicious, and the triglycerides are high, it can't be accepted as the final word on your blood sugar control.

"It's been my experience that itching with no other discernible cause frequently is associated with otherwise nonsymptomatic cases of adult-onset diabetes or hypoglycemia. Remember, you said there's diabetes in your family. Also, there's the Hemoglobin A1c test, which helps screen for diabetes, too."

"So, what was my test?"

"Nine percent. The normal is from 4 to 9 percent."

"That's not high."

"True, but right at the upper end. Since there's diabetes in your family, your mineral pattern was suspicious, your triglycerides were high, the blood sugar and Hemoglobin A1c were high-normal, and most importantly since you're still itching, I think a glucose tolerance test should be done."

"But I don't have any other symptoms of diabetes."

# Mild Diabetes May Have No Symptoms

"Remember, sometimes mild diabetes has no symptoms. It's like some cases of high blood pressure—no symptoms. But, maybe you do. Remember you told me you wake up at night a lot? That's one of the symptoms that happens frequently with hypoglycemia. Sure, most of those times you itch, but blood sugar problems could be causing the itching and waking up all at once. Also, you said you've been having a few more headaches. That sometimes is caused by blood sugar difficulty, too. So maybe you're not entirely asymptomatic after all."

"I guess I don't want to have diabetes or hypoglycemia because it's such a hassle getting all the sugar out of the food. But Mother's been telling me that for years. And if it'll get rid of this itching, it's worth it."

Mrs. Carson's six-hour glucose tolerance test showed mild diabetes mellitus combined with hypoglycemia, a frequent combination. By very strict criteria, it was only slightly abnormal.

At her next appointment, Mrs. Carson reviewed what she had read about blood sugar problems and decided to put herself on a high-protein, low-carbohydrate diet, the kind with lots of meat, eggs, cheese, fish, salads, and low-calorie vegetables. She also eliminated all refined sugar, refined carbohydrate, and junk foods.

I gave her a list of vitamins C, B, and E (basic for all blood sugar problems). I also suggested the minerals chromium (in its organically derived form, especially important for blood sugar control), zinc, potassium, manganese, and dolomite (source of calcium and magnesium).

Six weeks after she started her blood sugar control program, her itching was completely cleared. It only returned when she "slipped," eating too much sugar or junk food.

# Itching Has a Number of Causes

Itching has so many causes that a book could be written about it alone. Among the more common ones are allergy, infection, liver disease, kidney disorders, and chemical sensitivity. There's definitely no single cause.

Cancer of various types are among the more unusual causes of persistent itching. If no other cause can be found, cancer screening is always wise, particularly if there are other grounds to suspect it.

I can't explain why blood sugar disturbances sometimes lead to itching, but when they do, control of the blood sugar problem controls itching, as it did in Mrs. Carson's case. Itching, however, accompanies diabetes and hypoglycemia in only a small minority of cases.

## REFERENCES

**Itching**

Flaxman, B. Allen. "Pruritis: Identifying and Treating Causes." *Postgraduate Medicine,* May, 1981, pp. 177–186.

"Itch." *Lancet,* September 13, 1980, pp. 568–569.

Krupp, Marcus A., and Chatton, Milton J. "Gastrointestinal Tract & Liver." In *Current Medical Diagnosis and Treatment 1978.* Lange Medical Publications, 1978, pp. 385–386, 1038.

**A 14-year-old boy is disappointed because he can't play sports like other kids. He has Osgood-Schlatter disease, which he will probably outgrow, but the pain needs attention now. A little-known—yet helpful— treatment with vitamin E and selenium eliminates his pain and gets him back to basketball, gym class, and just plain running around.**

# 41 A CASE OF TEENAGE KNEE PAIN

"It's a shame, because Andrew's such an active boy. He wants to play basketball in high school like his older brothers. He didn't play soccer or baseball all summer, resting his knees as he'd been advised to do. The pain did improve, but as soon as he started basketball this year, his knees got really sore again. He had to stop."

"I was doing really good, too. Coach said I had a shot at making the high school team next year."

Andrew was in for the first time, along with his mother. She'd been able to take care of some of her own health problems with diet change and exercise, so she'd decided to see if something similar might help Andrew.

"Can't understand it. Andrew's been healthy for years. Except for this, the last time he saw a doctor was before junior high school, for a school physical. We eat right at home, now, and he certainly tries to get his exercise."

"How old are you, Andrew?"

"Fourteen."

"When did your knees start to hurt?"

"Seventh grade."

"What grade are you in now?"

"Ninth."

"So you were twelve?"

"Yeah."

"More like twelve and nine months, doctor. A little over a year and a half ago. He'd had a really rapid growth spurt just before that, over two inches. We thought it had something to do with growth, so we just ignored it for two or three months. But then his knee started to swell a little in front, and hurt worse, so we took him to the pediatrician."

"Which knee was it, Andrew?"

"Left one. But they both hurt now, unless I just don't do anything."

## Told to Avoid Sports

"What did the pediatrician say?"

"He said it was Schlatter disease."

"Osgood-Schlatter disease, dear. He said there wasn't anything to do for it, except take aspirin when it hurt bad. Andrew was told to stay strictly out of sports that summer, and hope it healed."

"So he did?"

"After a painful reminder or two. That was the summer before this last one. He tried to play baseball, got a flare of pain in the other knee, so he believed the doctor and quit."

"Really a drag," Andrew said. "The year before that I hit .387, best percentage on the team. I wanted to try for .400."

"Then when school started, they had volleyball in gym class—"

"Pain city," Andrew broke in. "I lasted only two weeks."

"So we went to see an orthopedic doctor. I know the pediatrician said there wasn't anything to do, but Andrew was so discouraged."

"What happened?"

"The orthopedic doctor told us the same thing, that usually the pain goes away for good when full growth is reached. Most of the time it doesn't go away sooner, it just gets better or worse."

"By that time I'll be clear through high school," Andrew grumbled.

"The doctor tried a cast on his worst knee, the left. He said complete immobilization for a few weeks and anti-inflammatory medicine might take the pain away."

"I had a cast on from here to here," Andrew said, indicating an area from midcalf to midthigh. "Crutches, too. I took a real strong medicine . . . I think it's called phenylbutazone . . . for ten days, then aspirin the rest of the time. All I got out of it were some neat pictures on my cast, and some of the girls carried my books for me. But my knee started to hurt again once the cast came off."

"After that, the orthopedic doctor said the only thing left to do was try a longer rest period from any sports."

"I stayed out half of this spring and absolutely all summer," Andrew said. "Felt pretty good when school started, but I still didn't exercise until basketball practice. No gym at all. Coach said that would be best; he's seen a lot of this over the years. I should just exercise in the sport I really wanted to do, not risk setting it off in anything else."

"It may be Andrew will just have to wait until his bones are fully grown," his mother said, "but those vitamins I took helped me so much I decided to try coming here this year."

"Second annual get-my-knees-better visit," Andrew remarked.

"Andrew! Don't be smart. Besides, it hasn't been two years, yet."

"I should look at your knees, Andrew. I know you've had that done a lot already but I'd like to check for myself. Please come into the examination room."

"Should I come too, doctor?"

"Aw, Mom . . . "

I looked at Andrew's mother. She smiled, sat down again. "I'll just wait," she said.

As Andrew had not been in before, I checked everything over, but as his mother had said, he appeared physically quite healthy, except for his knees.

## Tender to the Touch

They were both sore, right where the large tendon from his kneecap attached to the prominence of bone below. This area, called the tibial tubercle, was tender to pressure, more on Andrew's left knee than his right. The tubercle was definitely enlarged on the left, and a little on the right.

"Have you had an x-ray taken?"

"Sure, the orthopedic doctor did that. Both knees. He said there was a little calcium deposit on the left side, but there wasn't any permanent damage."

"Fortunately, Osgood-Schlatter disease is never permanent. It can be a problem for a few years, though."

"Yeah, darn it."

I finished checking Andrew over. We went back to my office.

"Just as you said," I started. "About an average case of Osgood-Schlatter. Everything else looks OK, but as Andrew's not been in before, I'd like to have a blood count, urinalysis, and mineral analysis done."

"Think you might find something on those?"

"Not specifically about the knee problem. They're routine screening tests for good health. After all, his last blood count and urinalysis was probably at the pediatrician's two or three years ago."

"No tests for his knees?"

"None I know about." Since Andrew and his mother both looked disappointed, I hurried on. "But that doesn't mean there's nothing to try."

# Selenium and Vitamin E

"Please have Andrew take selenium, 50 micrograms, three times a day, and vitamin E, 400 international units, twice daily. If you can, check back in a month. I'd like to see how he's doing." I wrote the recommendations out, and handed them to Andrew's mother.

"Selenium? Vitamin E? What will they do?"

"Usually, they take away Osgood-Schlatter pain. They have for most teenagers who've tried it the last few years."

"How does it work?"

"I don't know. I've never found any documentation, except for an unrelated type of knee problem. It works somehow though, as the pain usually goes for good in two to six weeks. Either it's the selenium and vitamin E, or an unusually large number of coincidental disappearances of the pain at the same time."

"What you're saying is that this isn't a proven remedy, but it seems to work," Andrew's mother observed.

"Usually."

"It's worth trying. There's nothing else to do."

"Except wait until it's too late to play basketball, or anything else anymore," Andrew said.

"What about side effects?"

"I was just going to mention that. Except for very rarely causing hypertension in adults, I've not seen any with vitamin E. Selenium in very large doses can be potentially dangerous, but all the evidence I've been able to find indicates this dose is much safer than the phenylbutazone he tried last year. In fact, I've not seen or been able to find any evidence of side effects at this dose. High doses can be toxic, though, so don't overdo it.

"Furthermore, we usually can cut back the amount to 50 micrograms of selenium twice daily in a month, then once a day for the third month. Then none."

"Why so long, if the pain goes away sooner?"

"To make sure it stays away."

"It won't come back even if I exercise?" Andrew asked.

"Once it's gone with the selenium and vitamin E, usually not. In the few cases where it has, repetition has taken it away again."

"What about exercise?"

"It's probably wisest to wait until the pain seems gone, or nearly so, to allow time to heal. Then, like any other recovery, starting slow and building up is best."

"I might be back at basketball before the first of the year!"

"Probably. Remember, I didn't say it's foolproof. Occasionally, there are no results. But your chances are good."

"Sure hope it works on me." Andrew turned to his mother. "Won't have any trouble getting me to take my vitamins this time, Mom."

"You couldn't tell him that vitamin C and a good multiple vitamin would help him get back to sports, could you, doctor?"

"Afraid not. Selenium and vitamin E are usually enough. However"—I turned to Andrew—"vitamin C and a multiple vitamin are a good idea for staying healthy."

"OK, OK, I'll take anything . . . for a while, anyway."

Andrew and his mother left, making an appointment to come back in a month.

# Playing Soccer Again

By the time he returned, Andrew's knees were much better. There was much less tenderness over his tibial tubercles. Andrew's mother reported he'd been out playing soccer during the previous week without telling her. "I wouldn't have let him if I'd known," she said.

"It's hard to keep kids down once their knees start getting better. But stop right away if the pain gets worse with exercise," I told Andrew.

There wasn't much else to say. I reminded Andrew to cut the amount of selenium back, and return or call back only if his knees didn't improve.

I didn't hear from Andrew or his mother until she came in for a problem of her own several months later. She reported that Andrew's knees were pain free shortly after his second visit to the office. She'd let him go back to basketball, gym class and "just generally running around." Like most teenagers treated with selenium and vitamin E, his Osgood-Schlatter knee pain has not returned.

# An Unproven Treatment That Works

Selenium and vitamin E have continued to be very effective in eliminating the pain of Osgood-Schlatter disease. Although I'm sure it will happen sometime, I haven't yet seen anyone not improve with selenium and vitamin E treatment.

I can't claim any great biochemical insight in developing the treatment: It was one of those "educated guesses" several years ago that after passage of time appears to have been accurate. Hopefully, an orthopedic department or sports-medicine clinic will do a "controlled study" on Osgood-Schlatter disease with selenium and vitamin E soon.

Meanwhile, adolescents with whom I work continue to improve. After several years, I'm inclined to believe it's more than coincidence. Even teenagers I've never seen appear to be helped, as the following letter from a reader says:

*Our son Eric has had it for two-and-a-half years. He continued playing soccer, basketball, and baseball. His coaches were very understanding and patient because he is a fine athlete. It was not unusual to have to help him up stairs and ice pack his knees after practices and games. Just sitting in the car after activity was agony for him.*

*The last time he saw a doctor and had x-rays was in July and we were told possibly up to a year more of pain in his left knee and perhaps two more years in his right.*

*A friend brought our attention to your vitamin E and selenium program which he started September 19. On October 23 he was running with no pain—a miracle!*

*Eric was 14 years old October 2. He tried out for and*

*made the high school basketball team and is running up to
30 laps of the gym a day. He will finish your program
January 19.*

*Eric will be a big man since at 14 years he is 5'11" tall
and wears an 11½ shoe. I have heard the children who grow
rapidly have this problem. It seems to me that it's a
combination of fast growth and extreme activity since I
have observed both separately in children with no knee
problems. Since Eric was six years old he has been in all
three sports all year with no season off. This was his choice
and we were told he could not do permanent damage. He
just lived with the pain. He never did give his knees a rest
before your program.*

*Once again we cannot thank you enough.*

Toxic amounts of selenium for adults appear to be 1,500 to
2,000 micrograms daily or more. Although vitamin E experts such
as Wilfrid E. Shute, M.D., have noted that high doses of vitamin E
occasionally are associated with high blood pressure, I've not seen
it happen in adolescents using vitamin E and selenium treatment.

## REFERENCE

**Selenium**
Faelten, Sharon, and the editors of *Prevention* magazine.
"Selenium." In *Complete Book of Minerals for Health*. Rodale
Press, 1981, p. 112.

**Some three-and-a-half years of suffering from irregular spotting and heavy menstrual bleeding come to a halt once this 40-year-old woman incorporates vitamin A, bioflavonoids, and other changes into her dietary plan. That once-feared hysterectomy, her only alternative to excess bleeding, is happily avoided.**

# 42 A CASE OF HEAVY MENSTRUAL BLEEDING

Rita Sanchez was 40, with black eyes and straight black hair showing an occasional strand of gray. Her complexion was dark, and appeared well cared for. She seemed relaxed, but showed an undercurrent of worry.

"I am here to find out if there's anything else I can do besides have a hysterectomy. I try to take care of myself, but this is beyond my control. I've had all my children, I know the uterus isn't an essential organ, but I don't like the idea of major surgery. There's always the possibility of complications." She paused for breath.

"You haven't mentioned exactly what the problem is yet."

She laughed. "I'm getting ahead of myself again. It's bleeding, way too heavy. My periods go on for eight to ten days, and heavier all the time. I actually get weak; I have to take iron all the time because I'm anemic. Also, I have some bleeding in between menstrual periods, sometimes just spotting, sometimes a little more."

"How long has this been?"

"Really heavy like this almost a year, but actually it's been nearly this bad for about three-and-a-half years."

"That's quite awhile for heavy bleeding."

"Don't I know it! But, I had a D & C a year and a half ago . . . maybe I should start at the beginning.

"My menstrual periods were always very regular through my teens and twenties. In fact they still are. They always lasted three to five days, and as far as I could tell were medium heavy, nothing unmanageable. I did take birth-control pills for a few months, but I got a minor case of phlebitis and had to stop. I have three children, no problems there.

"When I was 31, I started having a little spotting in between periods, but nothing much, and not always every month. It went on for a couple years, then stopped. I didn't have any trouble again until I was 34."

I made a few notes; she continued.

## Symptoms Kept Worsening

"First, I noticed my periods were getting heavier. I had to use more pads and tampons than before. That went on for a while, then they started getting longer, too, from five days at most to six, then seven or eight. I'd started spotting again some months, too.

"I went to see my gynecologist. She suggested trying hormones or birth-control pills to control the cycles, but I recalled the phlebitis, and she said hormones were out. I understand they don't always work, anyway. So she put me on iron, and said if it kept up or got worse, I could have a D & C.

"Well, it did keep getting worse. I didn't like the idea of surgery, even 'minor' surgery like a D & C, so I tried to put up with it. But by a year and a half ago I was having to stay in bed two or three days every month, and had to stay around the house most of the rest of the time. Going out was just out of the question ten days, one-third of each month. So I gave up and went in for the D & C."

"What happened?"

"Well, in the first place, I didn't have cancer or anything. I have to admit I was worried, even though my gynecologist told me that was really rare with the type of bleeding I was having."

"That's true. Unfortunately, it's much more likely in bleeding after menopause."

"I sure wasn't having menopause! Anyway, she gave me a really good examination when I was anesthetized, said I was normal, and the report from pathology on the D & C was normal, too. So I stopped worrying about cancer."

## Only Temporary Relief

"And your periods?"

"They were less for four months after. Still more bleeding than when I was younger, and lasting five to six days, but tolerable. I wasn't in bed, and I could go out. It didn't last, though. The fifth and sixth months got worse, and by a year ago, back to as bad as ever. Nine, ten days a month, three days in bed, tired all the time. That's been going on again for a year now."

"You've checked back with your gynecologist?"

"Several times; I was just there last week. Same thing, normal examination, no other problems, just too much bleeding. She said I could get another D & C—she's been telling me that all year—but as far as I can see, the whole thing would probably come back again. She agrees; she can't say for sure whether another D & C would work any better than before.

"So, we talked about a hysterectomy. As she said, that would take care of the problem. I am 40—I don't really 'need' my uterus anymore, I suppose." She shifted uneasily in her chair. "But still . . . is there anything I can do with my diet, or vitamins and minerals, to stop all this bleeding without surgery?"

"Possibly. Let's talk about what you eat."

"At breakfast, I have coffee and a piece of toast. For lunch, usually cottage cheese, or a piece of cheese and an apple. Dinner is really variable. Quite a bit of Mexican food, as you might expect, tacos, tortillas, refried beans, corn, but we do have the usual kinds of meals as well—beef, chicken, peas, corn, lettuce and tomato salads. . . ."

"How about desserts, snacks?"

"I eat mostly nuts, cheese, or apples when I want a snack, but I'm watching my weight, so I don't have many snacks."

"Do you use refined sugar, white flour?"

"Yes . . . but I know I should stop."

"How about lemons, oranges, grapefruits, green peppers?"

"I never have eaten much citrus. I think I'm allergic. I do use red pepper in cooking."

"How about carrots, yams, broccoli, spinach, squash, liver?"

"Carrots sometimes. Can't stand broccoli or squash. Sometimes spinach, but not much."

"Do you take any vitamins?"

"A multiple, but that's all."

I made a few more notes. We went over the rest of her health background. However, as she'd just been checked by her gynecologist a week before, we both decided another pelvic examination couldn't be useful.

# Extra Vitamin A

"I'd like you to try using 25,000 international units of vitamin A three times daily. That's about three times as much as a person should take on their own. Before we're done, let's go over the side effects so we can both watch for them. However, they're very unlikely as this dose is only temporary." I wrote this out on a small notepad. "Take it with meals. Also, to make sure it has the best chance of working, take 200 international units of vitamin E daily and 50 milligrams of zinc. Also, a blood test for pancreatic digestive enzymes, to make sure the vitamin A is likely to be absorbed."

"You wrote that all down for me?"

"Yes."

"Good, that's a lot to remember. What does the vitamin A do?"

"Hopefully, stop the bleeding problem. Drs. Lithgow and Politzer reported that in a group of 40 women, 92.5 percent had either substantial improvement or a complete return to normal with vitamin A."

"That sounds like a good percentage. How long does it take?"

"They reported they asked women to use vitamin A for 35 days."

"That's all?"

"Yes. However, when the vitamin A works, and I've found it usually does, I recommend taking a lesser dose for several months, to build up storage, and prevent further problems."

"Sounds simple enough . . . but are you sure it'll work?"

"Can't be sure until you try. But I've been using the treatment since I first read about it, and it works in a large majority."

"What if it doesn't? Then I'd have to get a hysterectomy, wouldn't I?" She still looked worried.

"No, there'd be at least one more thing to try. But let's see how this does first. Please make sure to call back in two or three days about your pancreatic enzyme test. If your levels are too low, then the vitamin A isn't likely to work."

"What do I do if my test is low?"

"Take pancreatic enzymes. But the nurse will tell you about that, if necessary."

# A Question of Toxicity

Mrs. Sanchez got up to go, then remembered something else. "What about vitamin A being toxic? Isn't this an awfully large dose?"

"No, it isn't. I've never seen an adult suffer vitamin A toxicity at that amount. According to a pharmacology textbook, *The Pharmacological Basis of Therapeutics*, even in children all reported cases of toxicity have been long-term doses of 50,000 to 500,000 international units daily. I don't want to give the impression that vitamin A is completely safe—it isn't. But most of the talk of vitamin A toxicity is overdone, more propaganda than accurate information.

"Besides, the symptoms of toxicity are very noticeable, and go away once vitamin A is stopped. They include hair loss, headaches, nausea, bone and joint pain, and lumps developing on the bones of the arms and legs. Not exactly the sort of thing that sneaks up with no warning."

"I guess it would be pretty obvious, and I could just stop, couldn't I? But you said you've never seen toxicity in an adult at 75,000 international units?"

"Never seen it, or heard of it, either, when taken for short periods of time."

"Good enough."

"Before you go, I should mention that your diet is fairly low in vitamin A. Besides taking the vitamin A supplements, you should also pay attention to food sources."

"OK. I'll check into that."

## "I Couldn't Believe It"

Three months later, Mrs. Sanchez was back. "I couldn't believe it, even after you told me," she said. "Even the first month, my period was down to seven days and noticeably less heavy. This last one was normal. What a relief! Does it usually work that fast?"

"Frequently, but not always. I'm glad it worked that quickly for you."

"I cut the vitamin A down to 50,000 international units daily after two months. I asked the nurse. I didn't need those pancreatic enzymes. Should I continue the zinc and vitamin E also?"

"For another few months yet. Then you could gradually cut back."

"You know, I'm surprised, but even with my last period normal I still had a tiny bit of spotting at midcycle. Won't the vitamin A stop that?"

"I'd think so. But remember I mentioned there was another treatment you could try if the vitamin A didn't work?"

"Yes. What was it?"

"Bioflavonoids. Your diet is rather low in them, too. The main sources are citrus; other sources are fruits or vegetables where vitamin C is found. There've been reports in France of correcting abnormal uterine bleeding with bioflavonoids. I usually recommend one gram of mixed bioflavonoids, containing rutin, hesperidin, and other bioflavonoid factors."

"I do drink orange juice occasionally."

"Well, occasionally isn't enough for your circumstances."

"I'll add some bioflavonoids, and see what happens."

I didn't see Mrs. Sanchez again for over a year, when she came in with one of her children. She reported that her periods were back to "just like when I was 25," and no spotting at all. She had continued small amounts of vitamin A, bioflavonoids, zinc, and vitamin E.

# Vitamin A Is a Conservative Treatment for Excess Bleeding

A conservative approach to health care clearly dictates that vitamin A treatment should be tried first for menorrhagia (heavy bleeding), before the more risky measures of hormone therapy, or D & C (surgical scraping of the uterus). An even more conservative approach would be to try large amounts of vitamin A-rich foods before taking supplemental vitamin A. There's no excuse at all for performing a hysterectomy to stop overly heavy menstrual bleeding without trying vitamin A, particularly if it isn't tried because "vitamins aren't likely to help."

Certainly vitamin A won't work every time: two South African researchers, Drs. D. M. Lithgow and W. M. Politzer reported that for 40 women, menstruation returned to normal in 57.5 percent, and substantial improvement occurred in another 35 percent. I've found the percentages to be accurate: Less than 10 percent of those for whom I've suggested vitamin A treatment have failed to improve or correct their menorrhagia.

For those few where vitamin A treatment isn't satisfactory, bioflavonoids are the next thing to try. Only if these specific measures fail (and general nutritional improvement doesn't help) is there any need to proceed to hormones or surgery.

Drs. Lithgow and Politzer also proposed at least one reason why vitamin A treatment might work. They point out that enzymes necessary for the internal production of hormones are underactive in vitamin A deficiency, even when the deficiency is mild. Supplementing vitamin A stimulates enzyme activity, normalizing hormone production. Thus vitamin A can help the body to do naturally from the inside what synthetic hormone pills or injections do from the outside.

Bioflavonoids are said to decrease capillary fragility. It isn't known, however, whether that's why they help to correct abnormal uterine bleeding.

Heavy menstrual bleeding can indicate a more serious problem, particularly for older women in the decade before menopause. In Drs. Lithgow and Politzer's group, 2.3 percent had cancer; another 3.5 percent had fibroids or polyps. Vitamin A won't cure these problems. However, when vitamin A is successful, it usually only takes a month, or two at most. Furthermore, no one needs to wait until menstrual bleeding becomes exceptionally heavy before trying a little extra vitamin A. (If there's any uncertainty, it's wise to check with your physician.)

Since 1981, I've heard of only a single case of vitamin A toxicity when using 50,000 international units daily. Compared to even over-the-counter drug toxicity, the hazard from vitamin A is small.

If you're having excessively heavy menstrual bleeding, check with your doctor. If nothing serious is found to be the matter, try vitamin A for a few weeks before proceeding to other measures. The uterus you save could be your own.

## REFERENCES

**Bioflavonoids**

Bourne, Geoffrey H. "Citrus Fruits and Processed Citrus Products in Human Nutrition." In *World Review of Nutrition and Dietetics.* Vol. 6. Hafner Publishing Company, 1966, p. 208.

"Flavones Used in Functional Uterine Bleeding." *Family Practice News,* March 1–15, 1974, p. 66.

**Vitamin A**

Burton, Benjamin T. "Vitamins I: Fat-Soluble." In *Human Nutrition*. 3d ed. McGraw-Hill, 1976, pp. 89–90.

Goodman, Louis S., and Gilman, Alfred, eds. "Fat Soluble Vitamins." In *The Pharmacological Basis of Therapeutics*. 5th ed. Macmillan Publishing, 1975, pp. 1573–1574.

Guthrie, Helen A. "Basic Principles of Nutrition." In *Introductory Nutrition*. 5th ed. C. V. Mosby, 1983, p. 336.

Lithgow, D. M., and Politzer, W. M. "Vitamin A in the Treatment of Menorrhagia." *South African Medical Journal*, February 12, 1977, pp. 191–193.

Concern about a family history of osteoporosis brings a 50-year-old woman in for a checkup, hoping to prevent the impending problem. Cutting back on protein and acid-forming foods, maintaining a high calcium to phosphorus dietary ratio, and getting plenty of exercise is offered as the plan of attack.

# A CASE OF OSTEOPOROSIS PREVENTION 43

Alice Burton had come in for discussion of her recent checkup and laboratory tests. She was a strong, vigorous-looking woman, 50 years old, five feet six inches tall, and overweight at 148 pounds. Her physical examination had disclosed no obvious abnormalities and no diseases. As she had noted on her first visit, she didn't think she was ill, but came in for preventive reasons. She had this in mind as she sat down.

"John and I went to see Mother in Iowa last month," she said. "It's the first time since she broke her hip four years ago. She's as alert as ever, but she's not getting around as well, of course. What I noticed this time is she's started to get a definite hump in her back, just like Grandmother used to have. That's a sign of bone loss, isn't it?"

"It certainly is. A dowager's hump is caused by the collapse of spinal vertebrae, usually more than one. That means bone loss, osteoporosis, is fairly well advanced. Of course, her hip fracture at age"—I looked at my notes—"71 is usually a sign of osteoporosis, too."

"I know, I've read that in a lot of places. Another thing, Mother's shorter than just a few years ago. It's odd, but Grandmother, Mother, my daughter, and I all measured 5 feet 6 inches at age 18. I've lost a little fraction, but Mother's 5 feet 3½ inches now. Grandmother was scarcely 5 feet in her nineties, before she died."

Mrs. Burton smiled. "I remember her telling me, 'Age takes its toll, Alice; we grow in youth and collapse in old age.' She even willed me her cane; she told me we were so alike I'd need it if I made it to 90." She became more serious again. "But that's what I'm here about. It seems the women in my family are destined for osteoporosis; I want to do everything I can to prevent it. It is possible, isn't it, with good diet? It's not strictly hereditary?"

"No, it's not strictly hereditary. There may be some hereditary component—that can't be denied—but most of the evidence points to environmental factors, particularly diet and exercise, as being extremely important in the prevention of osteoporosis."

## Difficult to Detect

"Did I show any osteoporosis on my checkup?"

"No, but remember it can't easily be found with a physical examination, anyway. It's usually only found on x-rays or other special examinations."

"We didn't do any x-rays, though."

"There didn't appear to be any need. Also, it'd be really unusual to have significant bone loss at age 50, anyway. That usually starts showing up on x-rays, if it's going to, after 60."

"So I should have x-rays at age 60, then?"

"Not at all, unless there's good indication. Waiting until osteoporosis arrives, then trying to correct it, is much less successful than doing as you're doing, and preventing it in the first place."

"That can be done for sure?"

"Very few things are absolutely for sure in medicine, like the rest of life. But I'd say there's a high degree of probability. Let's take a look at your diet, first." I looked at what I'd recorded at her checkup, which went as follows:

**Breakfast:** eggs, bacon or sausage (no nitrites), granola with milk, whole-grain toast, herb tea

**Lunch:** cheese (frequently cottage cheese), salad, apple or orange

**Dinner:** beef, pork or chicken (fat removed), potato, whole-grain bread, corn, peas, or beans. Occasionally carrots or celery, usually salad

**Desserts:** fresh fruit, sometimes ice cream (natural type with honey)

**Snacks:** cheese, rye crackers, sunflower seeds

**No refined sugar, white flour, artificial sweeteners, or caffeine. Alcohol on social occasions**

**Supplements:** one gram vitamin C, 800 international units vitamin E, bone meal, lecithin, brewer's yeast, multiple vitamin and mineral.

# Too Much Protein

As I scanned the list, Mrs. Burton remarked, "I know that's a big breakfast, and I'm overweight. But I go to work every day, and it definitely helps me get through the day better."

"Breakfast is the best time of day for your largest meal, and for at least some protein. You're right about helping to keep you working at your best. But we definitely need to talk about protein, overall. Before we do that, though, I should tell you that you've done a much better than usual job of watching your diet for good health. All whole foods, no refined sugar, no synthetic chemicals, no caffeine—that's very good."

"Thank you. I've really tried. I'm glad you didn't see what I ate regularly 15 years ago. But there's still a problem with all the protein, isn't there? I suspected as much. You know, when I was changing from eating junk foods to a good diet, I discovered I didn't have enough protein. I read how important it was for staying strong and healthy. I guess I kind of went overboard. I hope I haven't done any damage."

"Let me tell you about some dietary-pattern studies. Scientists have compared the bone mass of older Eskimo women, who eat an extremely high-protein diet, with that of older women with a lower meat intake. The older Eskimo women had a lower bone mass. That did not show up in younger women, however.

"Bone loss studies have been done comparing women on lacto-ovo-vegetarian diets (milk, eggs, vegetables, no meat) and women on omnivorous diets (which include meat). While no great difference in bone loss is found in the twenties, thirties, and forties, there's definitely a difference in the fifties and older, accelerating with age. The omnivorous women had more osteoporosis at each decade past 50, and progressively worse with time. One of the studies by Dr. Alice Marsh showed that lacto-ovo-vegetarians lost 18 percent of bone mass between 50 and 89 years of age, while the omnivorous women lost 35 percent."

"That's definitely a difference, all right, but removing meat protein can't be the only factor. After all, there's lots of protein in eggs, milk, and cheese."

"An excellent observation; the meat protein isn't the only factor. High-protein diets of any sort have been shown to cause excess calcium loss. Unfortunately, a study, published in the *American Journal of Clinical Nutrition*, shows that even high-calcium intake along with the high protein doesn't correct the problem. However, when meat is eliminated from a diet, the overall protein is usually less."

# Acid-Forming Foods

"Protein isn't the only potential problem in your diet, though. There's considerable evidence that a diet which is more 'acid forming' also increases calcium excretion and increased bone loss."

"Which foods are acid forming?"

"In general, meat, other high-protein foods, most cereal

grains including wheat, and other starches. By contrast, most vegetables and fruits are less acid forming, or more alkaline."

"And I eat quite a lot of whole wheat and other starches. It doesn't help that it's whole grain?"

"Whole grains are definitely better than refined, for innumerable aspects of good nutrition. But for acid forming, it doesn't help that much."

Mrs. Burton looked glum. "I bet that's not everything, is it?"

"Unfortunately not. The dietary calcium to phosphorus ratio is very important, too. Even if the foods you eat are high in calcium, if they're as high or higher in phosphorus, the calcium is overwhelmed, in a manner of speaking, and doesn't help much."

"What foods are particularly high in phosphorus, compared to calcium?"

"Some of them are a familiar list: meat, poultry, fish, whole wheat, cereal products. On your particular food list, sunflower seeds are also high in phosphorus; so are peas. Of course, most processed foods are higher in phosphorus than calcium, too. But you've excluded those."

"Isn't lecithin high in phosphorus?"

"Yes; so is bone meal and brewer's yeast."

"Good grief. Practically my whole good diet is working against me, at least in the phosphorus to calcium department. But don't I need those supplements? Don't I need lecithin to keep my cholesterol down?"

"Most vegetarians, even those who eat eggs and milk, have no trouble keeping their cholesterol levels under control."

"So you're telling me I should become a vegetarian, and stop taking lecithin, bone meal, and brewer's yeast?" She crossed her arms and sat upright, not smiling at all.

"No, I think you're overreacting. It's a matter of relative proportions and balance. There are a lot of modifications you can make without doing immediate drastic revisions. And remember what your goal is, too. Maybe osteoporosis, fractured hips, and a dowager's hump aren't so bad after all, considering this news about your diet?"

Mrs. Burton laughed, and relaxed a little. "I guess I was getting too defensive. Give me some suggestions."

## Some Easy Substitutions

"Well . . . protein at breakfast is still a very good idea. Why not have eggs or sausage, not both? You could substitute vegetables for cheese sometimes. In the evening, you don't always have to have an animal protein. Some nights you could substitute more raw vegetables and fruits.

"Whole grains and starches such as peas and corn are good foods, but remember that along with meats, they're acid forming." You are using quite a bit of whole-wheat granola and toast . . . why not substitute root or leafy vegetables sometimes? Not always, just sometimes.

"Besides high-protein and acid-forming foods being a problem, there's calcium-phosphorus balance. Most deep green leafy vegetables have a high calcium to phosphorus ratio. Use them more often. Try yogurt as a snack instead of sunflower seeds sometimes. It has a better calcium to phosphorus ratio."

"Looks like I've got some studying to do."

"That's right. I really can't discover, even in several years, what all your food preferences and dislikes are. You may not even know yourself. Get a book that lists the approximate calcium and phosphorus content of foods, and put together a program with at least an equal amount of each; if possible, more calcium than phosphorus is even better. Watch out for too much protein, and for too many acid-forming foods."

"Sounds reasonable. By the way, since you can't tell osteoporosis by looking, and x-rays at my age won't help, is there any evidence on my tests that I might be getting into problems? What about blood tests for calcium and phosphorus?"

"Even in women with severe osteoporosis, blood tests for calcium and phosphorus are usually within normal limits. They're just not helpful for detecting calcium deficiency. However, your hair test is showing some problem: the calcium and magnesium are too high."

"Too high? I thought my problem was that I didn't have enough calcium intake. Doesn't too high mean too much?"

"Only occasionally. Usually it means too much phosphorus, too little calcium in the diet, causing secondary hyperparathyroidism, which probably causes the hair  ̣lcium and magnesium to go up."

"That's a little too involved for me. I'll take your word for it: There's probably a study done on that, too. So I'll go home, cut the protein back some, eat fewer acid-forming foods, and make sure my calcium to phosphorus ratio is good. Is that it? Oh, what about supplements?"

"The ones you're using are good ones, but probably it would be best to correct the calcium to phosphorus ratio by using less bone meal and more calcium, possibly the type derived from oyster shells. At least one gram of extra calcium daily would be a good idea, particularly in your case, with osteoporosis in the family. Don't forget vitamin D, especially here in the Northwest. Why don't you stop the lecithin for a while, and keep track of your cholesterol and HDL cholesterol after you've made your diet changes. Brewer's yeast is a high source of phosphorus, but it has so many other good things in it . . . why not try continuing it, maybe a little less, and see if you can fit it into your overall calcium-phosphorus balance? Actually, you could do that with all the supplements, if you wanted. Remember, it's not the absolute amounts, but the balance that's important. More calcium than phosphorus, overall."

# Exercise Can Help

"Before you go, I should mention one other thing. From what you told me, I gather you don't exercise much. It's been observed repeatedly that inactivity leads to bone loss; the more inactive you are, the worse it is. Recently, a study was done to see if perhaps exercise could actually increase bone mass in a measurable way.

After one year of exercise three times a week, postmenopausal women were found to have gained in total body calcium."

Mrs. Burton thought for a minute. "Not only no loss, but actual gain?" She got up to go. "Well, that settles it. Diet change, and back to tennis, too." She turned around at the door. "If I do all this and still get a dowager's hump, you're in trouble."

I laughed. "Remember, very little's for sure in medicine. You could go skiing at age 80, hit a tree, and still break a hip, good bones or not. But chances are you'll be a lot closer to five feet six inches than your mother or grandmother was."

# Preventing Osteoporosis

Osteoporosis is a major health hazard for women following menopause. Decreased hormone secretion is obviously one contributory cause, and many studies have shown that supplemental estrogen after menopause is useful in its prevention and treatment. Enthusiasm for estrogen replacement therapy has been dampened somewhat, however, by demonstrating its association with an increased risk of cancer. Fortunately, enough information has been accumulated about osteoporosis to make it preventable for most women. For a few for whom prevention may not be successful, hormone and other more risky treatment is still possible.

Is it absolutely necessary to become a vegetarian at the time of menopause to maximize chances of osteoporosis prevention? As I mentioned to Mrs. Burton, it isn't *absolutely* necessary, but certainly would make it simpler. Vegetarianism combines several osteoporosis prevention factors into one dietary program.

Protein is definitely decreased. Although entirely adequate for good health in a well-planned vegetarian program, there's not enough protein to cause excess loss of dietary or supplemental calcium. There's also much less phosphorus in a vegetarian diet, provided that unprocessed traditional foods are used. The acid/alkaline balance is automatically favorable unless more than half of the diet is grain derived.

Despite the many other health benefits of a vegetarian diet

(less cancer, heart attacks, strokes, high blood pressure, diabetes, diverticulitis, and gallbladder disease), I don't urge all those I work with to become vegetarians. Although that might seem inconsistent with maximum disease prevention, it's very consistent with sound medical practice. In addition to its status as an inexact science, medicine is an art; some of that is the art of what's practical. Early training, social circumstances, and long-developed personal preferences usually preclude serious consideration of vegetarianism, which is seen by most Americans as a radical dietary change. So although a properly planned vegetarian diet is best for anyone's health in almost any circumstances, including osteoporosis prevention, it may not be appropriate.

Another major factor in osteoporosis appears to be, in many cases, a failure of adequate calcium absorption. In a long-term (one-and-a-half to four-year) study by Herta Spencer, M.D., of calcium supplementation under carefully controlled circumstances in a metabolic research ward, investigators found that women with osteoporosis have decreased ability to absorb calcium from the intestine. Sixty-seven to 82 percent of dietary and supplemental calcium was excreted unabsorbed by the women studied. When all calcium losses from the body were considered, only 3 to 7 percent of the calcium from diet and supplements was retained in the body by the women with osteoporosis, compared to 42 to 50 percent by supplemented nonosteoporotic individuals. The majority of other studies of calcium absorption in osteoporotic individuals cited by these investigators lead to the same conclusion: People with osteoporosis don't assimilate calcium well.

These researchers don't indicate why calcium is poorly absorbed. If the reason or reasons could be found, it might be helpful in prevention and treatment of osteoporosis. Although medical literature documentation is very scarce, observation has convinced me that one major reason for calcium malabsorption by women with osteoporosis (as well as the much smaller number of men) is our old friend, hypochlorhydria (or low stomach acidity).

No, I'm not going to tax your patience with yet another discussion of the problem. I'll just mention the data leading to the conclusion that low stomach acidity is a major contributing factor to osteoporosis, and you can read about it in more detail in the chapter "Good Digestion: Why We Can't Take It for Granted."

The most important data come from direct testing of women (and men) with osteoporosis, and bone loss from the jaw, a condition of great concern to dentists. Our laboratory finds that nearly all have varying degrees of low stomach acidity. That has also been the case for the few young people with osteoporosis we've tested. Their degree of stomach acidity is lowest and the worst of all.

Individuals with osteoporosis and low stomach acidity usually improve their calcium assimilation by taking hydrochloric acid supplements. That can be demonstrated by follow-up x-rays (bone density increase), by hair mineral analysis (calcium levels improve), and by symptom improvement (fingernails become stronger and muscle cramps disappear with less supplemental calcium).

Considering the large percentage of individuals past 55 with low stomach acidity, it's obviously a major factor in osteoporosis, and almost always overlooked and not even tested for. As with iron assimilation, the relationship may not be exact since there's not enough data at present to say, but it's important, too.

There's no question that calcium is the principal dietary and supplemental mineral needed for osteoporosis prevention and treatment. Studies using calcium alone in treatment, though, have had variable results, some good, some termed disappointing. However, there are no authorities who recommend against calcium supplementation for osteoporosis; all agree it should be used. A paper by Robert Marcus, M.D., of the Stanford University School of Medicine, recommends that total daily calcium intake should be one gram daily before, and 1,500 milligrams daily after menopause.

Remember, however, that no nutrient functions by itself in our bodies. Supplementing with calcium alone (or perhaps with vitamin D) ignores the possible role of many other nutrients in bone metabolism. While it's extremely important to the scientific study of osteoporosis to figure out exactly which nutrients do what, goals for personal health care are different. Each of us has only one set of bones, one body to take care of for only the space of one lifetime. Science may not find all the answers while each of us is here. For these reasons, a study of osteoporosis conducted by Anthony Albanese, Ph.D., a prominent calcium and osteoporosis researcher at the Burke Rehabilitation Center in White Plains, New York, is very important.

Dr. Albanese's group compared changes in bone density occurring in a group of women supplemented with 700 to 800 milligrams of calcium alone with those of a group supplemented with at least the Recommended Dietary Allowance (RDA) of 6 other minerals and 12 vitamins (in a "multiple" tablet form). Evaluation of bone density before and after 12 months of supplementation showed improvement two to three times greater in the calcium-multivitamin-and-mineral group compared to the calcium-alone group.

Dr. Albanese didn't indicate which, if any, of the other vitamins and minerals should be considered most important, besides calcium. Much more research will be required to answer that question, if indeed it's answerable. Scientists may finally conclude that an adequate supply of all nutrients is essential not only for bone health, but for the entire body, a key concept of nutritional biochemistry, and one that holistic practitioners have been promoting for years.

Other developing knowledge elsewhere in medicine supports the multiple-mineral-with-calcium approach. Research into heart disease is increasingly showing that an oversupply of calcium without sufficient offsetting quantities of magnesium, manganese, potassium, and other minerals may actually cause some types of heart problems.

One other fact of importance noted in Dr. Albanese's study: A 1959 United States Department of Agriculture survey of 5,500 women said to be in good health showed that in the 45-and-older age group, the average calcium intake was 450 milligrams daily, far below the RDA of 800 milligrams. Particularly if you're female, do you know how much calcium you're getting each day? And don't forget the other minerals.

Emphasizing further the other mineral point, recent studies have shown magnesium deficiency in 16 of 19 women with osteoporosis, and a reverse correlation between zinc levels and jawbone loss in 51 individuals. That means the less zinc in your diet the greater your potential for bone loss.

Before leaving the topic of minerals and osteoporosis, I'd like to comment on phosphorus. Nearly all observers agree that the average American diet contains more than enough phosphorus, especially with its heavy contribution from processed foods. However, there's increasing research to indicate that the ratio of calcium to phosphorus may be just as important to the development of osteoporosis as the absolute amount of calcium. Even added calcium may not help if there's too much phosphorus.

In my practice, I've found hair analysis to be a very useful tool in the detection of calcium to phosphorus ratio problems. When unexpectedly high calcium and magnesium levels are discovered on a routine screening hair mineral test, I ask the individual to correct her calcium to phosphorus dietary ratio, and to use supplemental calcium. Nearly every time, a follow-up test shows a drop in hair calcium and magnesium levels toward normal.

Unfortunately, that finding is all too frequent, especially in younger women. Hopefully, by correcting the calcium problem before menopause, much osteoporosis can be prevented. In older women with already advanced osteoporosis, the hair mineral analysis more often shows low calcium and magnesium levels. It appears that abnormal or false-positive elevations are a more frequent phenomenon in the earlier stages of the problem.

Two final observations. Most experiments show that exercise is beneficial in the prevention and treatment of osteoporosis. Almost always, that's true. Very preliminary findings from Christopher Cann, Ph.D., of the department of radiology at the University of California (San Francisco) School of Medicine, however, indicate that women with exercise-induced amenorrhea (loss of menses) may be at risk for osteoporotic bone loss. CAT scans of a group of women runners between ages 19 and 49 with amenorrhea for five to ten years showed significantly less bone mass than a similar group who didn't run. One researcher speculates that such bone loss may be due to a decrease in the production of the menstrual hormone, estrogen, caused by low levels of body fat.

All the scientific evidence regarding osteoporosis may not be in for a long time, but there is enough available information to give you an excellent chance to prevent osteoporosis personally. One bit of data on which all authorities agree is that prevention is far preferable, and easier than after-the-fact treatment. You have only one set of bones: If you haven't already, why not keep them intact when you're *80* by starting preventive measures now?

## REFERENCES

**Acid-Forming Diet**

"Acidogenic Diet May Be Among Factors Causing Osteoporosis." *Family Practice News*, May 1–15, 1976, p. 18.

Barzel, Uriel S. "Acid Loading and Osteoporosis." *Journal of the American Geriatrics Society*, September, 1982, p. 613.

**Calcium**

Albanese, Anthony A. "Effects of Calcium and Micronutrients on Bone Loss of Pre- and Postmenopausal Women." Paper presented at American Medical Association meeting, January, 1981.

Lee, C. J.; Lawler, G. S.; and Johnson, G. H. "Effects of Supplementation of the Diets with Calcium and Calcium-Rich Foods on Bone Density and Elderly Females with Osteoporosis." *American Journal of Clinical Nutrition*, May, 1981, pp. 819–823.

Marcus, Robert. "The Relationship of Dietary Calcium to the Maintenance of Skeletal Integrity in Man—An Interface of Endocrinology and Nutrition." *Metabolism*, January, 1982, pp. 93–101.

Spencer, Herta et al. "Absorption of Calcium in Osteoporosis." *American Journal of Medicine*, August, 1964, pp. 223–234.

**Calcium Absorption and Stomach Acidity**
Hunt, J. N., and Johnson, C. "Relationship Between Gastric Secretion of Acid and Urinary Excretion of Calcium After Oral Supplements of Calcium." *Digestive Diseases and Sciences*, vol. 28, 1983, p. 417.

Ivanovich, Peter; Fellows, Harold; and Rich, Clayton. "The Absorption of Calcium Carbonate." *Annals of Internal Medicine*, May, 1967, pp. 917–923.

Mahoney, Arthur W., and Hendricks, Deloy G. "Role of Gastric Acid in the Utilization of Dietary Calcium by the Rat." *Nutrition and Metabolism*, vol. 16, no. 6, 1974, pp. 375–382.

Mahoney, Arthur W.; Holbrook, Reid Scott; and Hendricks, Deloy G. "Effects of Calcium Solubility on Absorption by Rats with Induced Achlorhydria." *Nutrition and Metabolism*, vol. 18, no. 5–6, 1975, pp. 310–317.

Personal Communication with Walter Mertz, M.D., Director of the Human Nutrition Center, United States Department of Agriculture, 1983.

**Calcium/Phosphorus Ratio**
Bland, Jeffrey. "Dietary Calcium, Phosphorous and Their Relationships to Bone Formation and Parathyroid Activity." *Journal of the John Bastyr College of Naturopathic Medicine*, May 1, 1979, pp. 3–7.

Lutwak, Leo. "The Role of Dietary Calcium Phosphorous Ratio in Human Nutrition." *Proceedings of the Meat Industry Research Conference*, March 21, 1975, pp. 63–66.

Massey, Linda K., and Strang, Mary M. "Soft Drink Consumption, Phosphorous Intake, and Osteoporosis." *Journal of the American Dietetic Association*, June, 1982, pp. 581–583.

**Exercise**
Aloia, John F. et al. "Prevention of Involutional Bone Loss by Exercise." *Annals of Internal Medicine*, September, 1978, pp. 356–358.

Gonzalez, Elizabeth Rasche. "Premature Bone Loss Found in Some Nonmenstruating Sportswomen." *Journal of the American Medical Association*, August 6, 1982, pp. 513–514.

Smith, E. L.; Reddan, W.; and Smith, P. E. "Physical Activity and Calcium Modalities for Bone Mineral Increase in Aged Women." *Medicine and Science in Sports and Exercise*, vol. 13, no. 1, 1981, p. 8.

## Hair Analysis

Wright, Jonathan V., and Severtson, R. Bradley. "Observations on the Interpretations of Hair Mineral Analysis in Human Medicine." *Journal of the International Academy of Medicine*, April, 1982, pp. 13–16.

## Magnesium

Cohen, L., and Ketzes, R. "Infrared Spectroscopy and Magnesium Content of Bone Mineral in Osteoporotic Women." *Israel Journal of Medicine*, December, 1981, pp. 1123–1125.

## Osteoporosis

Albanese, Anthony A. *Bone Loss: Causes, Detection and Therapy.* Alan R. Liss, 1977, pp. 88–90.

Albanese, Anthony A. et al. "Problems of Bone Health in Elderly." *New York State Journal of Medicine*, February, 1975, pp. 326–336.

## Protein

Allen, Lindsay et al. "Protein-Induced Hypercalciuria: A Longer Term Study." *American Journal of Clinical Nutrition*, April, 1979, pp. 741–749.

Licata, Angelo A. et al. "Acute Effects of Dietary Protein on Calcium Metabolism in Patients with Osteoporosis." *Journal of Gerontology*, vol. 36, no. 1, 1981, pp. 14–19.

## Vegetarianism

Ellis, Frey R.; Holesh, Schura; and Ellis, John W. "Incidence of Osteoporosis in Vegetarians and Omnivores." *American Journal of Clinical Nutrition,* June, 1972, pp. 555–558.

Marsh, Alice G. et al. "Cortical Bone Density of Adult Lacto-ovo-vegetarian and Omnivorous Women." *Journal of the American Dietetic Association,* February, 1980, pp. 148–151.

Sanchez, T. V. et al. "Bone Mineral Mass in Elderly Vegetarian Females." Paper presented at the Bone Mineral Measurement Conference, 1978.

**Zinc**

Frithiof, L. et al. "The Relationship Between Marginal Bone Loss and Serum Zinc Levels." *Acta Medica Scandinavica,* vol. 207, no. 1, 1980, pp. 67–70.

Priscilla Clifford is two months pregnant, but nauseated and throwing up all the time. Combinations of vitamins C and K—a relatively unknown treatment—relieve her of her miseries within only one week's time.

# A CASE OF SEVERE PREGNANCY NAUSEA 44

"I've got to stop this throwing up all the time. My obstetrician says I might have to go in the hospital on IVs if it gets much worse. I don't want to do that, but I can hardly keep anything down and that's not good for the baby either, is it?"

Priscilla Clifford was two months pregnant with her second baby. She'd been a patient of mine for other reasons, but as I don't deliver babies, I hadn't seen her since she'd become pregnant. However, she'd come back to see if there was anything to do about her nausea and vomiting.

"How long have you had this much of a problem?"

"Practically since the first day I was pregnant. Well, actually, I did get nauseated before I missed my first menstrual period, but all this throwing up didn't start until after that. It's been every day since."

"Have you tried doing anything about it so far?"

"Sure. I read in ... I think it was Adelle Davis ... that vitamin B$_6$ might help. I took 50 milligrams of that a day, had to really struggle to keep it down. It didn't do a thing. So I happened to be talking to Kathy Voegtlin—she had her baby last year, you know, she's a patient here, too. She said you told her it was safe to use as much as 200 milligrams, three times a day, if necessary.

"So, I tried it. But that doesn't seem to help me, either. I tried for a whole week, too, with no relief." She suddenly appeared worried. "That is safe, isn't it? I haven't done anything bad to my baby?"

"Not as far as I know. I've seen many women have to use that much to control nausea and vomiting, or get rid of edema fluid. Dr. John Ellis, who's had much more experience with $B_6$ treatment, hasn't seen any problems, either.

"There are two possible hazards after the baby's born, though. Six hundred milligrams of pyridoxine daily has been found to shut off nursing, so the amount has to be cut back. Secondly, if the baby is exposed to high amounts of $B_6$ before it's born, and then very little immediately after birth, for example in a commercial formula, it possibly could have withdrawal seizures. However, both these theoretical hazards are easily avoided by nursing the baby while continuing to take 20 to 30 milligrams of pyridoxine a day. Of course, it's best to do all this under the supervision of a doctor experienced in the use of vitamins and minerals.

"But excuse the digression—that may not apply to you if we can't get the $B_6$ to work."

"Can't get it to work? I've already tried, and it doesn't! Also, I've tried this"—she held out a bottle of a commonly prescribed medication for nausea and vomiting of pregnancy—"and it doesn't work, either. I don't know what to do." She suddenly looked almost green. "Excuse me." She rushed out.

When she got resettled, I said, "I'm really surprised that the vitamin $B_6$ didn't work. It usually does. But occasionally, when swallowing it doesn't work, injections do. I don't know why that is; possibly an absorptive problem of some sort during pregnancy. I'd like you to try a $B_6$ injection every day, for the next few days. You can get them here, or you or your husband can learn to give them to you. Let me know how you do."

Four days later, the nurse came into my office. "Priscilla's back. She says the injections didn't help. I don't understand it . . . injections usually do. Could you come and talk to her?"

I went to the examination room where Priscilla was waiting.

"I was supposed to get another shot today," she said. "But they're just not helping. If anything, I'm getting worse. Maybe I'll just have to go on IVs in the hopital. If the shots haven't helped by today, even a little, there's no point continuing, is there?"

## Vitamins C and K Work Together

I agreed there probably wasn't. "But don't give up yet. A few months ago I came across another article about a way to help stop nausea and vomiting in pregnancy. The doctor who reported it said it helped in 64 of 70 consecutive cases, with complete relief of symptoms in three days. Three more cases had vomiting relieved, but not nausea."

"Why didn't you try that before? Sixty-four of 70 is pretty good! Is it a drug, or dangerous?"

"No, not a drug. It's vitamin K along with vitamin C. As far as I know, in the doses used, it's not dangerous."

"Is this something new?"

"No, it was reported in 1952."

"Why didn't you tell me before?"

"I just found the information recently, as I said. I haven't had much chance to try it. As you know, I don't deliver babies anymore."

"But you think it's safe?"

"Safer than that drug you've tried. Also, the doses are small. In fact, vitamin K is the same vitamin given to all infants just after they're born to prevent hemorrhagic disease of the newborn, which is nothing more than bleeding from vitamin K deficiency. Since I found this article about vitamin K stopping nausea and vomiting in pregnancy, I've been wondering if there isn't a connection. Why else should so many babies require vitamin K, if their mothers get enough? Of course, I'm just guessing. . . ."

Mrs. Clifford started to look nauseated once more. "I'll be glad to prevent trouble for my baby, if that's the case," she said. "But right now, how about some for me?"

"I'm sorry. I've been carrying on too long again. The quickest way of getting it in you is an injection." I asked the nurse to get an injection of vitamin K and vitamin C.

"I've been trying to take a little vitamin C every day; it hasn't helped. But I've never seen vitamin K in the health food store in anything but a tiny dose."

## Modest Doses Used

"I know. There hasn't been any public demand for it; besides, as a fat-soluble vitamin, it theoretically could be toxic in very large doses. However, the doses reported effective are fairly small, and were necessary, on the average, for only 30 days. You're right about the vitamin C not working by itself. Dr. Richard Merkel, who wrote the report, pointed out that neither vitamin C nor vitamin K worked by itself. They had to be taken together. The dose of vitamin C, by today's standards, was very small: 25 milligrams."

"That's not much at all. I've been taking one gram when I can. Is that OK?"

"Should be. Take it right along with the vitamin K." I wrote out a prescription for five-milligram vitamin K tablets. "This is a small dose, five milligrams, but you'll still have to get it at the drugstore."

"This prescription says vitamin $K_1$. What's the difference?"

"Vitamins $K_1$ (phytonadione) and $K_2$ (menaquinone) are the naturally occurring forms. Pharmaceutical textbooks say that vitamin $K_1$ appears to be safe to use. Vitamin $K_3$, menadione, a synthetic form, is theoretically toxic in very large doses. $K_3$ is the type used in Dr. Merkel's report, but I'd still rather stick with $K_1$."

"Will it work as well?"

"It should, although it's harder to absorb than $K_3$. Of course, we could if necessary get around that with injections. But if it just doesn't work, which I doubt, small doses of $K_3$ should be OK."

Priscilla called back one week later to report that all her nausea and vomiting were gone. She tried to stop taking vitamin $K_1$ in two weeks at my recommendation, but found she had to continue for six weeks before she could stop without return of symptoms.

I don't have an obstetrical practice, so I haven't recommended vitamins K and C for nausea and vomiting of pregnancy very often. Those few times, it's worked well. However, given the impressive statistics in Dr. Merkel's report and the apparent safety of this treatment, I thought it would be appropriate to pass this case history along.

# A Medical Mystery versus a Nutritional Marvel?

A persistent minor mystery of routine medical practice is that a possibly dangerous, entirely synthetic chemical continues to be the most widely prescribed remedy for nausea and vomiting of pregnancy, while the very effective and much safer treatment described above is entirely ignored. That might be excusable if therapy with vitamins K and C had been described in an obscure or foreign medical journal, but that wasn't the case. It was published in the *American Journal of Obstetrics and Gynecology*, where it should have been noticed by nearly every practicing obstetrician.

Certainly it was "only one study," but the results were impressive. At the very least, the report of Richard L. Merkel, M.D., should have stimulated several follow-up evaluations of his treatment program. I've never found any; apparently his extremely promising work sank into the "vitamins aren't important" swamp of opinion without a trace. Hundreds of thousands of pregnant women and their unborn infants in the subsequent three decades have instead been dosed with possibly more dangerous synthetic drugs, never having been informed of a safer vitamin alternative.

It's been suspected that the most widely prescribed drug for the nausea and vomiting of pregnancy, called Bendectin, may also cause birth defects. Although not proven one way or another, the evidence has been sufficient to provoke lawsuits against its manufacturers. As we go to press, the manufacturer has ceased production of Bendectin.

Vitamin $B_6$ is also very effective for many women. Years ago, John Ellis, M.D., pioneered its use and demonstrated its safety. Even with passage of time, no one has found vitamin $B_6$ unsafe during pregnancy. Interestingly enough, the same most widely prescribed synthetic drug also contains ten milligrams of vitamin $B_6$; the manufacturer's product description states: "Studies indicate $B_6$ has an antinauseant activity." It's a matter of speculation why vitamin $B_6$ is combined with the synthetic drug: One obvious question is whether the drug or the $B_6$ is doing the work. If the drug is effective, why combine it with $B_6$, and if it's the $B_6$, why use the drug at all? There's no evidence that the drug and $B_6$ "work together," as is the case with vitamins K and C. Unfortunately, ten milligrams of vitamin $B_6$ is often an inadequate amount.

The type of vitamin K used by Dr. Merkel is a synthetic form known as vitamin $K_3$. According to one authoritative textbook of pharmacology, small doses of vitamin $K_3$ are considered safe, but "moderate" doses have caused hemolytic anemia and high bilirubin levels in the newborn, especially premature infants, which could lead to very serious complications. Other sources say that doses of vitamin $K_3$ producing side effects have been "large" and "extraordinarily high"—100 milligrams daily in one report.

A natural form, vitamin $K_1$, is routinely given to infants for prevention of "hemorrhagic disease of the newborn." According to the same textbook, it appears to be safe. A scientific study of 204 infants demonstrated that giving five milligrams of vitamin $K_1$ daily to expectant mothers for one or two weeks before delivery had the expected beneficial effect on the newborn infant's clotting time, and caused no undesirable side effects. Logically, prenatal administration of vitamin K might be a better preventive for neonatal hemorrhage, before the stress and trauma of birth rather than after. As a side benefit, a few cases of maternal postpartum hemorrhage might be prevented, also.

Although the five-milligram vitamin $K_3$ dose used by Dr. Merkel is definitely small, and almost certainly safe (not to mention safer than a synthetic nonvitamin drug), I've used vitamin $K_1$ because it's the natural form and has an even better reputation for safety.

On two occasions in my experience vitamin $K_1$ hasn't been effective when swallowed, but injections have succeeded in stopping the nausea and vomiting of pregnancy. The explanation is probably to be found in the more difficult assimilation of vitamin $K_1$ (as compared to vitamin $K_3$). $K_1$ is fat soluble, absorbed in the upper small intestine only if bile salts are present. Commercially available $K_3$ is water soluble, and absorbed in the lower small intestine and colon with or without the presence of bile salts. Injections of $K_1$ avoid problems with assimilation which may be present in individuals unresponsive to swallowing it.

Unlike other fat-soluble vitamins, there is little vitamin K stored in the body. What limited stores exist are slowly destroyed; vitamin K deficiency can develop in weeks when circumstances interfere with its absorption.

Since yet another form, vitamin $K_2$ (menaquinone), is produced by intestinal bacteria, it's sometimes thought that food sources of vitamin $K_1$ are unnecessary. However, in one experiment, volunteers who ate a diet devoid of vitamin $K_1$ developed abnormal blood clotting tests in just three weeks. Adding food sources of the vitamin reversed the abnormality, leading the researcher to conclude that foods rather than intestinal bacteria provide more vitamin K. So little vitamin K research has been done that most tables of food composition don't list it. In nature, vitamin K accumulates in the chlorophyll-forming parts of plant leaves; deep green leafy vegetables are thus an excellent source. Cabbage, tomato, peas, carrots, soybeans, and pork liver are said to be good sources.

In case it's confusing, the various K vitamins appear to have essentially the same functions in the body, unlike the B vitamins (each of which performs very different functions from the others even though they frequently work together).

At present, there's no data regarding deficiency of vitamins K and C in nauseated, vomiting pregnant women. The apparent effectiveness of these two vitamins together, but not taken separately, implies some other effect than correction of simple deficiency. Whatever the effect, five milligrams of either vitamin $K_3$ or $K_1$ and 25 milligrams of vitamin C taken simultaneously appear quite safe.

There's absolutely no reason for vitamin K and C treatment of the nausea and vomiting of pregnancy to be neglected any longer (or vitamin $B_6$, either). Why use drugs if vitamins are effective? Drugs can and should be used when necessary, but always when more conservative measures aren't effective. This basic principle is taught to all medical students, but all too often is ignored in present routine medical practice.

## REFERENCES

**General**

Cochrane, W. A. "Overnutrition in Prenatal and Neonatal Life: A Problem?" *Canadian Medical Association Journal*, October 23, 1965, pp. 893–899.

Gilman, Alfred; Goodman, Louis S.; and Gilman, Alfred, eds. *The Pharmacological Basis of Therapeutics*. 6th ed. Macmillan Publishing, 1980, pp. 1592–1596.

**Vitamin $B_6$**

Ellis, John M., and Presley, James. *Vitamin $B_6$: The Doctor's Report*. Harper & Row, 1973.

Foukas, Matthias D. "An Antilactogenic Effect of Pyridoxine." *Journal of Obstetrics and Gynecology of the British Commonwealth*, August, 1973, pp. 718–720.

Marcus, R. G. "Suppression of Lactation with High Doses of Pyridoxine." *South African Medical Journal*, December 6, 1975, pp. 2155–2156.

**Vitamins C and K**

Hill, Reba M. et al. "Vitamin K Administration and Neonatal Hyperbilirubinemia of Unknown Etiology." *American Journal of Obstetrics and Gynecology*, August, 1961, pp. 320–324.

Merkel, Richard L. "The Use of Menadione Bisulfite and Ascorbic Acid in the Treatment of Nausea and Vomiting of Pregnancy." *American Journal of Obstetrics and Gynecology*, August, 1952, pp. 416–418.

Owen, George M. et al. "Use of vitamin $K_1$ in Pregnancy." *American Journal of Obstetrics and Gynecology*, October 1, 1967, pp. 368–373.

Udall, John A. "Human Sources and Absorption of Vitamin K in Relation to Anticoagulation Stability." *Journal of the American Medical Association*, October 11, 1965, pp. 107–109.

**The pain and swelling of a rash is eliminated in just two days once this young post-doctoral student begins taking potassium iodide supplements and avoiding artificial food chemicals.**

# 45    A CASE OF PAINFUL "RED BUMPS"

Amy Robertson looked a little feverish as she came in. She sat down, and promptly rolled up her trousers to the knees, her shirt to the elbows. Appearing on both shins and the outsides of both arms were red, raised nodules from one to three inches in diameter. She had at least a dozen, mostly large, scattered about both shins; a half-dozen or less, mostly smaller, on the outer forearms.

"That's the problem," she declared.

I bent forward to observe more closely. The nodules were very red; the one I touched was quite warm.

"Before you feel the need to press harder, let me tell you they all hurt," she said. "That's been established."

I withdrew my finger. "Looks like . . ."

". . . erythema nodosum." She finished for me. "Red bumps, in Greek or Latin. I know that. What I need to know is how to get rid of them."

"Even if we didn't do anything about them, usually they're gone in three to six weeks," I said.

She looked slightly disgusted. "And usually don't return.

However"—she tilted her head slightly, assumed a different tone—" 'perhaps 10 percent of the patients have continuing crop-like appearance or new lesions or recurrences after free intervals.' "

She returned to her original posture and tone of voice. "That's me, 10 percent or less. This is the seventh time in the last four years. It wouldn't be so bad if it was just red bumps, I can live with that. Trouble is, they hurt terribly for two weeks or so. Twice, it's been so bad I could hardly walk. It feels like it's going to get that way this time."

"Have you had other symptoms?"

"I'm a regular textbook case. I get a sore throat and swollen glands first, then a fever. I've got that now. Then all my joints start to ache, and these bumps break out. They do go away, usually in a month, but I'm tired of it."

"You must have had tests done before."

"Of course. Actually, I'm not being fair with you. I'm a post-doctoral student at the university; I'm in the libraries a lot. After the second attack of this erythema nodosum, I went to the medical library to do some research. Unfortunately, I only found a few details that the internist I saw hadn't mentioned."

"Such as?"

"Oh, about the fewer than 10 percent who have bumps that keep coming back, and that it occurs most frequently in women between 20 and 30 years of age. I'm 26."

"You've had tests?"

"Every one in the book. I've been chest x-rayed and skin-tested for tuberculosis and various fungal diseases. Negative. I've been cultured for strep numerous times. I don't have syphilis. I might have a chronic viral infection, but there's no way of proving or disproving that. I'm not taking birth-control pills anymore, and I haven't taken sulfa or any other drugs except aspirin since this thing started."

I noted her list.

"Sounds like a thorough investigation."

"Yes, I'm not unhappy with that. The internist explained to me that erythema nodosum is thought to be a delayed allergy or sensitivity reaction pattern to a wide variety of injections or drugs. Trouble is, we couldn't find any of them in me."

"What about birth-control pills?"

"Well, I was taking them when my first attack happened. But I stopped when the doctor told me to, and haven't had any since."

"The aspirin?"

"I only take it when they really hurt badly during an attack. No other times. It doesn't seem to make them worse."

She looked thoughtful for a moment. "I don't really expect you to find a cause. That's been checked out thoroughly. I thought well, maybe high doses of vitamin C or something like that might knock this down quicker."

"Since it's probably an allergic or hypersensitivity reaction, high doses of vitamin C might help a little, in fact. However, a study has been published about a high-dose natural-element treatment that is probably quicker and more effective. Before we get into that, though, let's go over causes a bit more.

"As you pointed out, you've been thoroughly checked for most of the infectious agents associated with this type of sensitivity, except the unprovable viral ones. You're not taking any drugs. But prescription and nonprescription drugs are only a small percentage of all the chemicals we're exposed to. I'm sure you've read that there are literally thousands of possible synthetic chemicals in food alone, as well as thousands more variably present in the environment?"

"Those can cause erythema nodosum? It's not in the textbooks I read."

"Not yet, but many practitioners have their suspicions."

"How could we possibly figure out if it was one of those? There aren't tests for chemical flavors, colors, preservatives, not to mention pesticides, insecticides, antibiotics and hormones fed to animals. . . ."

"Along with household and industrial chemicals, too. But you can make a start."

"How?"

"Try eliminating some broad categories, and see what happens. It won't help an acute attack like this, but perhaps you'll avoid recurrences."

"Well, I've moved twice in the last three years. Gas heat once, oil once, electric now. Hardwood floors twice, carpets once. Different furniture. Makes it less likely it's around the house. . . ."

"True, although not absolutely so. However, I'd recommend starting with a large group of food chemicals: artificial colors, flavors, preservatives."

"That's going to be a real chore. And I won't even know for sure if it's going to work."

"Not unless the problem doesn't return. But it's worked for others before, and besides, it'll be better for your health, anyway."

She sighed. "I know, I know. OK, I'll try it. Now, what's this about some quick relief?"

"It's not absolutely for sure, but worth trying. Drs. Schulz and Whiting, both of South Africa, published a report covering 28 cases of erythema nodosum. Relief of symptoms was reported within two days in 24 cases."

"Two days? What did they use?"

"Potassium iodide."

"Potassium iodide? Hmm . . . I thought I read the problem could be caused by iodides."

"One textbook does say that. But the right dose apparently helps. Helped 16 of 17 cases of nodular vasculitis, too."

"How does it work?"

"It isn't known, but the doctors' theory is that potassium iodide causes the release of heparin, a natural substance produced by the body, which can suppress delayed hypersensitivity."

"Whatever. Do I go get some kelp? That's a good source of iodine."

"Unfortunately not. Even if the iodine in kelp were effective—and remember there's a slight difference between iodine and iodide—you'd have to take approximately 6,000 kelp tablets a day."

"Good grief. How about the potassium iodide tablets in the stores?"

"Afraid not. Even with the newer, larger sizes, it'd take 3,000 to 4,000 daily. Fortunately, potassium iodide is available in adequate dose on prescription." I wrote one out.

"The whole problem will be gone in two days?"

"Not the whole problem . . . the pain and swelling. The doctors reported the rest of the healing took an average of two weeks. And in 24 of 28 cases, not all."

"That's good enough. If it works this time it'll probably work again if the nodules come back, won't it?"

"Probably, but we won't know anything until it's tried."

Ms. Robertson's erythema nodosum became pain free and much less swollen in the two days predicted. She took the time to eliminate all artificial food chemicals from her diet, even though it was a lot of trouble. She can't be absolutely sure which food chemical or chemicals she was reacting to—and we've decided that one or more of them were probably the cause, since she's had no recurrences of the erythema nodusum at all in the four years since.

# New Support for Potassium Iodide Therapy

Since Drs. Schulz and Whiting published their original report regarding potassium iodide, the treatment has been found to be usually successful by researchers in Germany and Japan.

The Japanese investigators reported: "Administration of . . . [potassium iodide] . . . showed a substantial effect in 11 of 15 patients with erythema nodosum [painful red bumps on the front of the legs], 7 of 10 with nodular vasculitis [inflammed vessels caused by an allergic reaction]. Relief of subjective symptoms, including tenderness, joint pain, and fever, occurred within 24 hours. Substantial improvement in the eruption occurred within a few days. . . . The patients to whom the [potassium iodide] was administered shortly after the initial onset of erythema nodosum seemed to respond most satisfactorily."

Unfortunately for self-treatment, the doses of potassium iodide used by the Japanese investigators were again high: 300

milligrams, three times daily. As noted in the same report, iodide treatment has been reported elsewhere to have side effects, including acne, eczema, bruising, and paradoxically (since these are the conditions it also helps) erythema nodosum and vasculitis. In the Japanese study, however, no side effects were observed during the therapy; duration of the treatment was relatively short.

Considering the relatively high dosage of potassium iodide required and the possibility of side effects, self-treatment isn't wise. However, there's no reason why these reports can't be called to the attention of your doctor. For a small fee, photocopies for strictly personal use can usually be obtained from any university medical library.

It's not known why iodide might work. Most explanations, while quite plausible, are at present still guesses.

## REFERENCES

**Erythema Nodosum**

Beeson, Paul B.; McDermott, Walsh; and Wyngaarden, James B. *Cecil Textbook of Medicine*. 15th ed. W. B. Saunders, 1979, p. 2295.

Farber, Eugene M., and Abel, Elizabeth A. "Drug Eruptions and Urticaria." In Section 2: Dermatology, *Scientific American Medicine*. Scientific American, pp. 1–2.

**Oral Contraceptives**

Bombardieri, Stefano et al. "Erythema Nodosum Associated with Pregnancy and Oral Contraceptives." *British Medical Journal*, June 11, 1977, pp. 1509–1510.

**Potassium Iodide Treatment**

Horio, Takeshi et al. "Potassium Iodide in the Treatment of Erythema Nodosum and Nodular Vasculitis." *Archives of Dermatology*, January, 1981, pp. 29–31.

Schulz, E. J., and Whiting, D. A. "Treatment of Erythema Nodosum and Nodular Vasculitis with Potassium Iodide." *British Journal of Dermatology*, January, 1976, pp. 75–78.

> Injections of vitamin $B_{12}$ change a confused, disordered, and forgetful woman back into her "spunky" self.

# 46 A CASE OF PREMATURE SENILITY

There's something fundamentally wrong with the attitude that nutritional therapy should never be tried, even if harmless, unless absolute proof of deficiency can be established, while drug therapy, with all its potential side effects, is OK to try first. Medical science and therapeutics are supposed to be conservative, trying the least harmful measures before those with more potential for danger. Unfortunately, when vitamin therapy is considered, it's looked upon by many physicians as radical.

Measures such as diet, vitamins, minerals, relaxation therapy, and exercise are conservative; drugs and surgery are considerably more radical. Not to say drugs and surgery don't have their place: They do, when and if more conservative measures don't work. This case, as you'd expect, illustrates these points.

"Mother's really starting to worry us," Mrs. Liebermann said. "After Father died, we were worried about her living alone. But she did just fine. Kept visiting her friends, shopping, calling us on the phone regularly. Of course, his death hit her hard emotionally, but she kept going, and seemed to bounce back in a few months.

"That's four years past. She had no problems until about eight or nine months ago, when both Sadie (that's my sister, she's two years older) and I noticed Mother was acting a little strange. Nothing definite, just not herself. More forgetful of things she'd never forgotten before. She's really gotten bad now. We're thinking she may have to go into a nursing home.

"I didn't mention that since Father died, I've offered to have Mother come live with us. So has Sadie, but she absolutely refused. She said she valued her independence too much. Besides, she had resolved never to burden her children. If she ever got that bad, she used to say, she had enough money saved to support her in a good nursing home, and that's where she wanted to go. She made us promise that's what we'd do. It looks like it's happening too soon. . . . That's why I'm here, to ask if there isn't anything else to do."

"You mentioned she's forgetful. What else? There must be other things bothering you, or her, or you wouldn't be so concerned."

## Signs of Confusion

"Other things? I can tell you lots of those. But let me finish about being forgetful. . . . I don't mean just a little. She'll write down a shopping list, take it with her, and forget she ever made it. I've found them in her purse later. For years she's gone to the same club on Wednesdays. I got a call from one of the ladies wanting to know if she was well—she'd missed three Wednesdays in a row. When I asked her about it, she said she kept forgetting it was Wednesday.

"Besides forgetful, she seems depressed. Sometimes when I visit her, she's just sitting there, not doing anything. She doesn't even come to the door, which by the way she leaves unlocked, frequently. She never used to do that. I've asked if anything's bothering her. She says no, she doesn't know what it is, she just doesn't feel quite right.

"Also, sometimes she's clear mentally, if you know what I mean, and sometimes confused. She'll stop in the middle of a sentence I could complete, not able to find the words. She can't find things at home that she's kept in the same place for years. She's been a crossword puzzle fan ever since I was a little girl, but in the last few months she hasn't done one. Says they're too hard these days.

"Sometimes she seems to understand that something's happening to her. She'll call, and discuss it in the most reasonable way, saying she must be getting senile, and laugh. Other times, when I try to talk to her about it, she looks blank and acts as if nothing ever happened."

# A Physical Problem

"Sadie and I don't think mother's going crazy. She's always been stable mentally; there's no history of mental problems in the family as far as we know. We think there's something physically the matter. So we took her to her regular doctor first. He examined her, did some tests, said she was fine, and referred us to a psychiatrist. As I said, we didn't think that's what the problem was, but we went."

"What did the psychiatrist say?"

"She diagnosed it as 'organic brain syndrome,' a physical, not psychological, disorder. The problem is that she can't say what causes it, just that many old people get this way. We could try a drug or two . . . a so-called 'psychic energizer,' or an antidepressant. If that helped, fine, if not, a nursing home was the only answer."

"Did you try the drugs?"

"Of course not . . . not yet, anyway. Mother's too young for a permanent sentence to drugs or a nursing home. She was 73 only a few weeks ago.

"Since the psychiatrist said it was 'organic,' we took her to the clinic [she named a large local referral center]. They put her through everything—x-rays, scans, blood tests, urine tests. Couldn't find anything. The supervising doctor there suggested the same sort of drugs the psychiatrist had.

"Well, all this time I'd been talking to friends and reading.

One friend told me the same thing had happened to her father ten years ago. Their doctor, who's since passed away, put him on vitamin $B_{12}$ shots, and he snapped right out of it in three to four weeks. He gives himself the shots now, because he won't give them up. So I read about vitamin $B_{12}$ deficiency; it really sounds like Mother: confused, forgetful, depressed, withdrawn. I asked the supervising doctor at the clinic if it could be a $B_{12}$ problem. He got mad, told me this vitamin thing was just a fad, but if I insisted he'd have a blood test done, anyway."

"How'd it turn out? Normal?"

"Yes. When we went back, it seemed like he couldn't wait to show me the lab slip. That proved it couldn't be a vitamin $B_{12}$ problem, he said. He pressed me to put Mother on drugs, but I said we'd wait. Fortunately Mother agreed, said she'd do whatever I said. Sadie was there, too, to back me up.

"We decided I'd come here to talk to you first. Even if it isn't a vitamin $B_{12}$ problem, maybe some other vitamin would help. The book I was reading listed those same symptoms for several of the other B vitamins."

"That's true. Many of the B vitamins are important for good mental function. But don't be positive it isn't a $B_{12}$ problem, yet."

"The lab test was normal."

## Test Can't Be Trusted

"Doctors who work with nutrition have observed for years that doing a vitamin $B_{12}$ blood test is useless. The thing to do is try $B_{12}$ when it seems indicated, and watch for any results."

"Why?"

"The absolute blood level of any nutrient is only one of many factors. It tells us nothing about the functioning of that nutrient in various tissues, such as the brain. Some people need more than so-called normal to function properly. Needs may vary at different times of life, or under different stresses.

"In addition to quantities of any nutrient, transport in and out of cells may be faulty. Some nutrients must be 'activated' before they're effective. Many nutrients work better in the presence of others, working poorly or not at all if something's absent. These are only a few reasons why a blood level of a nutrient is only part of the picture.

"Getting back to vitamin $B_{12}$. . . . There's another good reason to ignore the blood test. A recent report shows clearly that it's inaccurate and unreliable."

"Unreliable?"

"Right."

"So for who knows how many years, people have been told their vitamin $B_{12}$ levels were normal, based on a no-good test?" She shook her head.

"Exactly. Which is why, despite all the lab testing I recommend, I keep in mind advice repeated to medical students: Clinical observation is primary, laboratory determinations secondary. What we observe comes first. Sometimes accurate laboratory determinations are crucial, particularly when testing finer points of body chemistry, but direct observation should never be ignored. So, for example, when people keep reporting they feel better with vitamin $B_{12}$, and their doctors, friends, and relatives also observe improvement, then contradictory blood tests should be thrown out the window, since vitamin $B_{12}$ is usually harmless."

"So can I try vitamin $B_{12}$ for my mother?"

"Please bring her in first. $B_{12}$ is probably what we'll try, but I must talk to her, and check her over first. I know she's had extensive checkups lately, and no diseases were found. So I won't be asking her to repeat most tests already done. There are probably a few having a bearing on nutritional status that should be done. More important, I need to talk to her myself, make my own observations, before trying to do anything to improve her problems."

# "It's as If I'm Losing My Mind"

Mrs. Liebermann and her sister brought their mother in. She was a pleasant older woman who appeared as described by her daughter; sometimes clear, sometimes not. She agreed with her daughter's description of how she'd been, adding that she didn't understand it, and sometimes felt frightened. "It's as if I'm losing my mind," she said.

She added a few more details. She wasn't sleeping as well at night as last year. Her joints hurt, although they hadn't swelled. She had "tingly-like" feelings on and off in her hands.

As expected I could find no other diseases on examination. Instructions about giving vitamin $B_{12}$ by injection were given to Mrs. Liebermann, for use for her mother at home.

A few days later, Mrs. Liebermann phoned in to say her mother seemed better already. She phoned nearly every week at first, letting us know she was improving steadily.

Three months later, Mrs. Liebermann came in with her mother once more. The change was obvious. There was no sign of forgetfulness or confusion. Her mood was notably better, and her sense of humor seemed restored.

"I'm going to let my daughter ask the questions," she said. "After all, she's been doing most of the talking about me. Thank goodness, or I'd never have recovered my health."

Mrs. Liebermann's questions were few. Did the $B_{12}$ have to be given by injection or could it be swallowed? What about other B vitamins? Why did her mother need vitamin $B_{12}$ shots now, when she hadn't before?

I advised that to be sure of results, the injections should be continued for now. Many older people develop defects in absorption of vitamin $B_{12}$, either in association with hypochlorhydria (insufficient stomach acid, which is more frequent in older individuals) or for reasons presently unknown.

In addition, I recommend adding to the injection a small quantity of folate, almost always found in the body in association with $B_{12}$, as well as B complex vitamins. At least one study had shown that some older people who were swallowing vitamins daily still had deficient blood levels of individual B vitamins, corrected only by injection. After a few months, if Mrs. Liebermann's mother really disliked injections, she could try taking large quantities of these vitamins orally each day. Sometimes extra amounts will "force" absorption. If she remained well, fine. If not, she could always return to the injections. All B vitamins taken orally, except niacin ($B_3$), are generally considered safe even in enormous quantities (although thiamine can cause drowsiness). So trying this procedure would be perfectly safe.

Mrs. Liebermann's mother remains well. Vitamin therapy will not keep her or any of us healthy forever, but at least she can enjoy her older years much longer, with a clear mind and mental outlook unclouded by totally preventable malfunction.

Certainly not every case of deteriorating mental function in an older person will turn out this well. Some will still require drugs or institutional care. But it brings us back to my original observation: Conservative measures such as vitamin therapy should always be tried first. Even if laboratory studies seem to disagree, there's no harm in a period of trial, relying on clinical observation. If that doesn't work, we can always proceed to trying drugs or other more radical measures, to see if they're any more effective.

# Old Age Can Bring Deficiencies, but It Doesn't Have To

As noted by one group of investigators: "Intestinal malabsorption becomes increasingly prevalent with extreme old age." (Oddly, the ages of people that group studied ranged from only 65 to 92.) Using only standard measurements of malabsorption, and requiring abnormality on two of them or more to establish the diagnosis of malabsorption, that group found it present in 39 percent of these older individuals with symptoms, and in 12 percent of the control group (also older individuals, but without symptoms).

Using more sophisticated techniques, Herman Baker, M.D., and associates studied 228 ambulatory residents in a nursing home, with an average age of 87. All were said to be on a good diet, and all had taken at least one multivitamin tablet daily for three to five months before this study. Despite good diets and vitamin pill intake, 39 percent were deficient in one or more vitamins. The most common deficiency was vitamin $B_6$, followed by niacin, $B_{12}$, folate, and thiamine.

Sadly, even injected vitamin treatment doesn't reverse mental decline in some older individuals. And it's obvious that malabsorption of nutrients is an explanation in some but not all cases.

# REFERENCES

### Aging and Nutrient Absorption

Baker, H.; Frank, O.; and Jaslow, S. P. "Oral Versus Intramuscular Vitamin Supplementation for Hypovitaminosis in the Elderly." *Journal of the American Geriatrics Society*, January, 1980, pp. 42–45.

Baker, H.; Jaslow, S. P.; and Frank, O. "Severe Impairment of Dietary Folate Utilization in the Elderly." *Journal of the American Geriatrics Society*, May, 1978, pp. 218–221.

Kaufman, William. "The Use of Vitamin Therapy to Reverse Certain Concomitants of Aging." *Journal of the American Geriatrics Society*, November, 1955, pp. 927–936.

Montgomery, R. D. et al. "The Aging Gut: A Study of Intestinal Absorption in Relation to Nutrition in the Elderly." *Quarterly Journal of Medicine*, April, 1978, pp. 197–211.

### Diagnosis

Cohen, K. L., and Donaldson, R. M. "Unreliability of Radiodilution Assays as Screening Tests for Cobalamin (Vitamin $B_{12}$) Deficiency." *Journal of the American Medical Association*, October 24/31, 1980, pp. 1942–1944.

Donaldson, Robert M. " 'Serum $B_{12}$' and the Diagnosis of Cobalamin Deficiency." *New England Journal of Medicine*, October, 1978, pp. 827–828.

### Vitamin $B_{12}$

Elsborg, L.; Luna, V.; and Bastrup-Madson, P. "Serum Vitamin $B_{12}$ Levels in the Aged." *Acta Medica Scandinavica*, vol. 200, 1976, pp. 309–314.

The removal of 75 percent of his stomach has caused a 43-year-old man some serious problems with digestion, creating a whole host of ailments including fatigue, shingles, bone spurs, and bursitis. A series of vitamin $B_{12}$ injections (along with folate, $B_{12}$'s metabolic partner) help bring his energy levels back to normal and quickly quell his pain.

# 47    A CASE OF SHINGLES AND FATIGUE

"I'm 43 years old and feel like I'm falling apart," Mr. Kressels declared. "This case of shingles was the last straw. I remember my grandfather had shingles when he was 89. The other people I've known who had it were all in their sixties or seventies. So I decided to come in to find out what's going wrong in my system."

"That's a good idea at any age. Illness, especially repeated illness, usually indicates that a life pattern change is needed."

Mr. Kressels grimaced. "Don't I know! So where do we start this time?"

"Let's start with the shingles. Do you still have them?"

Mr. Kressels pulled up the right side of his shirt. Fifteen to 20 mostly healed sores formed an arc from back to abdomen, just above the waistline. "That's what's left. Still hurts, burns, though not as bad, and it's starting to itch like crazy."

"What have you done about them?"

"So far, suffered. I knew they'd go away eventually."

"Too bad you didn't get a series of vitamin $B_{12}$ injections, with thiamine. That makes them go away a lot more quickly, and cuts the pain and burning way down."

"I did talk my doctor in Spokane into giving me a B$_{12}$ shot just after they broke out. It definitely helped. Didn't realize that a series would do more."

"One thousand micrograms of B$_{12}$; 50 milligrams of thiamine every day until they're gone. It also helps to apply aloe vera and vitamin E."

"I'll do that part, but they're mostly healed, and going in for a shot every day now would be a real nuisance."

"We have everyone who needs repeated B$_{12}$ injections learn to give their own at home. That way it's simple and inexpensive."

"Maybe I don't need them anymore."

"Maybe not for shingles, but when a problem improves with a certain nutrient or nutrients, it's advisable to determine if there wasn't enough in the diet previously, if perhaps the individual requirement is higher than usual, or if the absorption or metabolism of the nutrient is faulty. Particularly in the case of vitamin B$_{12}$, it's often faulty absorption. I've learned to be suspicious of poor B$_{12}$ absorption in anyone who gets shingles or any other B$_{12}$-responsive problem, at any age."

"Doesn't B$_{12}$ help fatigue and tiredness?"

"Yes, for many people. In fact, Drs. Ellis and Nasser have even done a double-blind, crossover trial of vitamin B$_{12}$ against a placebo (fake pill) for tiredness."

"I've been tired all the time, no matter how much sleep I get, for at least ten years. Not that I don't get my work done—I do—but I don't have any extra energy, no get up and go."

"Besides shingles and fatigue, what else is falling apart? Or is that it?"

# Painful Bone Spurs

"No, there's plenty else. I've had pains in both heels on and off for two, three years. Two months ago, I could hardly walk, my left heel hurt so badly. I had x-rays taken."

"Bone spurs?"

"Both heels, left worse than right. I've taken some anti-inflammatory medication, so they're somewhat better now, but

I've been told I may need surgery eventually." He paused. "How did you know it was bone spurs?"

"They're not an unusual problem in sore heels. But actually, it fits a pattern. Have you had bursitis yet?"

"I've had that on and off for nearly ten years, one shoulder or the other. Once, in my left elbow. How'd you know?"

"Just quessing. What about sciatica?"

Mr. Kressels stared. "I was hospitalized for sciatica four years ago. Got so bad I couldn't walk. My chiropractor couldn't help."

"Is that the only time you've been hospitalized except for ulcer surgery?"

"Have you got my medical records somewhere?"

"No, I'm taking unfair advantage. When you pulled up your shirt to show me the shingles I couldn't help but see your surgical scar, too. It looked like the type that could be left by surgery for ulcers, among other things. Putting that together with shingles, fatigue, bone spurs, bursitis, and sciatica, it's an easy guess that you must have had part of your stomach removed for some reason. The most usual one is ulcers."

"You mean all those things are related?"

"Probably."

"When I was 27, I had three-quarters of my stomach removed; they called it a '75 percent gastrectomy.' They couldn't get the bleeding stopped any other way. Talk about a signal that change is needed! Losing 75 percent of my stomach made me think about what was going on in my life. I did some reading, saw a psychologist for a few months, and ended up reevaluating a lot of my goals and behavior. I was thinking of trying that route again with these problems I've had, especially the fatigue, if I couldn't find anything physically the matter."

"So far it sounds physical."

"All that stuff can be due to my stomach surgery?"

"Probably. More specifically, to the inability of your system to absorb adequate quantities of vitamin $B_{12}$, since three-quarters of your stomach's gone."

"$B_{12}$ helps bone spurs?"

"Almost every time. A 1,000 microgram injection every day

until the pain is gone, then repeated as often as needed to keep the pain away. It usually clears up bursitis, too, and helps prevent it from coming back. Same thing, along with thiamine, for sciatica.

"I don't mean to say $B_{12}$ treatment for those problems is foolproof. It isn't; no treatment is. But it works in the large majority of cases, even for people who haven't had stomach surgery."

"Wish I'd known that a few years back. Better late than never. You know, I've read that people who've had stomach surgery need $B_{12}$ shots sometimes, so I've asked about them occasionally. Each time after I explain about my surgery, the doctors say maybe. Then they do a blood count, and say no because I'm not anemic."

"That's an unfortunate but fairly common misunderstanding of the uses of vitamin $B_{12}$. Certainly anemia is part of the terminal phase of vitamin $B_{12}$ deficiency, but many people who have never been anemic are helped by vitamin $B_{12}$. In fact, all nutrients have uses other than relieving end-stage deficiency problems."

"Sounds like all I need is to learn how to give myself $B_{12}$ shots."

"Hold on, there are other things that normal stomachs do—besides helping to absorb vitamin $B_{12}$—that you may need. Besides, we haven't finished your health history and checkup yet."

Fortunately, aside from things previously noted and accidental injuries, Mr. Kressels had not had other health problems. Ulcers "ran in his family," as did diabetes. He didn't get much excercise ("makes my heels hurt"), ate more than a little junk food. Unlike many other Americans, he ate absolutely no beef.

## "Beef Makes Me Gassy"

"Doesn't feel right," he said. "Kind of heavy in my stomach. Makes me gassy. I'd read beef wasn't essential to health, so I gave it up."

"That might be an important clue. I was going to ask you to get a gastric analysis done for acidity, anyway, since you've had the stomach surgery. Your reaction to beef suggests your stomach acid is probably too low."

"Can't we just assume that? With 75 percent of my stomach gone, I imagine most of the acid production went with it. Isn't it a good idea for my stomach acid to be low?"

"There are just as many problems from too little stomach acid as from too much, just a different kind. They're usually due to poor digestion and absorption of a wide variety of nutrients."

"The surgeon told me it's been proven that stomach acid isn't necessary for digestion. Other doctors have told me that, too."

"I know, and most textbooks say the same thing. I disagree. Through experience in working with minerals, vitamins, and other nutrients, I've observed that many of these nutrients don't absorb into the body adequately if stomach acid secretion is insufficient. The mineral analysis often reflects this problem. We'll see if yours does.

"Besides practical experience, I have a theoretical disagreement. I can't believe our bodies would concentrate hydrochloric acid one million times greater in the stomach than anywhere else in the body, if it weren't necessary and important to proper body function."

"That's what I've thought, too," Mr. Kressels agreed. "Why go to all that work if it's not needed? Poor engineering design. Trouble is, my stomach was overdoing it, and now I don't have much stomach left to make acid with."

"Not only that, but your vagus nerves, which stimulate acid production, were in all likelihood cut. But we're getting ahead of things; let's wait until your examination and tests are done."

As we both expected, Mr. Kressels's gastric analysis showed practically no acid production. His mineral analysis showed a pattern typical of malabsorption; analysis of a stool specimen disclosed undigested meat fibers as well as an abnormally high percentage of "unfriendly" bacteria. Reflecting the bacterial situation, the urinalysis gave a highly positive reaction for indican, a frequent accompaniment of abnormal intestinal bacterial growth.

Despite these abnormalities, his blood count was within normal limits, although on the low side.

A series of vitamin $B_{12}$ injections (along with folate, $B_{12}$'s "metabolic partner") helped to bring Mr. Kressels's energy levels back to normal. Although he takes them on his own schedule, three times monthly, he reports he "can tell" when he misses one. Since starting $B_{12}$ injections four years ago, he's had no further pains from his bone spurs, no recurrence of sciatica, and just one beginning recurrence of bursitis which he quickly quelled by using injectable $B_{12}$ every day until it subsided.

To correct his problem with mineral malabsorption, poor digestion, and bacterial imbalance in the intestines, he's had to take supplemental hydrochloric acid cautiously with meals. He discovered early that betaine hydrochloride capsules (frequently recommended for individuals with insufficient stomach acid) gave him problems. We've settled on a prescription for dilute hydrochloric acid, along with a small amount of tablet-form pepsin, and regular doses of acidophilus bacteria. With these "digestive aids," the abnormal tests cited have returned to mostly normal.

Mr. Kressels reports he "can really tell the difference" in his digestion if these items, especially the dilute hydrochloric acid, are omitted.

Lastly, his blood count, while never "abnormal" by routine standards, has maintained an improvement of over 10 percent over his original "low-normal."

# The Intrinsic Factor Is Essential for $B_{12}$ Absorption

Surgical removal of part of the stomach also removes much of its ability to secrete the intrinsic factor—a substance essential for vitamin $B_{12}$ absorption. For that reason alone, part of postgastrectomy treatment should include self-administration of vitamin $B_{12}$ by injection, but it doesn't always. Like some diabetics, an individual with part of his or her stomach missing will need injections for the rest of his or her life, so self-treatment is therefore the best choice. Despite the logic and documentation of the need for injectable $B_{12}$ after gastrectomy, I still encounter individuals who, like Mr. Kressels, say they've never been advised about it.

More recent research shows that missing the intrinsic factor is not the only problem in postgastrectomy absorption of vitamin $B_{12}$. Acid and pepsin secretion are markedly decreased, too; that's the point of the surgery. In order for $B_{12}$ to be absorbed, it must first be separated from the food in which it's naturally present. Separation occurs during the process of digestion, which is performed in the stomach by acid and pepsin. If acid and pepsin are very low, as happens postgastrectomy, $B_{12}$ can't be separated from food, so it's not available to be bound to the intrinsic factor (if there is any) and can't be absorbed. Thus it's been shown that all three substances—acid, pepsin, and the intrinsic factor—markedly diminished by stomach surgery are important in vitamin $B_{12}$ assimilation.

In postgastrectomy individuals these findings, of course, raise a question about the occurrence of similar $B_{12}$ malabsorption by individuals with decreased secretion of acid, pepsin, and intrinsic factor for reasons other than gastrectomy. Although I've made a point throughout this book about the relatively high rate of natural occurrence of hypochlorhydria (low stomach acidity), there's another common medical cause of low stomach acidity, and low level of pepsin and intrinsic factor—the effects of cimetidine (Tagamet), which in recent years has become one of the most widely prescribed ulcer treatments in the United States.

The effects of cimetidine on vitamin $B_{12}$ absorption have been studied. Predictably, it decreases the absorption of vitamin $B_{12}$ naturally present in food, since acid and pepsin secretion are markedly diminished by this drug. In studies reported so far, the absorption of "crystalline" vitamin $B_{12}$ (unbound to food, the type found in vitamin pills) was not significantly decreased. Since crystalline $B_{12}$ is the type used in the Schilling test, the usual medical test of $B_{12}$ absorption, this effect of cimetidine on $B_{12}$ would go undetected in standard medical investigations.

At the very least, these data suggest that individuals taking cimetidine for any length of time should also take supplemental vitamin $B_{12}$. As stated by one group of investigators led by I. L. Salom, M.D.: "This impairment of $B_{12}$ absorption raises the possibility that long-term, full-dose therapy with cimetidine may produce $B_{12}$ deficiency similar to that seen in other hypochlorhydric states."

Not yet researched, however, is the effect of gastrectomy, cimetidine, and naturally occurring low stomach acidity and low levels of pepsin on mineral absorption in general. Poor assimilation of iron and calcium in naturally occurring low stomach acidity has been documented. In my office, a uniformly low level of minerals on hair analysis frequently uncovers asymptomatic individuals with this problem. But now that cimetidine is so widely prescribed, it appears that drug-induced mineral malabsorption will become even more prevalent. (Remember, antacids can also lead to this effect by excessively buffering gastric acidity.)

In the past year, some of the worst mineral analyses I've seen have been from a few individuals taking cimetidine for several months or longer. We've worked together to find natural alternative treatment and stop cimetidine treatment as quickly as possible, before the effects of various mineral deficiencies caused by malabsorption become serious.

## REFERENCES

### Cimetidine and $B_{12}$ Absorption

Salom, I. L.; Silvis, S. E.; and Doscherholmen, A. "Effect of Cimetidine on the Absorption of Vitamin $B_{12}$." *Scandinavian Journal of Gastroenterology*, vol. 17, 1982, pp. 129–131.

Steinberg, William M.; King, Charles E.; and Tuskes, Phillip P. "Malabsorption of Protein-Bound Cobalamin but Not Unbound Cobalamin during Cimetidine Administration." *Digestive Diseases and Sciences*, vol. 25, 1980, pp. 188–192.

### Fatigue

Ellis, F. R., and Nasser, S. "A Pilot Study of Vitamin $B_{12}$ in the Treatment of Tiredness." *British Journal of Nutrition*, vol. 30, no. 40, 1973, pp. 277–282.

### Malabsorption

Doscherholmen, Alfred, and Swaim, William R. "Impaired Assimilation of Egg $Co^{57}$ Vitamin $B_{12}$ in Patients with Hypochlorhydria and Achlorhydria and after Gastric Resection." *Gastroenterology*, vol. 64, no. 5, 1973, p. 913.

Lindenbaum, John. "Aspects of Vitamin $B_{12}$ and Folate Metabolism in Malabsorption Syndromes." *American Journal of Medicine*, December, 1979, pp. 1037–1048.

Williams, J. Alexander; Baume, P. E.; and Meynell, M. J. "Partial Gastroectomy: The Value of Permanent Vitamin $B_{12}$ Therapy." *Lancet*, February 12, 1966, pp. 342–344.

An overwhelming allergy to foods is suspected as the cause of a persistent sinus problem. Results of a special test called RAST confirms this patient's suspicion and helps him quickly discover just which foods are causing his problem.

# A CASE OF STUFFY SINUSES 48

"I know this sinus problem of mine is allergic. I'm tired of not being able to breathe through my nose for days at a time, or through only one side. Nights are the worst. I have to breathe through my mouth, which gives me a terribly dry throat. If I lie on my left side, I feel everything shifting over to block my left nostril. If I turn onto my right, it reverses. It's more annoying than not breathing at all."

Mr. Clanton paused for breath. I thought it was a good place to ask the obvious question.

"What's convinced you it's an allergic problem?"

"Several things, recently. I'd been on one of my every-few-years 'I'd like to breathe through my nose' campaigns, and was doing some reading. I decided to stop drinking milk. I also stopped eating cheese and other dairy products, and I found I could breathe much better for several weeks. At least 50 percent better. Then I gradually worsened again. I got to where I was a little less stuffed than before, but not much."

"Any allergy tests done?"

"Several times before, but none showed milk. In fact, I'd been convinced I wasn't allergic. But after I saw what happened with milk, I asked my regular doctor about the blood tests for allergies I'd heard about. He knows my history, and told me he didn't think I was allergic. He said that even in obviously allergic people the blood tests weren't that good anyway.

"But I insisted, so he told me he'd do a 'total IgE' blood test. He said it was a kind of summary, a total of all the types of allergens that were likely to cause my sinus and breathing problem. If my total IgE wasn't higher than the usual for nonallergic persons, then allergy couldn't be significant in my case."

"How did it turn out?"

Mr. Clanton rummaged around in his briefcase and finally pulled out a piece of paper, from which he read. " 'Total IgE,' 71, normal 40 to 100 units." He handed me the copy. "That got me discouraged again. If I didn't have any more IgE than nonallergic people, I couldn't be allergic. It must have been a coincidence. I was resigned to permanently stuffy sinuses again, but then I did two things that changed my mind."

"What were those?"

## A Drastic Step

"I got mad and decided to get back into milk and cheese in a big way. I always did like dairy products. After only two or three days, I was stuffed up worse than I'd been in a long time. I figured it had to be more than coincidence, so I decided on a drastic step, for me. I'd been reading about new methods for allergy testing and the idea of fasting was mentioned. It sounded logical that if you don't eat, and symptoms go away, food might be causing them."

"What happened?"

"Just like the books said: I felt no better—maybe even a little worse—on the first and second days. Only a little better the third day, but the fourth and fifth days I couldn't believe! I could breathe through both sides of my nose with my mouth shut. I fasted an extra day, it felt so good."

"Sounds like a good case for food allergies, all right." I made a few notes.

"That's why I'm here. I want to get those special blood tests for food allergies done."

"They're quite good, but nothing's as good as fasting and self-testing."

"That's what I understand, but let me tell you what happened when I came off the fast. First I got lucky, and just happened to decide to start with tap water instead of the distilled water I'd been using. I got a real surprise. The tap water stuffed my sinuses solid in 45 minutes. They took three days to clear. The books advised not eating anything else until the symptoms were gone. Otherwise how can you tell what's doing it? So I had to take another few days away from my job, as I was feeling weak. Once I got cleared, I thought I'd try eggs, as I needed some food. Bam! Solid sinuses again, this time for four days. By then my boss was getting impatient, and told me it was nice if I could breathe through my nose, but even nicer if I could do that and get my job done, too. I got the message."

# Not Enough Time

"So I decided to call the whole fasting thing off. I calculated that if I were allergic to a significant number of foods, say 20, just the 'not eating and waiting for my sinuses to clear' time would be 60 to 80 days. It could take another month or more to go through the nonreactive foods, even if I did it perfectly.

"Besides, I can't conduct a business that way. Can you imagine me having a plate of radishes at a business lunch, and then taking notes?"

"I suppose not. Too bad a simple explanation wouldn't do."

"Can't take the chance. People don't want to do business with someone who seems weird. If I turn out very allergic, it's going to be difficult enough designing a business meal to 'fit in.' "

"That's usually manageable, one way or another." I made a note to check for a fairly broad list of foods, as it seemed obvious Mr. Clanton was food allergic.

"Most people with food allergies have inhalant allergies, too, and vice versa," I remarked. "It's more unusual to have strictly one category or the other."

"I know, but my inhalant allergies aren't my major problem, apparently. Remember I said I had tests done before and my doctor knew my history? In the past 15 years I've been to three different allergists. The first one scratch tested me for inhalants and foods, and found I was mildly allergic to house dust, mold, and cat hair. He tried to desensitize me, but it didn't help. He found a few positive food reactions, but not bad ones. Milk wasn't one of them. I stopped eating whatever they were, but didn't get any better, so I lost interest and figured it wasn't allergy.

"I've tried two allergists since then, once on my doctor's recommendation. But it turned out much the same, except neither one would test me for food allergy. They both said scratch testing for food allergy wasn't reliable. The second allergist found the same thing: mild allergies to dust, mold, and animals. I tried desensitization again, but it still didn't work. The third allergist, after reviewing my records and the results of his own tests, said it wouldn't be worth the time or money to try desensitization again. He said I'd have to live with it, and implied it mostly wasn't an allergic problem."

"Do you get seasonal worsenings, too?"

"Only a little anymore, maybe in late spring. I forgot, pollen turned up on my skin tests, too. But as the last allergist pointed out, pollen desensitization probably wouldn't help a blocked-in-solid, all-year-round problem."

## More Specific Tests Needed

"Anyway, that's why I'm here. By now, my regular doctor's really convinced my sinus problem isn't allergic. I know it is, especially since I tried fasting, and I heard you did those RAST tests. Two of my friends really had good luck with them. Not perfect, but much better. What do they measure?"

"Antibodies—IgE antibodies actually—to individual food antigens."

Mr. Clanton sagged back in his chair, looking disappointed. "That means it won't work for me. I've already had my total IgE antibodies measured, and they weren't abnormal. You have the copy."

"That's not so. Even when the total IgE test is normal, it's been documented that clinically significant allergy to specific foods can be found. I've seen numerous cases of normal total IgE tests accompanied by positive tests for specific foods."

"How can that be?"

"I'm not sure myself. I've found the total IgE test a waste of time and money as an absolute predictor of allergy."

"I was told I'd saved a lot of money by not doing specific food testing, just the total IgE."

"Specific food allergy testing is expensive if many foods are done, and not always covered by insurance."

"My friends were told their insurance plan would cover ordinary scratch testing for food allergies, which even allergists say doesn't work, but not the RAST tests, which helped them a lot."

"That's one of the ironies. . . ."

"I know, like covering drugs, even if ineffective, and not minerals or vitamins, even if effective. But it's worth it to me to clear up this chronic stuffiness and breathe freely. Fasting just won't work out."

"You understand that even the best laboratory test, RAST or whatever, can't be guaranteed to work for you 100 percent. All lab procedures have some margin of error. For that matter, all doctors 'opinions have some margin of error, much as we don't like to think about it. At the present time, based on your experiences, and mine with similar situations and with lab testing, I'd recommend you get RAST testing done."

"I can't think of a more reasonable way to approach it. Put

me down for the tests." He paused for a minute. "Is there a difference between RAST tests?"

"Definitely. There are two very different ways of doing them, and then variations on those." I picked up his total IgE lab slip. "For example, this way of doing the test doesn't get as good a result as another lab would. That's true of many lab procedures, though, not just RAST tests. I make sure to evaluate and reevaluate lab procedures periodically to try to obtain the most accurate results possible."

# Allergic to Many Foods

When Mr. Clanton's tests returned, it was obvious why he'd had a problem for so long, and hadn't been able to pick out one or even a few foods that were responsible. He was highly allergic to apples, beef, Cheddar cheese, coffee, corn, eggs, honey, lemon, milk (cow's), oranges, peanuts, pork, rice, soy, wheat, and brewer's yeast. He was "only mildly" allergic to chicken, onions, potatoes, and tomatoes. As he pointed out, of 20 foods, 16 he shouldn't eat, and 4 he should eat not very often.

Over several months, he tested himself for 50 more foods. He found 17 "safe" foods, 13 more highly allergic, and 20 only mildly allergic. He discovered that by "rotating" his 17 safe and 24 mildly allergenic foods, he could keep his sinuses unstuffed, and he was able to breathe freely most of the time. Additionally, once the large majority of his allergenic foods (as well as tap water) were removed, he found he needed no further RAST tests, since he could then tell which food was causing problems.

As a bonus, he found his energy levels were much improved by allergenic-food avoidance.

A large number of highly allergenic foods, such as Mr. Clanton's 29, is really not rare. Sometimes symptoms are straightforward, as his were, but often they're not. At present, the best available nondrug treatments for food allergy appear to be avoidance of the food or sometimes desensitization as practiced by clinical ecologists. Research more closely approaching the roots of an "overwhelming allergy" problem appears promising, but no reliable solutions appear to be presently available.

## Food Allergy Is an Important Consideration in Sinus Problems

When stuffy sinuses are due to allergy, as they often are, inhalants such as dust, mold, pollens, and in some cases chemicals are the usual causes. Food allergy as a major factor is a cause in only a minority of cases. In addition, testing for food allergy is frequently inaccurate, so that minority has often been ignored.

If you're in that minority, though, it's very important. Fortunately, there's at least one type of food allergy testing available to family doctors that's sufficiently accurate to make a real difference. It's the radioallergosorbent test (RAST).

Most laboratory tests can be performed by a variety of procedures in different labs with relatively accurate and frequently interchangeable results. For some tests, though, it makes an enormous difference in how they're performed. The RAST test falls into that latter group.

Currently there are two RAST tests being performed at labs across the country. One is much more accurate than the other, as we found out when we compared the success track record for each test here at this office.

We asked individuals with chronic symptoms that didn't respond to standard therapy, who were suspected of being food allergic, to have blood drawn for testing. Each person's blood sample was then split in half, in order to accurately compare the two different methods. The first I'll call "L," which required testing be performed on the premises, and the second I'll call "P," which used a test kit available at commercial labs. To ensure accuracy, tests were run in duplicate.

What we found was that although procedure "L" left some room for error, it was far superior to procedure "P."

Subsequent experience has shown that test "L" is particularly weak in evaluation of cow's milk allergy. When a much broader range of foods is tested, test "L" has an even better record for accuracy.

Most physicians prefer to send their lab work to nearby laboratories. Unfortunately, most commercial laboratories rely on procedure "P" test kits instead of the more complicated "L" method. So if they order RAST tests, they're usually done using procedure "P." Since it rarely discloses food allergy, I'm sure that's the reason many practitioners have found the radioallergosorbent test (RAST) to be useless. When done by procedure "P," it is.

Even better testing procedures than the more accurate RAST system for disclosing food allergy are those followed by clinical ecologists. Evaluation in an environmentally controlled hospital unit by a clinical ecologist appears to be the absolute best, but can take several weeks and cost several thousand dollars. Even so, it's worthwhile for the most severely allergic individuals. Simultaneous testing (and desensitization) in the office by a clinical ecologist appears to be next best. However, for the average food-allergic person (and doctor not trained in clinical ecology) the more accurate RAST testing system is excellent for identification of foods causing problems.

## REFERENCES

**Allergy**
Grieco, Michael H. "Controversial Practices in Allergy." *Journal of the American Medical Association*, June 11, 1982, pp. 3106–3111.

Parks, Nancy. "Allergies: Winning the Battle." *Total Health*, January, 1982, pp. 20–21, 55–56.

**Diagnosis**
Moramarco, Sheila S. "A Doctor's Dispute." *Parade*, August 1, 1982, p. 15.

**General**
Berkow, Robert, ed. *The Merck Manual of Diagnosis and Therapy*. Merck Sharp & Dohme Research Laboratories, 1982, pp. 1966–1967.

Brace, E. R. et al., eds. *Good Housekeeping Family Health & Medical Guide.* The Hearst Corporation, 1979, p. 503.

**RAST Test**

Adkinson, N. Franklin. "Cost, Quality Control, Clinical Threshold Still Problems of RAST." *Family Practice News,* April, 1982, p. 49.

Hoffman, Donald R., and Haddad, Zack H. "Diagnosis of IgE-mediated Reactions to Food Antigens by Radioimmunoassay." *Journal of Allergy and Clinical Immunology,* September, 1974, pp. 165–172.

Moore, R. E.; Wright, J. V.; and Williams, B. F. "The Radioallergosorbent Test: A Comparison of Two Methods." March, 1982.

A relatively healthy man isn't feeling as good as he thought he should. Investigation reveals that his low stomach acid is the cause of his tiredness and digestive upset.

# 49 A CASE OF STOMACH ACID DEFICIENCY

"I guess I'm just a typical short-haired, middle-aged, health-food nut," Mr. Grisvold remarked.

"What do you mean by that?"

"It's a joke around our house. Our teenagers started it. Their mother and I are the short-haired, middle-aged, conservative health-food nuts, and the kids are the radical, long-haired, health-food freaks. They're into ecology and libertarian politics."

He smiled. "But they're good kids and it's all fun. That's not my problem, though. What I'm really concerned about is that I've been watching my diet and getting enough exercise for over 15 years, and I still don't feel as good as I think I should. There's nothing major the matter, just little things. Probably it's my age."

He paused. "I really don't know where to start because there aren't any major symptoms."

"Why don't you tell me what you've been doing about your health so far; we'll go from there."

"I guess I'll start at the beginning. Sometime in the early 1960s I read Rachel Carson's *Silent Spring*. That really started me thinking. Also, I'm a pilot. I'd been noticing more and more air pollution around the cities we were flying into—like a filthy brown cloud that just hangs in place.

"Our family was young then. My wife and I were talking about moving, and all of that helped us to make up our minds. We moved about 60 miles from the city, into what was a nearly rural area than. I put in an entirely organic garden.

"We started doing some more reading. We got rid of all the sugar in the house. My wife bought only whole-grain flour and breads. Of course, we'd already gotten rid of all the synthetic colors, preservatives, and so forth.

"It was worth it. Our three older children, who had chronic runny noses, frequent earaches, and tonsillitis, got over nearly all of that in the first year. Our second daughter was always pale and a little withdrawn. That all went away. We've had two more children—they've hardly ever been sick."

Mr. Grisvold caught himself. "But I came here about me, didn't I? Where was I? Oh, yes, I was about 35 then. I'd had a chronic skin condition—that cleared up. I'd had constipation and hemorrhoids; those went away, too. I was always a little bit tired; that got much better. My headaches disappeared, and so did my chronic sinus stuffiness."

## Tiredness and Digestive Problems

"Just after I turned 41, I noticed some of my problems were coming back a little. Particularly the tiredness and the digestive problems. So I did more reading and decided I needed more exercise and some supplements.

"Things got better again for another five or six years. We all started on a regular vitamin and mineral program, along with our organic foods. My wife really got herself going then. She's been zipping around ever since. You should see the kids!

"Well, three or four years ago, I started going downhill again. I'm a little tired most of the time, even if I get enough sleep. I'm constipated on and off, and have more gas than I think I should. I get indigestion sometimes. Even my skin is starting to break out a little.

"The kids say it's just middle age catching up with even health-food nuts. But I want to see if it's just age, or not."

"What sort of vitamins and minerals have you been taking?"

"Well, of course, vitamin C—two or three grams a day—and B complex. Vitamin E—400 international units a day. I make a protein drink every day, throwing in brewer's yeast, lecithin, and safflower oil. Five or six dolomite tablets a day and some zinc—my father had prostate trouble. Also, some cod-liver oil, desiccated liver, and kelp." He paused for a minute. "I think that's everything."

"Haven't you checked about your problems before now?"

"Oh, sure. I went to an internist. He gave me a complete checkup with upper and lower intestinal x-rays, a gallbladder x-ray, electrocardiogram, a whole quart of blood tests. He told me I was healthier than anyone he'd seen of my age in quite a while, and that I was worrying about myself too much. He told me not to take my vitamins because the FDA had proved they were just faddism. He wanted me to take an antidepressant."

By now, I felt I had a fairly clear picture of Mr. Grisvold's problem. As he said, it sounded like "nothing major" but it wasn't normal, either. Even though he'd had a fairly complete gastrointestinal workup done the year before and all was found normal, I had an idea that his gastrointestinal symptoms might be very significant.

"Tell me about your digestive problems again," I said.

"I have more gas than I think I should, both in my stomach and otherwise. Sometimes, when it's especially bad, the food in my stomach feels like it's just sitting there. But other times it's OK."

"Do you have diarrhea or constipation?"

"Constipation—but not all the time. That comes and goes."

"No nausea?"

"No."

"No bleeding or mucus?"

"I haven't had that since I had hemorrhoids years ago. With all the roughage from our garden, I've never gotten those back."

"Any foods particularly hard to digest?"

"I don't really know. Sometimes I think beans seem a little difficult—but I can't tell."

"I can't be absolutely certain, but I don't think we're going to have to look very far for the source of your health problems. I'd like you to get three tests done—a mineral test using a specimen of hair, a blood test for enzymes, and a self-test for stomach acid."

# Testing for Stomach Acid Deficiency

"What do you mean, a self-test for stomach acid?"

"Until recently, there was a relatively inexpensive and generally reliable lab test for stomach acid. That's unavailable now. There is a very exact test that involves putting a tube through the nose or mouth, down the esophagus into the stomach, and sucking out all the contents. Somehow, most people would rather not do that."

"I can see why," Mr. Grisvold replied. "What's the self-test?"

"Get some betaine hydrochloride tablets, five grain, at your health-food store. On three consecutive mornings take one, then two, then three on an empty stomach. If you have no bad reaction, take one or two before each meal for a week, and see how your digestion feels. If it's better, we can safely assume that your stomach didn't produce enough acid for proper digestion."

"I'm not sure I understand. Do I take just one the first day, or six altogether that day? What's a bad reaction?"

"One the first day, two the second day, and three the third day you're testing. After that one or two according to how much you eat and how your digestion feels. A bad reaction is anything that feels bad. Heartburn, worse gas, pain in the stomach—anything."

Mr. Grisvold thought for a minute. "Isn't taking acid dangerous?"

"Not unless you have an ulcer. If it hurts, don't take any

more. Neutralize the reaction with milk or baking soda in water. Somehow, though, I don't think you're going to have a problem."

"All right, I'll try it. What's the enzyme test?"

"That's for pancreatic enzymes. Many persons who don't have sufficient stomach acid don't have sufficient digestive enzymes either. This is probably related to the finding that one of the stimuli for pancreatic enzyme production is a hormone released from the duodenum (the uppermost part of the small intestine) when the acidified stomach contents empty into it. So: less acid, less hormone stimulus, less enzymes."

"That seems fairly simple. But you said this was a blood test? Aren't those digestive enzymes?"

"Yes, they are. But they're also present in the bloodstream. The tests I ask the laboratory to do are two of the most common and oldest enzyme determinations, called 'serum amylase' and 'serum lipase.' Usually they're done as a test for elevated levels, as in acute pancreatitis. I've observed that decreased levels are usually correlated with insufficient enzymes for proper digestion, frequently leading to symptoms of gas and constipation."

"That seems logical, also. What about the hair test? I've read that's for minerals. But why not take a blood test?"

"Blood tests are simply inaccurate as a measure of total body mineral content. It's possible to be 10 to 15 percent or more deficient in the total body content of a mineral, and still have a normal blood test. For example, most women with osteoporosis—a severe deficit of calcium in the bones—have a normal blood calcium. Hair tests aren't perfect, either, but if used by someone familiar with them, they're quite revealing."

Mr. Grisvold got up to go. "When should I come back?"

"In about three weeks. Your tests should be back by then, and you'll be through your self-testing."

When Mr. Grisvold returned, he appeared quite pleased. "I think we're onto something here, Doc," he said. "I took that acid test like you said, and didn't feel a thing. So I started taking the betaine hydrochloride supplements before every meal. I finally settled on two at a time. My digestion is practically back to normal already. Much less gas, and less constipation, too. No more heavy feeling in the stomach. This last week, it even feels like my food is getting into me better. Is that possible?"

"Lots of people have told me that same thing. Of course it's possible. Without enough acid in the stomach, protein-digesting enzymes don't function properly, and minerals don't absorb properly, either. Let's look at your mineral test."

Mr. Grisvold's mineral test showed decreased calcium, magnesium, sodium, potassium, copper, iron, manganese, and chromium. Only zinc and phosphorus were normal. It was a classic picture of gastric acid deficiency.

"That's a regular disaster," Mr. Grisvold commented. "Even with all those mineral supplements and good food for years! That doctor was partly right about me wasting my money—but not the way he thought. What if I hadn't been taking them? Well, what should I do? Oh, what about my other tests? The pancreatic enzymes?"

His serum amylase was definitely decreased. The serum lipase was borderline on the low side.

"So I need those, too?"

"Yes, I'd like you to continue using two betaine hydrochloride tablets before each meal. Also, one to three pancreatin tablets before or during the meal. Adjust this according to your food intake and the way your digestion feels, also."

"What about minerals?"

His test showed so many deficiencies that I suggested he get separate supplements for the two or three worst, and use a multiple for the rest, for now.

"That certainly looks good to me," Mr. Grisvold said. "Otherwise, I'd have nothing but mineral pills. I suppose we'll retest later to see what I still need."

"Right. But that's not quite everything."

"No?" Mr. Grisvold looked puzzled. "But that's everything we tested for."

"That's true. However, since it now appears fairly definite that you have a lack of stomach acid, I'd like to try an injection of vitamin $B_{12}$."

"What's that for? Why can't I swallow it?"

"I've found that the majority of my patients with decreased or absent stomach acid feel much better—less tired, a little calmer, a little clearer mentally—if they take vitamin $B_{12}$ injections regularly. Swallowing the vitamin doesn't work for them, either. Apparently most stomachs that don't produce acid can't assist vitamin $B_{12}$ absorption."

"Why is that?"

"I don't know for certain. It doesn't work in all cases. But injections work so often, I always suggest trying them once or twice. It's not known to be harmful."

"I knew someone who took $B_{12}$ shots for anemia. Do I have that?"

"That's pernicious anemia—an end stage of not enough vitamin $B_{12}$. It would take years still to get anemia. I'd prefer you take the injection before that happens."

"Me, too. Anything else?"

"No. Check with the nurse who gives you your shot about establishing a schedule. And—if all goes well—come back in three to four months to let me know how you're doing."

# Tiredness Gone

Mr. Grisvold returned in six months instead. "I've been so busy and feeling so well I just didn't get around to it," he said. "I finally decided I'd better let you know how I was doing. When I added that pancreatin to the betaine hydrochloride supplements, the last trace of digestive trouble disappeared. It's been fine ever since.

"My tiredness is gone—unless I stay up too late! My skin isn't broken out at all. I guess I must be digesting and absorbing what I'm eating better now. At the beginning, I needed to take the vitamin $B_{12}$ injection every three weeks. Now I'm down to every six weeks.

"I'm feeling so good I beat all my teenagers at tennis. I'm not hearing as much about 'middle-aged health-food nut' from those kids anymore. I have just one question. When can I stop taking some of these things?"

"The enzymes and minerals, probably soon. Remember, the need for them traces back to your lack of stomach acid. You're taking that regularly now. So, as soon as we retest you and find normal levels, you can stop the extra supplements."

"What about the acid?"

"I can't tell you that for sure. Some people's stomachs tell them by starting to burn or hurt when the acid's taken. Other people stop taking it when they're feeling better, and restart if their digestive symptoms return."

"Are there any harmful effects from taking it when you don't really need it?"

"I can't answer that for you for sure. I've not observed any. But I don't have data on many people who've taken it for 20 or 30 years."

"I guess I'll have to go according to how I feel. Considering how much better that is—especially my energy—I'll just take my chances."

I asked him to stop by at least every year as long as he was taking it. He agreed, and got up to go.

"Oh, what about the vitamin $B_{12}$ shots?"

"I can't tell you that. Blood tests won't help, either. A level that 'feels good' to one person isn't enough for another. But since there's no record of overdose, taking one when needed is felt probably not harmful."

"Looks like there are a few loose ends where more research is needed," Mr. Grisvold observed.

"Yes, there are," I agreed. "But weighing the risks of taking the acid indefinitely—which are probably small—against the risks of not taking it when needed, I'd definitely recommend that you continue. After all, with insufficient acid, protein digestion doesn't proceed properly. Furthermore, carbohydrate and fat digestion isn't normal if the pancreatic enzymes are down. Most mineral absorption is faulty, too."

"One last question. I'd been doing everything right for my health for years, and it wasn't working because of no stomach acid, or not enough. What happened to it?"

"I wish I could answer that, but I don't know. I don't know if anyone does. But I can tell you it's a source of a lot of nutritional problems for many people. All the minerals and good food in the world won't help very much unless it's compensated for."

# A Treatment That Works with Caution

I first worked with Mr. Grisvold in 1975 and 1976; his case (with a changed name, of course) was published in 1977. Since then, both he and I have learned more about his particular health problem.

At present, there's no organized training in nutritional biochemistry. Those who practice it are sometimes covering known ground, but sometimes we're working at the edges of our medical school training. When that is the case, it's always wisest to proceed slowly and cautiously until experience is gained, both with a particular individual and in general.

As noted in the chapter "Good Digestion: Why We Can't Take It for Granted," The average normally functioning stomach is capable of producing the equivalent of 25 to 30 or more betaine hydrochloride or glutamic acid hydrochloride capsules, with pepsin, per meal. Initially, two to three of these capsules were enough to relieve Mr. Grisvold's symptoms. But when follow-up testing on overall digestion and mineral absorption was done over the next few years, it was found that eight to nine of the ten-grain capsules were more effective. As in Mr. Grisvold's case, the symptom-relief dose in symptomatic cases of low stomach acidity is frequently less than the digestion-improvement dose as demonstrated by follow-up testing.

When Mr. Grisvold first came in, we didn't have available the radiotelemetry system (Heidelberg capsule) to test stomach acid. We could have used the older style stomach pumping, but it's never been widely acceptable to individuals having it done. It's also much more cumbersome for the laboratory doing it. Although the self-testing system recommended to Mr. Grisvold is sometimes helpful, I no longer recommend it since a much more precise diagnostic system is available. Self-testing can be deceptive, sometimes leading to the conclusion that supplemental hydrochloric acid capsules with pepsin aren't necessary when they really are, and sometimes indicating a need when none exists. Occasionally, individuals who don't really need supplemental hydrochloric acid capsules take them anyway because they don't seem to hurt, at least initially. It's unlikely, but remotely possible (I've seen it happen once) that a peptic ulcer and bleeding can be accidentally caused this way. It's very necessary to make absolutely sure hydrochloric acid capsules are needed before they're used, and to work with a physician familiar with their use.

Mr. Grisvold's case is a fairly typical example of the very numerous group of people with low stomach acidity except in one aspect: The majority of individuals with that problem have one or more significant food allergies. Mr. Grisvold didn't appear to; he wasn't tested for them as he did well without an allergy investigation.

A family history of heart disease and diabetes leads to suspicions of sugar susceptibility in an apparently healthy 35-year-old man. Follow-up testing shows both an increase in his weight and a significant effect on his platelets clumping.

# 50  A CASE OF SUGAR SUSCEPTIBILITY

Donald Nielsen was in to go over the results of his checkup and laboratory tests, which he'd had done the previous month. He was 35 years old, feeling well, but had come in mostly at the urging of his wife and his mother for a preventive-type check. Physically, no problems had been found. His laboratory tests were generally good, showing only slightly high triglycerides, and a few trace element deficiencies. I'd given him a brief list of supplements to "make up" the deficiencies as well as for general health maintenance. I'd also gone over the importance of whole unrefined foods, minimization of salt intake, and elimination of refined sugar. This last point seemed to bother him.

"No offense meant, but you sound like a tape recording of my mother about no sugar. The whole time I was growing up she had a running battle with my father. She wouldn't let us kids have any, but he'd sneak us candy occasionally, and ate it all the time himself."

I look at my records. "What did you say your father died of?"

Mr. Nielsen looked uncomfortable. "I know, I know, a heart attack when he was only 51. But that doesn't prove it's going to happen to me, does it? It doesn't even prove that sugar had anything to do with it. He was a heavy smoker, and never exercised. I don't smoke, and I jog seven miles a week.

"I guess what I'm trying to say is this sugar thing is another generalization which might or might not apply to me. For instance, I've read that eggs and animal fat raise some people's cholesterol, not everyone's, and salt only affects blood pressure in genetically susceptible people. Isn't sugar the same? How do I know it really makes a difference to me personally?"

I looked at Mr. Nielsen's diet history. He ate out a lot, and obviously liked sugar and sweets in general.

"There are so many reasons not to eat refined sugar, it would fill volumes," I answered. "As far as I'm concerned, the evidence indicates that total elimination of it would be best for everyone's health. However, a family history is a good indication for each person. In your case, besides your father's heart attack, your uncle and one great-aunt had diabetes. I definitely recommend against any sugar consumption at all with that kind of family health history."

Mr. Nielsen sighed. "Now you sound like my wife. She didn't say much when we were younger, but now she's sounding like my mother. They're ganging up on me. But I keep telling her I'm not my father or uncle. My mother's father is 89 years old, drinks six cups of coffee with two teaspoons of sugar every day, and he's just fine. How do you know I'm not like that side of the family?"

"Obviously, I don't. You have a good point about biochemical differences in response to sugar. That point's been demonstrated very well by Dr. John Yudkin, at Queen Elizabeth College in London."

# A Predictive Test

"I have a suggestion for you, if you really want to check yourself individually. We can follow suggestions made by Dr. Yudkin, run a predictive set of tests, and see what happens."

"What do you mean?"

"Dr. Yudkin studied 19 men, 21 to 44 years of age. They followed high-sucrose, no-sucrose, and 'normal' diets for alternating two-week periods. At each time period, body weight, cholesterol, triglyceride, glucose and insulin tolerance, and platelet aggregation were measured. There was no appreciable change in cholesterol in anyone studied; triglycerides rose in all 19. However, 6 of the 19 men had a distinct change in insulin levels, platelet aggregation, and body weight. The other 13 didn't.

"Based on similar studies in men with known atherosclerotic disease, Dr. Yudkin concluded that the six men showing significant change in plasma insulin, platelet aggregation, and body weight were 'sucrose susceptible.' For those individuals sugar was a definite risk factor for atherosclerosis."

"And for the other 13, it wasn't?"

"Probably not as much of a risk—for atherosclerosis, anyway. Dr. Yudkin couldn't predict about other problems."

Mr. Nielsen considered for a moment. "I think I'd like to try that type of test. Before I give up a lot of food I like, I want to make sure it's necessary for me, and not just a generalization."

"Remember, Dr. Yudkin's testing was relevant to atherosclerosis and probably maturity-onset diabetes. It doesn't take into account other effects of sucrose, such as interfering with resistance to infection."

"OK, but I'm mostly concerned about heart attacks and diabetes. That's what's in my family, at least one side of it. What do I do?"

"I'd like you to use a slightly longer trial period than Dr. Yudkin used, just to be sure. For one month, please eat absolutely no refined sugar at all. For the next month, approximately 14 ounces of sugar daily. At the end of each month, we'll measure your plasma insulin in response to sugar, your platelet aggregation, and weight."

"Fourteen ounces of sugar daily? That's almost a pound! Isn't that an unusually large amount?"

I looked at his diet history again. "Actually, you were coming close. There's considerable sugar in the soft drinks, pastries, and ice cream you eat. However, there's much more than commonly recognized in other foods. Here's a listing you could use."

He inspected the list. "Doesn't look like 14 ounces a day would be much of a problem. At least it'll be fun. My mother will have a fit, though."

"Explain to her the purpose of the test periods. One other thing: What do you intend to do if it turns out you're sugar susceptible?"

"Cut out all the refined sugar, I guess. I'm not stubborn or stupid. If I can see the handwriting on the wall, I'll do it. I just want to make sure it really makes a difference to my health, and that I'm not just giving in to my mother and wife."

Two months later, Mr. Nielsen was back to go over his sucrose test results.

"After the no-sugar month, your plasma insulin was 41 two hours after glucose challenge, and 21 three hours after. Your platelet aggregation time was three minutes, seven seconds; your weight 167 pounds.

"After the high-sugar month, your plasma insulin was 77 and 38; platelet aggregation two minutes, 17 seconds; weight 173 and a half.

"At least on these parameters, I'd say you're clearly sucrose sensitive. Not only that, but the insulin figures indicate you may be latent diabetic."

"What do you mean?"

"Dr. Joseph Kraft of Chicago has done extensive work on insulin response to glucose challenge. He's identified criteria for detecting persons who will probably become diabetic, even though their glucose tolerance tests are presently normal. Unfortunately, your plasma insulin response after the high-sugar month puts you in that group."

"I was afraid of bad results based just on my weight change. In the no-sugar month I lost four pounds; the next month I gained six and a half. Isn't that indicative, alone?"

"Probably. In Dr. Yudkin's study, the 6 'sucrose-susceptible' individuals gained over five pounds each in two weeks on high sugar; the 13 'nonsusceptible' gained a half-pound each or less."

"Well, I guess that's it. If sugar upsets my insulin and platelets, no sugar for me. If nothing else happens, maybe I'll make it past 51 years old." He got up to go, but sat down again. "Just one other thing: Aren't those forced results in a way? Not many people eat that much sugar a day."

"Remember, to 'bring out' the problem in just a month instead of over a lifetime requires a heavier-than-usual sugar load. Also, remember that in Dr. Yudkin's study the 'nonsusceptible' individuals didn't respond even to the extra-large sugar load. So the results are very real, not forced.

"Also, present statistics show that the average person consumes 125 to 126 pounds of sugar and other sweeteners per year, about 5½ ounces daily. Considering that my family and many others don't use any sugar, there must be some people eating close to 14 ounces daily."

Mr. Nielsen got up to go again. "I don't know about that arithmetic," he said. "What I do know now is that sugar is no good for me, personally, and not just a general consideration."

He smiled. "My mother and wife will really be happy. I'm in for several months of I-told-you-so, for sure."

# Refined Sugar Belongs in the Junkpile

Refined carbohydrates in general and refined sugar in particular have no place in an optimum diet. Our bodies' biochemical systems are still best adapted to whole, unprocessed foods, the types that could have been eaten by primitive man at nearly any time in the last million years or two. Refined sugar doesn't fit into that category; the sooner it's relegated to the junkpile of human dietary history, the better.

However, as with any other substance generally detrimental to health, some of us are more susceptible to it than others. As demonstrated in Mr. Nielsen's case, some of the specific biochemical effects are easily measurable. Individuals who demonstrate their sugar sensitivity biochemically need to be the very most vigilant about keeping refined sugar out of their diets.

Without putting yourself through the special testing that Mr. Nielsen required, how can you tell if you're particularly sensitive to refined sugar? Remember family history: You should be careful if there's a family problem with diabetes or atherosclerosis. However, as noted by Dr. Yudkin, there's another tipoff as close as your bathroom scales: Weight changes with and without refined sugar in the diet.

Dr. Yudkin's group noted that the 13 individuals who appeared not especially sugar sensitive gained from zero to two pounds after two weeks on a high-sucrose diet. The six individuals who were found to be sugar sensitive on other biochemical measurements gained from three to six pounds on the same program. (The difference is statistically significant.) The extra weight gained was lost again with sugar elimination.

If you're not yet convinced you should eliminate refined sugar totally from your diet, a sugar challenge with observation for weight gain is something you can do at home with very little hazard, except to the waistline and possibly the wardrobe. If you're still not sure after a self-challenge, the same specific biochemical testing done by Mr. Nielsen might also give you very worthwhile information.

However, changes in weight, serum insulin, platelet aggregation, and triglycerides are only some of the specific ill effects of refined sugar. By now, everyone agrees that dental cavities are largely attributable to sugar, but reactive hypoglycemia (low blood sugar) and behavior disturbances in some children are too.

Emanuel Cheraskin, M.D., D.M.D., professor of the University of Alabama, has devoted a considerable part of his career to documenting the effects of refined sugar on health. In one of his more publicized demonstrations of the adverse effects of refined sugar, he measured the germ-eating ability of white blood cells. Blood was drawn from volunteers before and 45 minutes after they drank a sugar-sweetened soft drink. White cells from the after-sugar blood specimens were found capable of destroying only half the germs that the before-sugar white cells could destroy. This effect can last for up to five hours. Therefore, if sugar is eaten at breakfast, lunch, dinner, and bedtime, either by itself or as part of a meal, the only time that white cells would have their full germ-destroying capacity might be between three or four in the morning and breakfast.

I could go on for pages about the specific bad effects of refined sugar and refined carbohydrates, but the most important reason not to use them at all remains the same: Our bodies' biochemical systems aren't adapted to them, since they haven't been a feature of human diets for more than a few generations, no time at all in the long span of human history. Look what happened to the health of the northern Canadian Eskimos, the Maori, and the Israelis from Yemen, largely because of a great increase in the consumption of refined sugar (see "The Case for a 'New Traditional' Diet").

It's true that refined sugar is worse for some people than others. But basically, it's not good for anyone at all.

## REFERENCES

**Diabetes**

Kraft, Joseph R. "Detection of Diabetes Mellitus *In Situ* (Occult Diabetes)." *Laboratory Medicine*, vol. 6, no. 2, 1975, pp. 10–22.

**Diet**

Yudkin, John. "Why Blame Sugar?" *Chemistry and Industry*, September 2, 1967.

————. "Evolutionary and Historical Changes in Dietary Carbohydrates." *American Journal of Clinical Nutrition*, February, 1967, pp. 108–115.

**Hyperactivity**

Prinz, Ronald J.; Roberts, William A.; and Hartman, Elaine. "Dietary Correlates of Hyperactive Behavior in Children." *Journal of Consulting and Clinical Psychology*, vol. 48, no. 6, 1980, pp. 760–769.

**Immunity**

Ringsdorf, W. M., Jr. et al. "Sucrose, Neutrophilic Phagocytosis and Resistance to Disease." *Dental Survey,* December, 1976, pp. 46–48.

Sanchez, Albert et al. "Role of Sugars in Human Neutrophilic Phagocytosis." *American Journal of Clinical Nutrition,* November, 1973, pp. 1180–1184.

**Sucrose**

Szanto, Stephen, and Yudkin, John. "The Effect of Dietary Sucrose on Blood Lipids, Serum Insulin, Platelet Adhesiveness and Body Weight in Human Volunteers." *Postgraduate Medical Journal,* vol. 45, no. 527, 1969, pp. 602–607.

Yudkin, John, and Szanto, Stephen. "Sugar Intake, Serum Insulin and Platelet Adhesiveness in Men with and without Peripheral Vascular Disease." *Postgraduate Medical Journal,* vol. 45, no. 527, 1969, pp. 608–611.

A 38-year-old woman suffering from an unusual allergy to the sun finally finds relief through injections of vitamin $B_6$ twice a week.

# 51  A CASE OF SUN ALLERGY (PHOTOSENSITIVITY)

"I haven't been able to go out in the sun for years now. Every time I do, I break out in hives on my arms and legs. It's very frustrating for me and my family. We used to like to get out a lot, camping and swimming especially. Now, if I want to go, I either have to keep all covered up, and stay hot and uncomfortable, or stay in the shade. Of course, it's cloudy or rainy a lot here, so I can go out then; but still, it's such a bother in the summertime that mostly I end up staying home."

"How long have you had this problem."

"Really bad, three or four years. But it was starting to cause problems six or seven years ago."

"Do you have lupus erythematosus?"

"No, no, I've been checked for that several times. I'm perfectly well other than these hives. All the doctors I've seen tell me, 'You're perfectly healthy, just stay out of the sun.' "

"You're not taking medications?"

"Just some vitamins. That's only been the last two or three years. I know some drugs can cause reactions in sunlight, because one of the first things I was told to do was stop my birth-control pills. But that didn't help. I've never taken any other drugs for any length of time.

"In fact, one allergist four years ago told me to get off all artificial flavors, colors, and preservatives because that had helped a few of his patients with sun sensitivity. At the time, I didn't know much about nutrition, so it didn't make any sense to me, but I tried anyway. That didn't help either, but I did learn a lot in doing it. Now, I wouldn't go back to artificial stuff for any reason. They're just like drugs."

"That's true in many ways."

From what Mrs. Wilson had told me already, I guessed she'd had herself thoroughly tested. However, to be complete, there were a few other questions left to ask.

"Have you been tested for porphyria, or has anyone in your family had this problem?"

"No one in my family has, as far as I can find out. And, yes, I've been tested for porphyria, twice, and my tests turned up negative. I should have told you I've been to the university about this, and had lots of tests, some of which I can't remember. It was all negative. They were very nice, and told me to come back in a few years when they might have something new."

"Were you given any treatment?"

"Just an antihistamine for the itching. It also seems to help make the hives go away a little quicker, but I can't tell for sure."

## "Little Red Hills"

"What happens when you go out in the sun? Do you break out right away?"

"No, nothing happens for an hour or so. Then my skin starts to itch. The itching gets worse and worse, even if I get out of the sun. The antihistamine helps some. Several hours later, I break out. When it first started, I might not break out until the next day, but the last few times it's been the same day."

"What does the rash look like?"

"Just like hives, you know."

"Could you describe them, anyway?"

"Well . . . they can be anything from the size of a dime to a half-dollar."

"Flat or bumpy?"

"Definitely bumpy. Just like little hills."

"What color?"

"Bright red—sometimes almost purple."

"Where do you get them?"

"Just about anywhere the sunlight strikes: arms, legs, neck. Somehow, I never get any on my face though."

Her description certainly was a typical case of hives. I went on to ask about other basic health information. She was 38, had two children, had never been hospitalized for illness, had no other allergies. Although she'd eaten an "average American diet" for most of her life, she'd been, as she said, "lucky," and suffered no detectable ill effects. In the past three years she'd switched over to a more healthful diet primarily as a result of her reading.

Aside from childhood illnesses, colds, and occasional flu, the only health problem she'd actually had other than the "sun allergy" was brought on by a drug. When she'd first started on birth-control pills, she'd become very nauseated, gained weight, and developed breast soreness. After her prescription had been changed to a low-dose type, her symptoms had subsided, except for some minor fluid retention. She didn't consider this a problem, as most of her friends "had the same problem." As she said, she was generally healthy.

## The Pill Increases Need for B$_6$

However, her problem with birth-control pills provided a clue about her metabolism. As many health-conscious readers know, women who have birth-control pill side effects, fluid retention, or premenstrual problems usually need more vitamin B$_6$ than others.

Writing in the *New York State Journal of Medicine*, Dr. Edward Mandel reported a treatment using vitamin B$_6$ for photosensitive skin eruptions. Since Mrs. Wilson apparently was "sensitive" in her vitamin $B_6$ metabolism, that seemed a logical place to start.

Because vitamin $B_6$ is generally safe, I asked her to start with the highest dose recommended by Dr. Mandel to his patients: 100 milligrams every hour while exposed to the sun. (Don't take that much without medical supervision.)

Mrs. Wilson was encouraged; after two or three questions, she left.

It was apparent that her experiment had not been a complete success when she returned six weeks later. She had fading hives on both arms.

"Well, I must give the vitamin $B_6$ a little credit," she said. "At least, I didn't itch as much, and I have a little less water retention. But I'm disappointed; I'd hoped for more. Have you had this work for anyone else?"

"As you know, your problem is a very rare one. I've treated only two other people for it. They both did well."

"Now what?"

"Tell me—when you were pregnant with your children, did you have nausea or vomiting?"

"Not with Jamie—he's the first. But I really did with Jennifer. It finally went away the fourth or fifth month."

"Most frequently nausea of pregnancy will clear up with enough vitamin $B_6$, sometimes several hundred milligrams daily. [Author's note: *AMA Drug Evaluations*, prepared by the American Medical Association, says vitamin $B_6$ is not helpful for nausea in pregnancy. Obviously, I disagree.] Sometimes, though, vitamin $B_6$ doesn't work for this condition when taken by mouth, but works just fine when injected. I don't know why, as vitamin $B_6$ isn't known to be a difficult vitamin to absorb, like vitamin $B_{12}$. However, those are the observed facts. So, before you give up, why not try it by injection?"

"How do I do that? I can't come in here for shots all the time."

"I don't want you to, either. You can learn to give your own, or have your husband give it."

"How much do I use? How often?"

"You'll probably have to experiment with dosages, if it does work out, to find exactly how much you need. I'd suggest 300 milligrams twice daily as a starting point."

# Why Injections?

"Why would it work by injection, and not when I swallow it?"

"As I said, I don't know. It must have something to do with absorption—obviously—if it does work. That happens rarely with other nutrients, also. At least it can't hurt, as long as the shot is given properly."

"Well, I'm not doing anything else, so I'll try."

I didn't hear anything from Mrs. Wilson for the rest of that summer. Four months later she came in again, in October. This time she looked happier.

"What happened?" I inquired.

"In the first place, I had to wait three solid weeks for the first sunny day. I thought my problem would be solved just by the weather. But seriously, the first time I took 500 milligrams by injection twice a day. I know that's a little more than you said, but I knew it couldn't hurt, and I wanted to make sure I got enough. You know, I didn't have an itch or a bump all day. I couldn't believe it. But it worked again the next day, and again no problem. I also noticed I lost about three pounds of water.

"Well, we spent the rest of the summer working on the right dose for me. It turns out that lately, if I take a shot of just 300 milligrams twice a week, I don't have any problem. If I let it go longer than that, and I'm exposed to sunshine, I start to get a little itchy. But you know what—if I take a shot right away, I don't get hives. Now, does that make any sense?"

"I don't know exactly what you mean by 'sense,' but if it works, stick with it. Dr. Mandel's patients required variable amounts of vitamin $B_6$, and usually stopped taking it with no recurrence of their hives."

"You mean, they stopped their treatment, and the hives stayed away? That certainly hasn't happened to me yet. I can tell, by the itching."

"No, but remember, his patients all were able to get it to work by mouth, also. So apparently your problem is slightly different. But you are needing less now than you were two or three months ago, so maybe you'll be able to quit treatment in a few months, too."

# A Simple Remedy for an Unusual Problem

Vitamin $B_6$ is generally regarded as safe to use. Even though the quantity recommended by Dr. Mandel could be as much as 900 milligrams daily, no one has reported adverse effects at that level. Some individuals who've had occasion to take as much as 4,000 milligrams daily have told me they "just didn't feel well," and cut the dose back. Others have no untoward effects even at this high dose. In general, the conservative approach would be to take no more than several hundred milligrams.

Mrs. Wilson's case was unusual since injectable $B_6$ was required. All of the people reported by Dr. Mandel got results with swallowing the $B_6$. Even better, it was only required for two to three days at most, following which the sun-induced hives didn't recur.

It's not necessary to "balance" extra vitamin $B_6$ by taking the exact same number of milligrams of each other B vitamin. It's wise to "back up" a large quantity of any B vitamin with extra B complex, perhaps one to three capsules or tablets daily, but precise matching of the dose is not necessary to enable the individually therapeutic B vitamin to function.

## REFERENCES

**Photosensitivity**

"Antiemetics." In *AMA Drug Evaluations*. 3d ed. PSG Publishing, 1977, p. 1091.

Mandel, Edward H. "New Treatment for Photosensitive Skin Eruptions: Results Obtained with Vitamin $B_6$." *New York State Journal of Medicine*, July 15, 1963, pp. 2097–2100.

A special test designed to determine vitamin $B_6$ needs calculates the exact amount to relieve a woman who's suffering from carpal tunnel syndrome (pain or numbness in the hand or fingers caused by pressure on a nerve).

# 52 A CASE OF VITAMIN $B_6$ DEPENDENCY

"I was really happy when I read that carpal tunnel syndrome is treatable with vitamin $B_6$. You see, I'm a typist and have to use my hands all the time, to support myself. Then I read Dr. Ellis's book, all his cases, and decided to start myself on vitamin $B_6$. I've been really disappointed. It hasn't cleared up after three months." Jane Horton looked as disappointed as she sounded.

"I added the other vitamins you mentioned," she continued, "still not much better. But I decided to come in anyway because I really don't want surgery on my wrists. Besides, I can't afford to take time off work, and right now I have no insurance. I figured maybe I wasn't doing something right, or I needed other vitamins, too. Maybe I wasn't absorbing them. I don't know."

"You're sure it's carpal tunnel syndrome?"

"That's what the orthopedic surgeon said. Besides, I had that electro-whatever test. It was positive."

"Electromyography?"

"That's it. Actually I figured it out myself before I even saw a doctor. Looked up all the symptoms. I started having tingling sensations in both hands that came and went, but after a while they came more than they went. About that time, I got numbness, particularly at the tips of my fingers. Once I got numbness, it didn't go. Then my hands started getting weak—first the left, then the right.

"By that time, I'd figured out the trouble. I didn't want to wait until the muscle near my thumb started to atrophy, as the textbook says. So I went to see the orthopedic surgeon. He made the diagnosis."

"Let me see your hands."

She held them up. They didn't look at all unusual. I asked her to bend her wrists as far forward as she could.

"The orthopedic surgeon had me do that too. Really made my hands hurt, tingling worse. Couldn't stand it for long, then. Since I started on vitamin $B_6$ I can do it a lot longer." She demonstrated wrist flexion and compression for three minutes. "It does increase the tingling a little still."

"Do your hands still hurt at other times?"

"Not really hurt, more like an electrical tingling. I don't mean to say it's not better—it is—but with my work, tingling is a real hindrance, and there's still some numbness."

"How much vitamin $B_6$ are you taking?"

"Two hundred milligrams, three times daily, like I read."

"That's usually more than enough for carpal tunnel syndrome; it certainly sounds like that's your problem. You have the symptoms and signs, and it's hard to argue with the nerve conduction test. Unfortunately, it does happen that treatment that works well for most people with the same problem doesn't work for a few. Sometimes there are unknown factors."

Ms. Horton looked more disappointed than when she had first come in.

## Try Vitamin $B_6$ Injections

"Before you get too depressed, there is a thing or two to try. You've been swallowing the vitamin $B_6$; perhaps it isn't being absorbed fully. Also, you've had partial symptom improvement. Perhaps you need a bigger dose."

"A bigger dose? Is that safe? I'm already taking 600 milligrams a day."

"Fortunately, vitamin $B_6$ is usually safe. Much larger doses than that have been given, even to children, particularly in orthomolecular treatment for mental problems."

"Why would anyone need so much vitamin $B_6$? I looked up the Recommended Dietary Allowance. It's only two milligrams daily."

"I can't say exactly. There are some clues: For example, medical textbooks recognize a category of illness called 'pyridoxine dependency,' in which cellular enzymes require much more vitamin $B_6$ to function properly in some persons than in others. Although textbooks don't say so, it's probable that there are 'dependency diseases' for each vitamin, not just $B_6$, since vitamins mostly function in the body as $B_6$ does, as coenzymes for various cellular enzymes.

"This is only one possibility. Given the relative scarcity of properly directed vitamin research, I'm sure there are other possibilities that haven't been found."

"So what do I do?"

"Quickest thing is to try an injection of vitamin $B_6$, or perhaps a series of injections."

"So if I get better with shots instead of pills, I can guess I wasn't absorbing the $B_6$?"

"Right."

"How much should I try?"

"Three milliliters daily is about as much as you could comfortably inject. It's 100 milligrams per milliliter, so that's 300 milligrams total. Please check with the nurse: She'll show you how to give yourself the injections."

"You want me to try one a day? For how long?" She didn't look pleased with the thought of daily shots.

"Better give it a good try: two weeks. If it's going to work, it should in that time."

She got up to go. "I sure hope it does," she said as she left.

Three weeks later, Ms. Horton returned. I could tell from the way she looked we probably hadn't gotten anywhere.

"Maybe a little better, but not much. For that, I can't see taking a shot a day. I went back to 600 milligrams daily, swallowed. Now what do I try? Maybe I have one of those B$_6$-dependency problems. Too bad there isn't some way of telling, other than just guessing."

# A Reliable Test

"Actually, there is. Luckily, there's at least one B$_6$-dependent enzyme that can be tested in the laboratory, and it appears to be a reliable indicator of how much vitamin B$_6$ a person needs."

"There is? You mean you can tell exactly how much vitamin B$_6$ I might need, individually, and not just go by average-person statistics?"

"That's the way it looks."

"Why not just draw a vitamin B$_6$ blood level . . . you know, check how much B$_6$ is in my blood."

"Because then we're back to average-person statistics. We'd know how much vitamin B$_6$ you have in your blood, but we wouldn't know what it's doing for you. The same amount of vitamin B$_6$ that's enough for someone else might not be enough for you. Actually that's obvious, since your carpal tunnel syndrome didn't improve like it does for most people injected with that much B$_6$."

"So this tells what the B$_6$ is doing for me, rather than how much I have?"

"Right. It's a functional test, rather than an absolute-level test. That makes it entirely individualized. Obviously, it's much more important to know what the vitamin B$_6$ is doing for you, rather than how much of it there is."

"Is it a blood test?"

"Actually two, or possibly more."

"Why more than one?"

"One is done to find the level of enzyme activity with your present level of vitamin B$_6$ intake. Then we increase your intake, wait ten days or so, and repeat the test. If the level of activity is significantly higher the second time, the increased amount of vitamin $B_6$ is necessary to 'saturate' the enzyme toward the maximum activity possible."

"You said maybe more than two tests?"

"If the enzyme activity isn't increased on the second test, then we stop, as that would mean the first amount of vitamin $B_6$ was enough to saturate, or fully activate the enzyme. There'd be no point going further. If the enzyme activity increases, then we keep raising the dose and repeating the test, until the enzyme activity doesn't increase anymore."

"I think I've got it. We just keep increasing the dose until the enzyme quits going higher. That's a full saturation dose. Right?"

"Right."

"What's the test called?"

"EGOT. That's for erythrocyte glutamic-oxaloacetic transaminase."

"I'll just go ask for the EGOT test."

I marked her lab slip.

"How much do I increase the vitamin $B_6$?"

"Double each time until the test stops increasing."

"That means 400 milligrams, three times a day?"

"Yes."

"Not too much?"

"Remember, this test individualizes for you. We'll find out if it's too much if your test doesn't increase from this test to the next."

# A Series of Increases

Ms. Horton's first EGOT determination was 808 units. Following her increase in vitamin $B_6$ to 400 milligrams three times a day, her EGOT ten days later was 1,713 units, a definite increase. She then increased her vitamin $B_6$ to 800 milligrams, three times daily. Her third EGOT test was 2,627 units, another significant increase.

With this last increase in the B$_6$ dose her symptoms disappeared entirely, so I asked her to increase the dose to 1,000 milligrams, three times daily, instead of doubling again. A subsequent EGOT determination was 2,703 units, not much of an increase. Obviously, 800 milligrams, three times daily, was enough to saturate her EGOT enzyme system and take away the numbness and tingling in her hands.

Obviously, Ms. Horton could have kept increasing the vitamin B$_6$ dose until her symptoms disappeared without running the EGOT test. However, the EGOT determination (which is relatively inexpensive) demonstrates biochemically that a much-higher-than-usual dose of vitamin B$_6$ is definitely needed to keep at least one of her enzymes functioning properly.

Functional enzyme testing (also called the "coenzyme-apoenzyme system principle" by some, "enzyme activation coefficient" by others) also has been developed for vitamins B$_1$ (thiamine) and B$_2$ (riboflavin). It's an improvement over just guessing what intake of a vitamin is needed. It's also an improvement over measuring the blood level of a vitamin, as it shows what the vitamin is actually doing for the enzyme involved, and of course for the person whose enzyme it is. It allows individualization of vitamin dosage.

Each vitamin is involved with more than one enzyme; it would be more helpful to measure as many enzymes as possible for each vitamin. Also, it's not been established for sure that maximal or "saturated" activity of each enzyme is always the best or healthiest level.

However, as demonstrated in Ms. Horton's case, functional enzyme testing can be a useful tool in evaluation of nutritional requirements. Although the development of functional enzyme testing is fairly new, it's already useful. Further developments should make individualization of vitamin dosage much more possible in the future.

Ms. Horton's functional testing was modified by having her take extra vitamin B$_6$ herself, rather than adding "activated" vitamin B$_6$ to her blood in the laboratory. Clinically, this modified procedure appears equally effective.

# Evidence for Vitamin B₆ Overwhelming

The evidence for a vitamin B₆ deficiency in the carpal tunnel syndrome is now overwhelming. In a landmark statement, George S. Phalen, M.D., the surgeon who originally described the problem and its surgical treatment, wrote: "Largely because of the efforts of Ellis and Folkers, vitamin B₆ (pyridoxine hydrochloride) in doses of 100 to 200 milligrams per day may, in the future, be the drug [sic] of choice in the medical treatment of carpal tunnel syndrome."

It's not known why many individuals with carpal tunnel syndrome (as well as other problems) require a much higher daily intake of vitamin B₆ than the two milligrams required for Recommended Dietary Allowances.

Care should be taken, however, not to add more than 500 to 1,000 milligrams of vitamin B₆ daily for specific conditions without advice and help from a physician knowledgeable in nutritional biochemistry. A report by Herbert Schaumburg, M.D., and others describing apparent nerve function problems in seven individuals who took 2,000 milligrams or more of vitamin B₆ daily is one cautionary example.

It's difficult to know how much is enough especially since vitamin testing is still in its infancy. When a variety of functional tests for each nutrient is available, laboratory evaluation of individual nutrient requirements will be much more precise.

Manufacturers have recently introduced another dimension in vitamin B₆ treatment as well as treatment with certain other vitamins—the active form.

Vitamin B₆ (pyridoxine) is not actually the form of the vitamin active in the body. A chemically active form is actually pyridoxal phosphate. (Some vitamins have one active form, others more than one.) The theory behind providing vitamins in these forms is that some individuals may have difficulty in metabolizing the vitamin from the way it's found in food into the form in which the body uses it.

Although it's much too soon to know for certain, and very little research has been published, it appears that in a few cases at least, using pyridoxal phosphate instead of plain (unactivated) $B_6$ can produce better results. I've observed one case where pyridoxal phosphate was effective and pyridoxine wasn't. I've also observed several cases where a lower dose of pyridoxal phosphate replaced a much larger amount of pyridoxine with the same degree of effectiveness. And I've seen several cases where there appeared to be no difference at all. Considering that pyridoxal phosphate costs much more as of this writing, it can only be recommended for trial when pyridoxine is ineffective.

## REFERENCES

**Carpal Tunnel Syndrome**

Ellis, John M., and Presley, James. "Rheumatism and the Carpal Tunnel Syndrome." *In Vitamin B₆: The Doctor's Report.* Harper & Row, 1973, p. 57–73.

Ellis, John M. et al. "Clinical Results of a Cross-Over Treatment with Pyridoxine and Placebo of the Carpal Tunnel Syndrome." *American Journal of Clinical Nutrition*, October, 1979, pp. 2040–2046.

Phalen, George S. "The Birth of a Syndrome, or Carpal Tunnel Revisited." *Journal of Hand Surgery*, 1981, pp. 109–110.

**Enzyme Measurements of Nutritional Deficiencies**

Kishi, Hiroe, and Folkers, Karl. "Improved and Effective Assays of the Glutamic Oxalocetic Transaminase by the Coenzyme-Apoenzyme System (CAS) Principle." *Journal of Nutritional Science and Vitaminology*, vol. 22, 1976, pp. 225–234.

Lonsdale, Derrick, and Shamberger, Raymond J. "Red Cell Transketolase as an Indicator of Nutritional Deficiency." *American Journal of Clinical Nutrition*, February, 1980, pp. 205–211.

Tillotson, J. A., and Baker, E. M. "An Enzymatic Measurement of the Riboflavin Status in Man." *American Journal of Clinical Nutrition*, April, 1972, pp. 425–431.

Williams, Roger J. *Nutritional Against Disease: Environmental Prevention*, Pitman Publishing, 1971, p. 79.

## Vitamin B$_6$ Deficiency

Gaby, Alan. "Why This Epidemic of Vitamin B$_6$ Deficiency?" *Prevention*, April, 1982, pp. 55–59.

## Vitamin B$_6$ Toxicity

Schaumburg, Herbert et al. "Sensory Neuropathy from Pyridoxine Abuse: A New Megavitamin Syndrome." *New England Journal of Medicine*, August 25, 1983, pp. 445–448.

# Appendix A
# EIGHT NEW CASES ON HEAL-
# ING WITH NUTRITION

## MAGNESIUM IF IT SPASMS

### The Esophagus

"I'm having more and more trouble swallowing," Judy Michaels said. "The neurologist said I had esophagospasm, but that just means my esophagus cramps, and I knew that already. That's why I was at the doctor's in the first place! All they could think of was to give me muscle relaxers, Valiums . . . my throat might relax but so would my brain. My friend said you might know what to do."

"What did your x-rays and other tests show?"

"They saw the spasm on x-ray, but all the other tests were negative."

"When do you cramp?"

"Mostly when I try to swallow something, but sometimes one just happens on its own. Those are the worst, they sometimes don't go away for half a day."

"How often?"

"Several times a day, sometimes one right after another."

"How long have you had these cramps?"

"5 years now, worsening all the time."

### Arteries: Fingers

"My fingers go all numb and white even when my hands aren't cold. When it's cold, they're white all time. Gets really bad. Even the warmest gloves don't help much." Jean Sutra held out both hands. "Naturally they're O.K. now. If you want a demonstration, though, cold water will do it."

"Raynaud's?"

"Raynaud's syndrome, that's what they call it. I've been checked for a lot of other stuff, too . . . you know, lupus, arthritis, all the stuff that's supposed to go with Raynaud's. None of those. They've got me on these pills" . . . she handed me a bottle of "calcium channel blocker" tablets . . . "that help some, but they make me tired."

"You're not a smoker?"

"Quit when this started. Didn't help."

### Arteries: Heart

"I'm taking these drugs for angina, and they do help, but I've been thinking they can't be doing any good in the long run," Tom Ivors said. "They're just symptom treatment, and don't do anything to restore the health of my heart, arteries, or the rest of me. In a way, they just postpone the day of reckoning, which is worth doing if correcting the damage is impossible. But I've been doing a lot of checking since my angina started, and the more I read, the more I think it might be. So here I am."

"How long have you had angina?"

"Let's see, I'm 58 now, so 3 years since it was actually diagnosed but I'd had chest pains on and off for a year or two before that."

"Any heart attack?"

"Cardiologist says he can't find any sign of one so far. It's the "so far" part I don't like."

"You've had artery x-rays, arteriograms?"

"When I first went to the cardiologist. He said I really wasn't clogged up as bad as usual, not enough for immediate surgery anyway. He thinks a lot of my angina may be due to spasms of my coronary arteries. That's what some of the drugs are for. He says that actually happens a lot, coronary artery spasm."

"How often do you have chest pains?"

"Before I went on these drugs, I was having them nearly every day, sometimes two or three times a day. But they were mostly light ones. It's when they started getting heavier that I decided to see the doctor."

"And now?"

"Sometimes I go two or three days without one, and when I do get one they're almost always mild. Don't get me wrong, the drugs are helping keep the pain away, and I'm grateful for that, but they're not rebuilding my health any, and I want to get at the problem that way."

### Lungs: Bronchial Spasm (Asthma)

"Eric is really wheezing today. He's already on a maximum amount of his bronchodilator, theophylline, and he's using his inhaler as much as he can. He had an adrenaline shot last week, it helped, but only temporarily. If he gets much worse, he usually has to take prednisone. We really hate to do that. I know it's the very first time we've been here, and you haven't done any tests or anything, but will vitamin B12 shots do anything to stop this?"

"Where'd you hear about vitamin B12 shots?"

"Two of our friends' children got rid of their wheezing that way when they came here. The first one we thought it was just a fluke, but after the second we decided to see if we could try it for Eric."

"Vitamin B12 shots do work remarkably well against

wheezing for children and teenagers. Approximately 80% have either elimination or substantial reduction of wheezing. But they take time . . . if you start today, you might not see any change for several days, a week, or more."

Eric's mom looked disappointed. "The way he's going, that might not be in time. When he's gotten this way before, most of the time he's had to go on prednisone temporarily. Oh well, maybe it'll stop the next one. . . ."

"Hold on, B12 takes time, but it's not the only thing you can do. For bronchial spasm and wheezing like this, there's at least one other nutrient. . . ."

### Back Muscles

"My back muscles have been going into spasms for several years now," George Franklin said. "I've seen two different chiropractors, an osteopath, an orthopedic surgeon, and a neurologist. Back adjustments don't seem to help, and all the others could suggest were muscle relaxers, which work, mostly, but they make me feel funny in the head."

"Have you tried acupuncture?"

"Yeah, that worked while I was getting the treatments and for a few weeks after, but then the spasms came back again. I don't want to do that again unless there's nothing else."

"Been checked for food allergies?"

"No. Allergies cause muscle spasms?"

"Sometimes. And when no other cause is found, allergies are one of the most commonly overlooked causes."

"Weird."

"Weird but true. There are a few other things to check for, too. And there's at least one non-toxic nutritional treatment that usually controls muscle spasms, even when no exact cause can be found."

### An Unusual Case: Severe Intestinal Spasm

Severe intestinal spasms are not at all unusual in emergency rooms, but Tahoma Clinic doesn't have an emergency facility, so we rarely·see them. When Emily Brouiller walked in bent over and clutching her abdomen, a nurse took her to lie down right away.

"I've just come from the emergency room," she said. "Two surgeons there want to admit me to the hospital, they say I've got a twisted intestine, a volvulus I think they said, and I'd probably need surgery to untwist it. They nearly killed me at that hospital with my last surgery, so I said no thank you I'd try over here first."

"You really should be back at the hospital," I said. "Something as severe as a possible volvulus, it's a lot safer. Besides, could be they'll just put you in bed, keep an eye on you, and it just might subside."

"I know, they said that too, and that's partly why I'm here. I figured I'd take that bed-time for something possibly more useful. Is there anything you can do?"

### If It Spasms . . . . Try Magnesium!

We gave Emily Brouiller 2 grams of magnesium sulfate (along with vitamin B6, which helps it work better) in an "IV push". Magnesium given intravenously abruptly relaxes the muscles in the walls of blood vessels, so they dilate rapidly, producing a feeling of intense overheating all over the body. As the overheating reached its peak, Mrs. Brouiller reported "my insides feel like they just relaxed". As her magnesium-provoked warmth faded, her intestinal spasm and pain faded, too, and she walked out pain free an hour later.

George Franklin didn't have allergies. We weren't any more successful than his other doctors at finding a cause for his back muscle spasms. However, a series of magnesium (with B6) IV's, followed by intramuscular injections (which he does himself at home), and then a combination of less-frequent shots and capsules of magnesium aspartate daily have kept the spasms almost 100% controlled.

Eric got magnesium, ascorbate and other nutrients IV before he left the clinic. (Relief of acute wheezing by IV magnesium has even been reported in the *Journal of the American*

*Medical Association!*) It reduced his wheezing by 90%, and when it started to return the next day, another IV "finished it off" along with continued use of his regular asthma medications. However, vitamin B12 "caught up" with his asthma after two weeks of daily injections, completely relieving his wheezing, so extra magnesium is only a part of an overall supplementation program.

Tom Ivor started with one week of daily self-administered 1 gram magnesium sulfate injections, and tapered through 3 a week, 2 a week to once weekly with an occasional "extra" injection when he thinks his angina might be coming back. Magnesium supplements taken orally don't work for him nearly as well as injections, a problem common to a substantial minority. He was able to discontinue his drugs after 6 weeks without any relapse. He says he can tell that the magnesium gives him more energy, too.

Jean Sutra also found that magnesium supplements taken by mouth help a little, but weekly magnesium injections prevent her Raynaud's syndrome spasms entirely, unless she plunges her hands in ice cold water.

After 4 months of weekly magnesium sulfate injections, Judy Michaels had no further problem with esophageal spasms. She continues to take a standard calcium-magnesium supplement "just to be sure, and besides it's good for my bones."

## Why Injections?

Some of the first clinical researchers in magnesium therapy noted that oral magnesium supplements often didn't work nearly as well as injections. For severe spasm, such as Eric's asthma (bronchial muscle spasm) or Emily Brouiller's emergency intestinal spasm, there's no question that IV injection of magnesium (preferably along with vitamin B6) is necessary. In less urgent muscle spasm situations, there's no harm done in trying oral magnesium. If swallowing it doesn't work, it's possible magnesium's not the answer. Certainly, we get leg muscle and uterine cramps and spasms because of insufficient calcium, or potassium.

However, magnesium treatment for muscle spasm of all kinds is so often effective that it should never be abandoned until injections have been tried.

Remember . . . . . if it spasms, try magnesium!

## PREVENTING CHILDHOOD INFECTIONS

Bruce Dennison was a veteran of surgery at age 5. Already tubes had been placed and replaced in his ears three times, and his tonsils and adenoids were gone.

"Enough's enough!" his mother said. "Even with all that, he keeps on getting earaches. Besides that, he gets one cold after another, coughs, runny noses . . . . seems like he's sick half the time. His pediatrician just says some kids are like that, and keeps on writing out prescriptions for antibiotics, decongestants, and referring him for more surgery. I just know there's got to be a better way!"

"Usually is," I said. "How'd you happen to bring him here?"

"His kindergarten teacher took pity on us, I guess. She says she's not supposed to give medical advice, so she didn't, but she said her sister's son had only one cold in two years since he'd been here, and no more drugs. We thought couldn't do much worse, so here we are."

"Fair enough. Let's get started. . . ." I asked Mrs. Dennison more questions about Bruce's health history, his surgeries, his medications. She told me about family health history. Then we got to questions about what Bruce ate.

"Well, we're in a hurry in the morning, his father and I both work, so he has toast and peanut butter, or cereal with milk. And I always make him drink a glass of milk. . . ."

"He eats lunch at kindergarten. They always make sure the kids get milk, too, it's school policy, and then the usual school stuff, you know, hot dogs, sloppy joes, carrot sticks, celery, jello. . . ."

"After school, I usually give him root beer and some crackers, or sometimes cookies or a granola bar. . . ."

"At dinner, we have beef or chicken, sometimes fish, potatoes or rice, and one or two vegetables. Corn, beans, broccoli, sometimes lettuce salads. Usually, some kind of dessert, pudding, ice cream, cookies.."

"Milk?"

"Oh yes, I always make sure he drinks his milk."

"What kind of cereal in the morning?"

"Usually something he's seen on TV."

"Whole wheat bread?"

"Sometimes, but mostly white. His dad doesn't like whole wheat much."

"Do you use many mixes or packaged foods?"

"Some."

I reviewed my notes. "Let's take a look at Bruce."

Mrs. Dennison got him from our waiting room where he'd been coloring. He climbed up on the exam table.

Some of his problems were obvious. He had dark circles under his eyes, and fine horizontal creases in his lower eyelids, which were slightly puffy. His nose was runny, and he looked a bit pale. The tube was still in his right eardrum, but it had slipped out on the left. The rest of his check-up was OK.

"I suppose you'll need to have some tests done?" Mrs. Dennison asked.

"Yes, but those are mostly for details. The basic problems are fairly obvious."

"Obvious? Are you sure?" Mrs. Dennison managed to look extremely skeptical and very hopeful at the same time. "Why hasn't his pediatrician told me? He's the expert on children, after all."

"That's true. But if his medical school was typical, it taught virtually nothing about nutrition and health. And after medical school, many doctors believe the "official line" that what we eat doesn't make a great deal of difference to most illnesses."

"All of Bruce's problems can't be due to what he's eating! That's hard to believe, especially after all this time. How is that obvious? What do you see?"

I sighed inwardly. "It's what I see, and what I hear. Also, please remember we've been at this at Tahoma Clinic since 1974, and have watched hundreds of children with recurrent infections of all sorts become nearly infection-free following the same basic principles. And those principles aren't original with us; doctors have written about them since at least the 1920's."

"So what's obvious about Bruce?"

"The dark circles under his eyes, and the way his lower eyelids look . . . he's allergic to some of his food."

"Allergic to food? He couldn't be. His pediatrician had him tested for that, when he was three."

"What kind of tests?"

Mrs. Dennison looked surprised. "Standard tests, I suppose. They made all those scratches on his back. They said maybe he was allergic to yeast, but that was about all."

"Scratch tests aren't accurate for food allergies. More importantly, Bruce's health history and physical exam almost scream allergy."

"So what kind of allergy tests do you do here? I'd hate to put Bruce through all those scratches again."

"Modern allergy testing requires only a single blood specimen for any number of food tests. The best available test is called an "IgG4/IgE RAST" test. But before we go on about allergy, we need to go over something more basic: refined sugar, and processed food."

"Sugar? What's that got to do with earaches?"

"Not just earaches, infections in general. Sugar significantly interferes with the ability of white blood cells to kill germs."

"But we don't give Bruce many candies and things like that. Doesn't it take a lot to cause a problem?"

"As little as a teaspoonful every few hours can do it." I looked at my notes. "Actually, Bruce is getting a substantial amount of sugar in his food. You'll find a lot of unsuspected sugar too, once you start reading labels carefully."

"All the sugar has to go? Even at birthdays and Christmas?"

"Why make him more susceptible to infections for his birthday?"

"OK, OK, good point. If this works, it's worth it." She

thought for a second or two. "Does refined food interfere with the white blood cells, too?"

"Not directly, like sugar, but it strips our bodies of minerals and vitamins needed for the best of health."

"Oh. Well, as long as we're changing, might as well do it right. You didn't mention food chemicals and additives, but I suppose you were going to get around to them."

"You beat me to it."

"We'll put them on the hit list, too. This better work, it isn't going to be easy. What else?"

"I realize Bruce hasn't had his allergy tests yet, but you'd probably better be making plans to forget milk and dairy products."

Mrs. Dennison said something semi-unprintable. "Sorry, but milk, too? This is getting unreal . . . are you sure?" She bit her lip. "I'm sorry. I've reminded myself we're not doing so well with what we're doing."

"No need to apologize. All these changes can be overwhelming to begin with, but you'll find they're worth it. You're right, I can't be absolutely certain about milk allergy yet, but milk is so usually a cause of recurrent infection in infants and small children that it's "guilty until proven innocent"."

"I hope you'll write this all down."

"Of course, and also a small group of supplements that helps to reduce the infection rate, too. Adjusted for a 5-year-old, of course."

The note I gave Mrs. Dennison read:

Please eliminate:  all refined sugar
      "      "     all refined flour
      "      "     all food chemicals

You'll probably need to eliminate milk, and dairy products, as well as other foods identified by Bruce's allergy test

Vitamin C (chewable, no sugar) 500 mg. morning and evening
Zinc picolinate 15 mg. daily
(Brand name) children's chewable multiple vitamin with 10,000
    units Vitamin A, daily

She read it through. "Only 3 vitamin-mineral supplements? Someone told me your vitamin lists are as long as my arm."

I laughed. "Well, Bruce's arms are shorter. Besides, one of those is a multiple vitamin-mineral combination. But don't worry, if things don't go well, there are other supplements we can add. These are just a "basic core group" for infection-prevention."

"Also, don't forget that there are many more vitamins and minerals in a whole-food diet, and no excess losses due to sugar and refined foods."

Bruce's allergy blood test (IgG4/IgE combined RAST) was positive for milk, wheat, beef, orange, peanut, lettuce, salmon, chicken, almond, sunflower seed, blueberry, broccoli, kidney bean, beet, and squash.

"No wonder his food was making him sick," his mom said. "But trying to plan around his food allergies and eliminate all the junk is making me sick!" With lots of help from books, her local health-food store, and Tahoma Clinic she got the job done.

Bruce is eleven now. The last time I spoke to his mother, she reported he'd had no earaches, no infections requiring antibiotics, and only 3 colds in the six years since she'd "completely and permanently changed our family's ideas about food."

## REVERSING MACULAR DEGENERATION

Enid Derwind was 72 the year her eyesight began to fail. At first she thought it was to be expected, like the change she'd had in her 40's, but the deterioration became more than just a little, and seemed to affect the very center of her vision the most, particularly in the right eye. It seemed almost as if she could see things more clearly if she didn't look right at them. She kept hoping the problem was temporary, but when it got so she couldn't read or see her television well, she went to her optometrist. He looked in Mrs. Derwind's eyes, did a test or two, and referred her on to an ophthalmologist to confirm his observations. The ophthalmologist agreed Mrs. Derwind was suffering from macular degeneration, deterioration of the part of the retina serving the center of the visual field of each eye. Her right eye tested worse (20/100) than her left (20/80).

"My ophthalmologist says there's nothing to do. I know you're not an eye doctor, but my niece with lupus says she's gotten so much better since she's been to Tahoma Clinic, off almost all her drugs, and feeling much stronger, and she kept after me to call your Hotline information number. The nurse who answered said you've worked with quite a few people with macular degeneration, and not all of them got better, but most did, so that was good enough for me. Might as well try as long as there's no harm done, particularly considering the alternative. Do you think you can do anything?"

"As you said, we can try. Let's see, it's been . . . . 7 months since this came on?"

"Nearly eight, but of course it could have started sooner and I didn't notice. At first it went slowly, but the last two or three months have been fairly rapid. Does it make a difference how long it's been?"

"Treatment seems to do best when it hasn't been more than 2 or 3 years, though one person got some benefit even though the degeneration had been going on for 7 years."

"Well, at least that's in my favor."

"How's your health otherwise?"

"Fairly healthy at 72, as far as I can tell. A little stiffness that comes and goes here and there, and of course I don't heal up quite as fast as I once did, but aside from my eyes, everything else is OK."

We went over the rest of her health history, and went through a check-up. Everything appeared normal except for thin, papery fingernails, and a slightly dry skin.

"We'll need to rely on your eye doctor for complete eye exams. We don't have the equipment here."

"I expected that. I'll keep you in touch about how those are going. What else do we need to get done here?"

"We should check your minerals, for sure. Other than that

and routine good-health screening tests, we should check your digestion and particularly stomach acid output."

"I heard about that test from my niece. She said she had hardly any acid in her stomach at all . . ."

"Yes, that's usually the case with lupus. In your case, thin peeling fingernails are a likely sign of low stomach acidity."

"Does that have anything to do with macular degeneration?"

"It might, but not necessarily. Low stomach acid leads especially to poor protein digestion and decreased mineral absorption. Since part of the treatment involves minerals, decreased mineral absorption could theoretically make it worse."

"But not necessarily cause it?"

"No."

"So . . . what minerals are we particularly interested in?"

"Selenium and zinc . . . and whenever we do something about zinc, we must pay close attention to copper. Actually, we routinely check 20 or more at once."

"Can I start any treatment now, or should I wait until the tests come back?"

"If you can, start now, or soon, anyway. Some of the treatment is given intravenously, though. You'll need to check with the nurse about that."

"Intravenous? What part? I can't just swallow it?"

"You can, and we recommend it, but just swallowing it sometimes doesn't work well at all."

"Why's that?"

"Probably poor absorption . . . why don't I just describe how our treatment came about, it'll make more sense."

"Sounds good, I was curious about that anyway."

"Over ten years ago, I came across a clipping from the *Yakima Herald* . . ."

"The Yakima what?"

"*Yakima Herald*, it's a newspaper. The clipping was a health column by a doctor Joseph Bittner. He described how he'd been losing his sight to macular degeneration, and how he regained it by taking supplementary selenium and vitamin E. Since there wasn't any other treatment for the problem, and vitamin E and selenium are relatively safe in supervised doses, I passed Dr. Bittner's observations along, and a few people had their vision improve."

"Of course, some didn't, and in exploring other ways to combat the problem, I had people add zinc, and later on taurine, an amino acid. Both zinc and taurine are very important to a normally functioning retina. The success rate improved with these additions, so that's what we were using for 2 or 3 years."

"Then someone came in with a very rapidly deteriorating macular problem. Her health history included a long list of supplements she'd been taking nearly every day for several years. Zinc, selenium, and vitamin E were all on the list."

"So maybe it was the taurine missing?"

"Could be a small part of it, but since she had signs of poor absorption, and her eyes were getting worse fast, we decided to try the selenium and zinc intravenously."

"Why not just a . . . you know, a regular shot? Like in the hip or arm?"

"Too much volume, too many cc's."

"Oh. What happened?"

"We were all very surprised. Right in the middle of the IV drip, she called the nurse and said her sight was improving! She said she could make out some of the print on a poster across the room that she couldn't read before the IV started. By the time the IV was done, she could see even more."

"Did the improvement last?"

"Good question . . . it lasted only a day, then got as bad as before. She was of course depressed by the time she came back for her next IV, but went ahead anyway . . . and her sight improved again. So we kept the IV's up twice a week until the improvement started to hold. Now she gets one every 3 or 4 weeks."

"How's her vision doing?"

"20/40, both eyes. It was over 20/200 when we started."

"Wow. But not everyone does that well, do they?"

"Of course not. A few don't improve at all."

"I guess I'll take my chances. Doing nothing sure won't get me anywhere. Oh, by the way, what happened to the vitamin E and taurine? You don't put them in the IV?"

"Absorption of vitamin E and taurine are rarely problems. Also, on the practical side, there's no individual taurine for IV use available, and vitamin E availability hasn't been reliable. So we have folks swallow those, along with extra zinc and selenium."

"I guess I misunderstood. Even though the selenium and zinc are in the IV, you swallow them, too?"

"Sure. Gives a better chance of slowing down or even stopping the IV treatment sooner. We ask people to get zinc in the picolinate form. Zinc picolinate appears to absorb and cross cell membranes best."

I wrote a list for Mrs. Derwind that included zinc, selenium, vitamin E, and taurine. She went to get her lab tests done, and to check with the nurse about the IV's.

Mrs. Derwind is now 75. Her vision is now 20/40 on the right, 20/30 on the left. She was able to discontinue the IV's without losing progress after 13 months, although she says she can tell a difference if she misses her oral supplements for very long. Since her stomach test showed very low acidity, she also takes a form of hydrochloric acid with every meal.

She checks her serum cholesterol, uric acid, and blood count periodically, since all can be adversely affected by a zinc-copper imbalance.

## PREVENTING COLON CANCER WITH FRIENDLY BACTERIA

"My mother had colon cancer, and my father and grandfather died of it," Mr. Allenton said. "I'm 57, older than my mother when she had hers. I'm doing everything I can to prevent getting colon cancer, too. I have regular check-ups, I've had that 'colon-scope' examination three times already. I get my doctor to check me for bleeding regularly. All that's been negative."

He looked at his notes.

"Ever since I read about high fiber diets and colon cancer, I've been eating more vegetables, taking wheat bran. Lately I switched to oat bran because of the cholesterol thing. I stopped buying anything with artificial color, flavor, or preservatives. Also, I've been taking calcium because I read a report it helps prevent colon cancer."

"I'm here to find out anything else I can about preventing colon cancer, as well as staying as healthy as I can."

"Good. It's much easier to prevent a health problem than to treat it later. When did you last have a general checkup?"

"About two years ago."

"Everything OK?"

"Yes."

"Any symptoms since?"

"None to speak of."

He told me the rest of his health history, then we did his checkup. I explained the lab tests I recommended. "One routine test specially pertinent to you is a stool and digestive analysis. It includes a measurement of butyrate, a non-toxic substance produced by normal intestinal bacteria mostly from dietary fiber. Butyrate's been found to help restore normal growth patterns to cancerous colon cells. Populations higher in stool butyrate have lower colon cancer rates."

"Mine should be fine with all the vegetables I eat."

When Mr. Allenson returned, the first thing on his mind was the stool butyrate test.

"Sorry to report that your butyrate level was low," I said.

"So that means I might have a higher risk of colon cancer?"

"All the research so far points in that direction."

"Can't understand it. I eat plenty of vegetables, use oat bran . . . . . should be plenty of fiber to make into butyrate."

"I can't be sure, but it could be the bacteria you have aren't up to the job."

"What do you mean?"

"You don't have the usual population of friendly colon bacteria. The lab reports the predominant aerobic bacteria is *Klebsiella pneumoniae*. There aren't any *E. coli* at all . . . they're usually a predominant type . . . . and no *Lactobacillus* either. Usually a lot of those, too."

"Shouldn't I have symptoms of some sort? Diarrhea or something?"

"Not necessarily. The lab tells me that in one test series of 642 specimens cultured for routine purposes, not specially because of symptoms, 5% had no *E. coli,* and 29% had no *lactobacillus.*"

"Everyone should have those two types?"

"Yes, and lots of them."

"And without them, the usual bacterial conversion of some of the dietary fiber to butyrate doesn't happen?"

"It's impossible to say what proportion of butyrate production each type of bacteria is responsible for. There's another large group of colon bacteria, the anaerobic ones, that this test doesn't even measure. The most accurate interpretation we can read from the data we have is that there's a major disruption of normal intestinal bacteria, and that's very likely why your stool butyrate test was low. We'll use that theory to start with, anyway."

"Can you tell why my friendly bacteria are missing?"

"Not really. Could be they were wiped out by antibiotics at one time or another. Other medications can affect them. Diets high in sugar and refined carbohydrate can contribute to the growth of the 'wrong' kind of intestinal flora. Sometimes it's a ph . . . acid-alkaline balance . . . thing, if there isn't enough acid being made by the stomach."

"So what do I do to get the 'friendly germs' back? Take some lactobacillus acidophilus from the health food store?"

"That's part of the program, putting the 'good guys' back. The other part is inhibiting the growth of the 'unfriendlies' until the 'good guys' can take over and crowd them out."

"But I shouldn't take any antibiotics to kill the bad germs, should I, or I could cause the same kind of problem all over again, with a different unfriendly bacteria."

"Exactly. Antibiotics aren't the answer to this germ problem. Fortunately, there are several relatively harmless natural remedies that usually do the job."

"What are they?"

"Let's start with just two, garlic and goldenseal. Both inhibit the growth of a variety of unfriendly micro-organisms, and promote the growth of many friendly ones."

"Goldenseal?"

"An herbal, or botanical. Health food stores have it. Sometimes it's called hydrastis."

"So I should use garlic, goldenseal, and both types of friendly bacteria, and if that works, the replacement bacteria should make more butyrate out of the fiber in my diet?"

"That's the theory. Often that's all that's needed. If it doesn't work, there are a few other relatively safe things to try. Sometimes we have to look for other complicating factors."

"Let's hope it works for me the first time around. Incidentally, if butyrate is natural and safe, isn't there a butyrate supplement?"

"Remember, butyrate appears to help prevent colon cancer, which is one of your goals, but the right friendly bacteria do supply butyrate and much more. For example, they synthesize a significant proportion of certain vitamins that we wouldn't get otherwise. And unfortunately there's no way of telling what harm the unfriendly bacteria might do. All in all, it's preferable to regrow the usual quantities of friendly intestinal germs, and persuade the others to go away. That way, the butyrate comes back as one part of the over-all normalization."

"Makes sense, and I'll try it. I was just thinking of alternatives in case it doesn't work."

Fortunately for Mr. Allenson, his second follow-up analysis showed a return to a more normal pattern of intestinal bacteria. At the same time, the level of stool butyrate rose to a more normal level, adding another significant factor to his colon cancer prevention program.

## A CASE OF INSOMNIA AND (A LITTLE) DEPRESSION

"I'm just not taking those drugs anymore!" Roger Coleman declared. "Every single one of them gives me trouble. Besides, when that last psychiatrist told me I had a biochemical illness, I decided Helen here's been right all along. I should have come over here years ago. She says you guys work on biochemistry with vitamins and minerals and things. Would have been here a lot sooner except my insurance covers drugs but not vitamins. But she said . . ."

"I said so what if it's covered if it doesn't do a lick of good! Roger hasn't had a good night's sleep without drugs in years, and all drugs do is give him side effects. Hangovers, dizzyness, heartbeat problems, nightmares, I can't remember what all."

"Well, that's all behind me, even if I never get another good night's sleep. Now I'm retired it doesn't matter if I have to take a daytime nap or two."

"Matters to me!" Mrs. Coleman exclaimed. "I want to do my sleeping at night, and when you can't sleep, you don't let me either, mostly. I've got too much to do daytimes to be up half the night. Besides, I can't get my housework done with you sleeping all over the place."

"You just don't want me cluttering up my own couch when you feel like having the girls over, that's really it."

"Let's not argue, Roger, we agreed we'd come to see Dr. Wright and give it a try. Here . . ." she pulled a paper out of her purse ". . . I've kept a list of every single drug Roger's been on over the last eighteen years." She handed it to me. "Fourteen different drugs on that list, almost one a year."

I read through the list. "All 'sleeping pills' the first few years, almost all antidepressants the last few."

"Yeah, it seems the older I got, the more they thought my insomnia was because of depression. I might be a little depressed here and there, but no more now than when I was twenty. The doctors' ideas change, not me. Got so they wanted me to go into regular depression counseling, but I drew the line there."

"I have to back Roger up on that," Mrs. Coleman said. "We've been married nearly forty years, and he just isn't a generally depressed person. It seems the worse his insomnia got, the more the doctors decided it must be due to depression, and gave him antidepressants. Sometimes I wonder if part of that isn't due to our age: it's almost as if older people are expected to be depressed." She paused. "At most, Roger's a little depressed now and again, but his big problem is really insomnia."

I looked at my notes. "You started having insomnia 18 years ago?"

"No, that's when it got so bad I started seeing doctors about it. Actually, I've had trouble getting a whole night's sleep most of my adult life. Also, at that time my job was particularly demanding, and I decided I had to do something."

"Trouble getting to sleep, or waking up and not getting back to sleep?"

"Usually some of both."

"How many hours sleep a night?"

"On my own, no drugs . . . it varies. Every once in a long time, 7 hours or more. Usually, before I retired, 2 to 4 or 5 hours a night. Definitely not enough to feel rested. So most of the time the last eighteen years I took something."

"Did all these medications put you to sleep?"

"All but one or two. The strictly 'sleeping pill' ones mostly put me right out, and if I woke up, another one put me under again. But all the sleeping pills made me groggy, just like I was hung over. Hard time getting going in the morning, practically needed coffee transfusions."

"And the antidepressants?"

"Well, I slept with those, too, but a different type of sleep, sort of restless. With some of them I had weird dreams and nightmares. Two gave me heartbeat trouble. Didn't seem to put me under like regular sleeping pills. On the other hand, I didn't get groggy hangovers either."

"Did you notice any difference in daytime depression?"

"I think so . . ."

"Roger and I talked about that a lot, doctor. Especially with the first antidepressant, he seemed, well, a little more cheerful at times when he usually wasn't. That was several years back, and was one of the things that made us go along with the depression idea for so long. But none of the other antidepressants ever did as well . . ."

"Why'd you quit the first one?"

"Same reason I quit all of them: side effects. If I remember, the nightmares got too bad with that first one."

"That was it, dear. Those nightmares also got me so curious I started reading about brain chemistry. I found out there's really not nearly as much known about brain chemistry as I thought: in fact, the package inserts for most of the drugs they were giving Roger said even the manufacturers didn't know how their own drugs worked."

"And all these other antidepressants gave you side effects, too?"

"Yeah, but I stuck with each one as long as I could because they mostly did help me sleep better, anyway."

"And now?"

"Like I said, since I retired this year, it doesn't matter so much whether I sleep at night or not. Helen's been after me to try this natural biochemistry thing . . . . . and like I said, that last doctor told me I had a biochemical illness."

"Most experts these days do say depression is a biochemical illness . . . and there's a lot of suspicion that insomnia is too."

"I was reading about that, doctor," Helen Coleman said. "So I thought I'd ask Roger to try some tryptophan. It's supposed to help insomnia and depression both, in case Roger does have any depression."

"And it didn't do a darn thing I could tell, even after a month of trying just like the books said, in between meals, no protein at the same time, and so on," Mr. Coleman said.

"Tryptophan was a good choice to try, though, for insomnia and maybe depression. You tried it with some vitamin B6 and B3, also?"

"The one I got had those things right in it and magnesium, too," Mrs. Coleman answered. "And Roger took three-and-half grams a day, half mid-morning, half before bed."

"So much for that. Well . . . since you've been reading up on brain chemistry, I'm sure you've read that the brain makes many of its neurotransmitters from amino acids, like tryptophan—"

"Helen knows more about that stuff, doc."

"—so let's just try something simple first. Even though there are literally hundreds of amino acids in our bodies, all but eight can be produced internally . . ."

"Those are called the "essential amino acids" aren't they?" Mrs. Coleman asked.

"Yes. Without sufficient quantities of each of the essential amino acids—"

"—our bodies can't make all the right neurotransmitters" Mrs. Coleman finished for me.

"That's right. Or sometimes there might be an imbalance . . . you know, too much of one, not enough of another. So, please come in for a fasting blood test for the essential amino acids, and we'll see if they might be the problem."

Mr. Coleman turned out to be deficient in the essential amino acids isoleucine, leucine, lysine, phenylalanine, and threonine. Only methionine, tryptophan, and valine were within textbook-normal standards. Using a "normalization formula", the lab computer calculated what percentage of each of the eight amino acids should be in an individualized blend for Mr. Coleman. After looking at his data, I recommended he take 10 grams (approximately 2½ tsp.) of the eight-amino-acid blend, stirred into applesauce twice daily.

Within 3 weeks, Mr. Coleman reported he was sleeping

considerably better. By 3 months, he had "no sleeping problems at all," and he and his wife noted he'd had "not even a little" depression. A repeat essential amino acid test showed only 1 of the 8 still deficient. One year later, he continues to need 1 tsp. of his individualized essential amino acid blend daily to keep his sleeping pattern normal.

Essential amino acid deficiencies are frequently found in association with hypochlorhydria (low stomach acid), food allergy, and other "malabsorption" problems, and often get worse in frequency and severity as we get older. Using all eight essential amino acids in individually-calculated blends insures that we don't get "out of balance" if we need to use them for a prolonged period of time.

## DISSOLVING A SALIVARY DUCT STONE

"I've had this sore area over the angle of my jaw on and off for several months now," Aaron Sampson said. "It's not extremely painful, but it does hurt. Lately it's been more on than off." He rubbed his jaw in front of his right ear.

"Just one side?"

"Yeah, just the right, never the left. Same area where I had the mumps when I was a kid, but that was both sides. Mumps doesn't come back in a low grade on-and-off form in adults, does it?"

"No. Besides, it's usually both sides, acute, and quite swollen. Have you had any swelling?"

"Not until lately, and it's more a puffiness than swelling. That's been there the last few times it hurt, but not before. Hurts a little to touch, but it's not real bad."

"Any fever?"

"No."

"How've you been feeling otherwise?"

"Fine as far as I can tell. No problems."

"How'd you happen to come in now? Has it been getting worse?"

"No, but my wife kept after me because it hasn't gone

away." He hesitated; I waited. "Also, I found something else. It's got me more worried."

"What's that?"

"Right here in my cheek, right in front of where it's been aching on and off all these months. I can grab it with my fingers . . ." he illustrated by pinching his cheek, thumb inside, index finger outside ". . . a lump."

"You hadn't noticed that before, when this all started?"

"No, but it doesn't hurt or anything, and I never thought of grabbing my cheek like that. My wife's worried the lump means cancer."

"Don't think so, but come down the hall to an exam room and we'll make sure."

I checked the area at the angle of Mr. Sampson's jaw from the outside, then got a rubber glove to check the "lump" he'd discovered. The area over his right salivary gland, in front of his right ear and downward over the jaw angle was all slightly tender and very slightly puffy. The "lump" was within his cheek just in front of the sore area, roughly opposite the upper rear molars. It was hard and about the size of a small green pea.

"Hasn't your mouth been dryer on this side the last few months?" I asked.

"Not really . . . . well maybe a little, now that you mention it. But it's not been a problem, so I haven't paid a lot of attention."

"That lump is a 'stone' in your salivary duct, that drains saliva from your right salivary gland into the mouth. You're right, it's one of the same glands that gets mumps."

"A stone?"

"Yes . . . like a kidney stone, or a stone in the gallbladder. Not made of exactly the same stuff, but still a hard accumulation that blocks the drainage duct."

"So when it blocks saliva, the gland hurts and swells?"

"Exactly."

"So it must not be completely blocked, or wouldn't it swell up really big and hurt a lot more."

"Right. It's an intermittent, partial blockage—"

"—which is why it comes and goes, right? It must be getting bigger because it's happening more, right?"

"Can't say for sure, but that makes sense."

"I've checked the other side, nothing there."

"Usually they don't happen on both sides at once."

"So what do I do about it?"

"The usual treatment is surgery."

"And that's what I'm doing here. My wife says you'll recommend the most conservative thing first, diet or vitamins or whatever, and surgery only if there's no alternative. So skip the usual for now, and tell me what else I can do."

"Iodide drops." I started to write a prescription.

"Iodine? Like my mother put on cuts when I was a kid?"

"That would probably work, too, but for a variety of reasons, I'd recommend you use these potassium iodide drops instead. Don't worry about prescription expense, they're quite cheap."

"What'll the . . ." he read the prescription ". . . potassium iodide drops do?"

"Dissolve the stone."

"That simple?"

"Simple if you know what to do. Can't give you a 100% written guarantee, but I can't remember anyone it hasn't worked for."

"How long does it take?"

"Hard to say, but several weeks to several months."

"Any side effects?"

"Too much iodide usually causes acne-like pimples. More than that, and folks report a persistent metallic taste, and a very persistently runny nose. Oddly enough, though, I've seen and heard of almost no side effects in people who've been taking it for salivary duct stones."

"Sounds good . . . . by the way, would it help to eat more seafood in the future? That's about the only food source of iodine, isn't it?"

"Really impossible to say, but it's logical. Very often, the same nutrient that will successfully treat a problem in big doses will prevent the same problem in small quantities."

"My wife keeps bugging me about eating seafood. I'm from the Midwest and just never got used to it. Sounds like it's time to start. . . ."

Mr. Sampson cancelled his follow-up appointment. Fortunately, his wife phoned in to say his salivary duct stone disappeared in 4½ months.

## A LOOK AT HAIR AND FINGERNAILS

"I used to have such a full head of hair. It's thinned out so much my husband's starting to notice" . . . . . "Look at these fingernails! They won't grow, they crack, they split, they peel and layer back. Gelatin and calcium don't help" . . . . . "I feel like a TV commercial: dull, lifeless hair. It's breaking a lot more than it used to" . . . . . . "I'm only 57, and I'm so thin on top you can see wide open spaces between each hair. I don't want to be a bald grannie!"

Even though fingernails and hair are common problem areas, there's not much "priority research" being done. We don't have a National Hair Loss Institute, and no politicians are declaring War on Split Nails. Trying to find answers to hair and fingernail problems isn't always easy.

What do you do when the bottle(s) of "hair vitamins" don't work, and your dermatologist says you don't really have a problem, but you know better? You say you've taken enough calcium to turn to stone, but your nails are as bad as ever? Nail hardener, silk or acrylic nails may "cover up" the problem, but wouldn't it be nicer, not to mention healthier, to grow your own?

What follows may give you further clues. Some items may be "self-help," but others require some assistance from a nutrition-oriented doctor.

Sorry, men, but there are no answers here for 'hereditary

male-pattern baldness'. When something's found for bald men that's non-surgical, inexpensive, and free of possible long-term side effects, it'll be written about, and surely in more places than just this magazine. If this month's discussion seems more directed towards women, it's partly because very few men ever say anything to doctors about fingernails or hair, even when there's an obvious problem. Whether that's due to hormones or "cultural conditioning" is a topic I'll avoid!

### "What Do You Mean, It's My Stomach?"

Or in the words of a clinic visitor: "Usually when they can't figure out what's the matter with me, they tell me it's all in my head. Now you're telling me it's all in my stomach. I suppose that's progress, but my stomach isn't bothering me. So what do you mean by that?"

One of the most common causes of excess hair loss and/or cracking, splitting, peeling, chipping fingernails is a malfunctioning stomach. When our stomachs don't make enough acid and pepsin (a major protein-digesting enzyme), a wide variety of nutrients are "lost". Amino acids (the "building blocks" of protein), minerals, vitamin B12, and folate head the list. With such a variety of nutrients impaired by a malfunctioning stomach, it's not a surprise that something has to 'give', and the hair and/or nails, being presumably less essential to health, are often the first to go.

But they don't always go together. While it's not unusual for thinning hair to be accompanied by weak, peeling nails, either can be separately affected by a malfunctioning stomach.

How to know if your hair or nail difficulty may be due to an unsuspected stomach problem? It's best to have your nutrition-oriented doctor's help on this one. Symptoms are frequently subtle, and self-treatment has occasionally resulted in a visit to the emergency room. If present, symptoms may include upper abdominal bloating and gas, mostly after meals. Constipation is common, but a few have diarrhea instead.

"Heartburn" can occur. (No, "heartburn" does not always indicate too much stomach acid!)

Unfortunately, it's not unusual to have low (or no) stomach acid and no symptoms at all. Although the older we get, the more frequent stomach malfunction becomes, it's relatively common even among people in their 20's and 30's—especially people with poor nails and falling hair!

### Folate and Hormones

"My hair got really thin during my last pregnancy. It's never come back!" . . . . . . "About six months after the baby was born, I started noticing lots more hair in the tub and sink!" . . . . . "Could it be birth control pills?" . . . . . . "What about the estrogen I've been taking?"

If you've lost hair during or after pregnancy or while taking hormones, think of folate first. Frequently, extra folate and a few months time are all that's necessary to reverse hormonally-related hair loss.

Though "hormones" are often related to folate deficiency, folate-deficiency hair loss can occur without any apparent hormonal association, simply through poor eating habits. So, before swallowing those folate supplements, it's not a bad idea to review the best food sources of this vitamin. Brewer's yeast, salmon, liver, lima beans, spinach, oysters, chicken, watermelon, potatoes, asparagus, kale, broccoli, and carrots are reported to have the most folate per portion. Most raw green vegetables are good sources of folate, especially since this vitamin is easily destroyed by heating, freezing, or exposure to light.

Once hair has started to fall, food sources usually need supplementation. 5 mg. daily is often enough, but for a very few individuals who need folate, even 50 mg. daily, swallowed, won't do the job. For these few, folate injections are needed. If your hormonally related hair loss doesn't improve with oral folate, check with your nutritionally-oriented doctor.

Folate is said to be non-toxic, but recent research indicates that folate and zinc probably interfere with each other's absorption, another point to check with your doctor if you're planning to take either one for any length of time.

### Thyroid

An underactive thyroid can be the cause of both hair loss and weak nails. Unfortunately, routine "thyroid blood tests" do not always uncover a weak thyroid. As more sophisticated (and much more expensive) thyroid function tests have become available, doctors are discovering that many individuals previously labeled "normal" are hypothyroid (underactive) after all.

This is very old news to any who have read of the work of Dr. Broda Barnes, or more recently Dr. Stephen Langer. Their books cover this topic so well that I've nothing further to write. Make sure the doctor you're working with doesn't rely completely on blood testing to evaluate your thyroid function.

### Essential Fatty Acids

Major drug companies are finally discovering that essential fatty acids may help prevent heart attacks, but it may be another fifty years before they get around to noticing that healthy hair and nails need them too.

"Dull" and "lifeless" are two adjectives that should send you in search of a bottle of linseed oil, not a bottle of the latest miracle shampoo. Don't dump it on your head; swallow about one tablespoon daily, and see what happens in a few weeks. Get a smallish bottle to minimize rancidity problems. (It's probably wisest to put a thousand or so units of vitamin E into any opened bottle of oil to retard rancidity. And don't forget to take vitamin E, 200 to 400 units daily, whenever you take extra oil for any reason.)

If you have dry, flaky skin and breaking nails as well as dull, lifeless hair, you're definitely a candidate for linseed oil treatment.

Linseed oil contains both "omega-3" and "omega-6" essential fatty acids. Fish oil contains the "omega-3" type, and almost all other vegetable oils contain only "omega-6". Human metabolism requires a balance of both types, making linseed the "preferred" supplemental oil for human use. (If you can't stand the taste, it's also sold in capsules.)

Best food sources of essential fatty acids are the sources of food oils: fish, unroasted nuts, seeds, and whole grains. Margarine and hydrogenated fats are detrimental to fatty acid metabolism, and should be strictly avoided.

### Biotin

Years ago, someone noticed that animals given biotin grew stronger hooves. Human nails (and hair) respond to biotin often enough that it's become a standard part of "hair-and-nails" supplement formulas. Used alone, 1 or 2 mg. daily is usually sufficient. Biotin is generally considered non-toxic.

Very specialized topical (rub-on) biotin preparations are in use at male baldness clinics. At present, most of these clinics are quite expensive, and the biotin preparations are not available for general sale.

Best food sources of biotin include liver, kidney, egg yolk, haddock, halibut, cod, salmon, and tuna. Vegetables generally contain much less: best sources are oat, orange, tomato, whole wheat, raspberries, cheddar, and grapefruit.

### Minerals

Many of us have observed on our own that taking calcium seems to improve nail quality. When trying calcium, it's usually wisest to "balance" it with magnesium; calcium in a "background" of magnesium plus a multiple mineral is even better. Remember that calcium and other minerals don't absorb well unless the stomach is making sufficient hydrochloric acid, and that as we grow older more and more of us have "underacidity" problems. Fortunately, "more absorbable" forms of calcium and other minerals (designed to "get around" underacidity and other assimilation problems) are starting to appear in nutrition stores.

For a few of us, too much zinc and/or too little copper can result in hair loss. Although this situation isn't common, it should be checked for when the more usual answers aren't working.

### "Balding Grannies" and DHEA

With "advancing age" and granny-hood, some women become "quite thin on top". When this is part of an over-the-whole-body hair loss (head, forearm, leg, pubic, and underarm hair all thinner) the problem is often hormonal. The "missing hormones" for hair are not estrogens, but rather androgens, the male-type hormones.

Women and men have both estrogens and androgens. Women have considerable estrogen and comparatively little androgen; for men, the balance is opposite.

Androgens are principally responsible for stimulating hair growth in both sexes. As women have only comparative traces of testosterone, no beards grow, but as is obvious from other body hair, women's bodies have larger quantities of other non-testosterone androgens.

Beginning at puberty, both sexes start to secrete more of the androgen dehydroepiandrosterone (DHEA). Usually, DHEA stays relatively high until the mid-30's, when levels begin a gradual descent towards very low in extreme old age. At our clinic, we've found that premature loss of both head and body hair in women is very often associated with prematurely low levels of DHEA. Improving prematurely low DHEA is accompanied by regrowth of normal head and body hair, and coincidentally for many women, an improvement in libido.

## PROSTATE ENLARGEMENT

"I'm not famous enough to have my internal anatomy spread all over the front page," Mr. Oelfred said "but my urologist says I've got the same problem as Ronald Reagan. He wants to do the same thing to me, too . . . cut! I'm allergic to surgery, so I checked at my natural food store, and they told me to eat pumpkin seeds, take zinc pills, and see this naturopathic doctor . . . ." he handed me a card. "She told me to keep eating the pumpkin seeds, take the zinc pills, and take some linseed oil, too. She also recommended this herbal concoction . . ." he reached into his pocket, pulled out and handed me a bottle ". . . that I've never heard of. I thought, O.K., they both recommended the zinc pills, so I took one, and got an upset stomach. Thought maybe it was a coincidence, so I took another one, and it happened again. 'Bout that time my wife told me she'd read an article of yours a few years back about prostate, and she thought it said zinc and linseed oil. She called your free clinic hotline, and the nurse said those are things you usually recommend, but of course she couldn't give specific recommendations over the phone. So here I am."

"How long have you had prostate trouble?"

"Started having trouble passing urine a year and a half ago. Wasn't too bad at first, so I ignored it. Got worse three-four months ago. Figured it was my turn, Dad had the same thing, only a few years older."

His expression changed suddenly. "Say, you aren't fixing to give me that prostate gland exam again, are you?"

"It should be checked if it's the problem."

"I understand that, but I just got checked at the urologists', and that's enough checking for me for a good long time. Why don't you and I just concentrate on fixing it if it's fixable, and if any more checking is needed, I plan to go back to the urologist, anyway. O.K.?"

"O.K. I'd appreciate it if you'd let me know how any future checking goes, if you don't get it done here."

"Oh, sure." He relaxed. "Now what do I do?"

"Answer a few more questions if you would. Health history, family health background, that sort of thing. And a few specific things . . . . you said your stomach hurt when you took the zinc tablet?"

"Yeah, tried it twice, did the same thing both times."

"Do you get any indigestion, much belching after meals, or bloating?"

"Now and again, but not all the time."

"Constipation?"

"If anything, just a little of the opposite. But that's not all the time, either. What's that have to do with the zinc pills?"

"Most people who get stomach upset from zinc have low stomach acid production, and aren't digesting and assimilating nutrients very well. Indigestion, bloating, and belching, and constipation are more usual symptoms."

"How's that connected with the prostate problem?"

"Same way it's connected with the health of every cell in the body. No part of our bodies can stay as healthy as possible without the best possible flow of nutrients for growth and repair."

"So if I don't digest it it won't get to the prostate to help fix it, or something like that?"

"Or to prevent trouble, either."

"Got it. What else?"

In addition to a gastric analysis, I asked Mr. Oeldorf to have a mineral analysis done, and "routine health screening" tests including cholesterol and high-density (HDL) cholesterol.

His test for stomach acid was quite poor. Following meal-time supplementation with betaine hydrochloride-pepsin capsules, Mr. Oeldorf noticed improvement in his digestion, less loose bowels, and almost-disappearance of indigestion and bloating.

"Those zinc pills don't bother me any more, either," he reported. "I've kept on taking one a day until my tests came back. Figured one a day wouldn't hurt, and both the natural food store and the naturopathic doctor recommended them. What about you? You know, I think the zinc might be helping a little tiny bit already."

"Wouldn't be surprised. Zinc is a key part of a prostate-improvement program. Please make sure to get the picolinate form of zinc . . . . that's zinc picolinate . . . . and use 30 mg., three times a day for now. Your tests show you could use that much for a few months."

"You also need some copper."

"I was low on copper?"

"Low end of normal. Probably not a problem now, but the extra zinc could "push out" enough copper to cause problems."

"Like what?"

"Too much zinc, too little copper, total cholesterol goes up, HDL-cholesterol goes down. Just the opposite of what's desirable."

"How was my cholesterol and HDL?"

"Looks good for now, but should be checked every few months if you're taking supplemental zinc."

"Shouldn't everyone who takes zinc take copper, then?"

"Nope, many of us have too much copper to start with. It's definitely an individual thing. With your tests . . . . please take 6 mg. copper daily for now. Separate the copper from the zinc by three to four hours, if possible."

"And keep an eye on your cholesterol and HDL tests as long as you're taking zinc. Every three to four months to start, less often if they stay OK."

"Cholesterol's that zinc-sensitive, huh?"

"For some of us."

"Now what's this my wife says about polishing my prostate with linseed oil? She read that in your article awhile ago?"

"It's true. In 1941, researchers reported that linseed oil alone was associated with normalizing 14 of 19 enlarged prostate glands."

"What's this 'associated with normalizing' stuff? Sounds like fancy talk for 'they took linseed oil and got better'. Isn't that what happened?"

"Yes, but it wasn't what's called a controlled study . . ."

"My prostate isn't controlled either, but I'll know if it's better. What do people tell you?"

"A very large majority tell me their prostate symptoms disappear or substantially diminish with zinc and linseed oil supplementation."

"Good enough for me. How much linseed oil?"

"One tablespoon daily to start. If you'd rather take it in capsules, 6 of the 1000 mg. size daily."

"Also, vitamin E . . ."

"My wife told me about that . . . something about taking extra vitamin E whenever you take a supplemental oil."

"That's right."

"She's got me on 800 units daily already. Is that enough?"

"Should be."

"Gee, you know I told her I didn't really need to come in here and pay you the money to tell me to take zinc and linseed oil. Could have given her the money instead!"

"Or maybe just invested it in pumpkin seeds the last few years. They're good sources of zinc and many of the fatty acids found in linseed oil."

"Figures. But I guess I needed to find out about that zinc-copper-cholesterol thing, and I never would have guessed my stomach wasn't making much acid at all."

"Could be just as important as getting your prostate better."

"I can see that . . . . now is that everything for the prostate, though? What about that herbal thing I brought in?"

"Usually zinc and linseed oil are enough. When they're not, there are other things, including herbal preparations, that can help in some cases. Try for the next few months and let us know."

Mr. Oeldorf phoned in to let us know that his prostate symptoms were almost entirely gone within seven months. His prostate was reported to be back to normal size when his urologist persuaded him to have it checked a month or two later. He was advised to cut his zinc back to 30 mg. daily, and his linseed oil to three capsules, as long as no symptoms returned. He also continues his vitamin E, and 2 mg. copper to keep his cholesterol-to-HDL ratio under good control.

# Appendix B
# DR. WRIGHT'S GUIDE TO CHOLESTEROL-CONTROLLING NUTRIENTS

**WARNING:** The individual nutrients listed below have been found useful and effective in the quantities given under Dr. Wright's supervision at Tahoma Clinic (Kent, Washington). It must be remembered that we are all different biochemically, not everyone reacting the same to even usually-harmless substances. For this reason, this GUIDE is meant as an exploration of possibilities only. Anyone wishing to apply any of the information contained herein to themselves should do so ONLY UNDER THE SUPERVISION OF A KNOWLEDGEABLE HEALTH CARE PROFESSIONAL.

## BEYOND (WAY BEYOND) OAT BRAN AND NIACIN

Cholesterol control is a national mania. Corner drugstores, health fairs, and Boy Scout troops offer cholesterol tests. "Low cholesterol" and "no cholesterol" are emblazoned everywhere. The lowly oat is transformed into advertising gold.

Yet most of the information about the "evils of high cholesterol" has been around for a generation or more. Sure, more studies have been done, but they've just shown more of the same, nothing brand-new. Cynics suspect that the introduction of several new patented "anti-cholesterol" drugs has more to do with the last few years of "cholesterol hype" than new scientific information.

Unfortunately, almost all of these patented medications do as much harm as good. It's not terribly helpful to lower the risk of heart attack while raising cancer risk by an equivalent figure. Similarly, if the risk of accident, suicide or violent death is significantly greater in the patent medication group, does it matter if there are fewer heart attacks? Dead is dead no matter what the cause. Patented drugs most often fail the test of lowering the overall death rate.

As you know, effective natural treatments not only help the problem they're designed for, but several others besides. For example, a permanent reduction in saturated fat intake while increasing dietary fiber lowers breast cancer, gallstone, and colon cancer risk at the same time heart attack risk goes down.

Many of us don't realize the truly remarkable range of natural and naturally-derived cholesterol lowering possibilities available. Most have been known as long as or longer than the now-well-worn oat bran and niacin routine; they simply haven't had as much press. A listing and brief discussion of 27 of them follows.

Let's start with foods: in addition to oat bran, research has shown that soy protein, raw carrot, yogurt, garlic, high-chromium brewer's yeast and onions all help to lower serum cholesterol.

It's difficult to say how much of each of these foods is needed to help lower serum cholesterol a certain amount. The best strategy is to include all of them in your diet, as much as you can tolerate, unless specific allergy makes it inadvisable.

Among botanicals and botanical extracts, alfalfa, ginger,

pectin, psyllium and guar gum have all been shown to have a cholesterol-lowering effect.

Alfalfa is available in capsules or tablets of varying sizes. If used by itself, 1 to 3 grams daily are usually necessary. Ginger and pectin can of course be used here and there in cooking; if taken as a supplement, at least 1 gram of ginger and 2 to 3 grams of pectin are needed. Psyllium is a common "bulking agent" found in many constipation-relief remedies; the daily "anti-constipation" dose stated on the containers appears sufficient. Guar is found increasingly as a food component, as it is not usually available as a supplement.

Before going over specific nutrients, it's again necessary to say that you should check with a health care professional about the use of specific supplementation. To continue:

Niacin does lower cholesterol quite effectively. It's also likely the most "hazardous" on this list. Individuals who've ignored the "early warning signs" (low grade nausea or queasiness) of too much niacin have sometimes landed in the hospital with "too-much-niacin" induced hepatitis (not the same as infectious hepatitis). IF ANY NAUSEA, STOP NIACIN. It can sometimes be resumed at a lower dose.

A few of us can't take niacin because of excess stomach irritation (different than nausea).

The well-known "niacin flush" while sometimes extremely uncomfortable always passes and isn't dangerous.

For these and other reasons, at Tahoma Clinic niacin is always recommended in a time release capsule (not tablet) in quantities ranging from 125 mg. twice daily to 500 mg. twice daily AS LONG AS THERE'S NO NAUSEA. Higher quantities are usually not needed if we take advantage of one or more other items mentioned in this report.

Vitamin C can be very helpful, but it takes more than present in the usual multivitamin. Three grams daily (not all at once) is a good "average amount". If you have a family or personal history of kidney stone, a lab test called "24-hour urine for oxalate" can help determine the maximum amount safe.

Lecithin has been used to lower total serum cholesterol

for years. It's often, linked with vitamin C. A component of lecithin, phosphatidyl choline, appears to be even more effective when concentrated. Choline/inositol supplements are also very closely related to lecithin in their action. One well-rounded tablespoonful or 6 of the "19-grain" capsules daily if you're using lecithin.

Magnesium not only helps lower total serum cholesterol, but can raise "HDL" (beneficial) cholesterol besides. 200 to 400 mg. daily in the aspartate form (partly depending on calcium intake) is our current recommendation. Too much magnesium can cause loose bowels or diarrhea.

Calcium can lower total serum cholesterol. 600 to 1000 mg. daily is usually adequate. When using calcium, it's almost always wisest to use a combination calcium/magnesium preparation.

Chromium has been found to reduce atherosclerotic plaque (in experimental animals), lower total cholesterol and raise HDL cholesterol (humans). We've observed that 500 to 1000 mcg. daily of the picolinate or polynicotinate form usually does the job.

Vitamin E can raise HDL cholesterol if enough is taken. 400 to 1200 IU is the range for most of us. However, more than a little vitamin E can raise the blood pressure for a very few individuals. Fortunately, blood pressure is easy to monitor.

Copper can help lower cholesterol for copper-deficient individuals. When using copper, keeping track of copper/zinc interactions is very important. We currently recommend 4 to 8 mg. daily of copper sebacate.

Chondroitin sulfate can help lower cholesterol, 1 to 3 grams daily.

Pantethine (a pantothenic acid metabolite) has been shown to lower total serum cholesterol in several studies. It also has a favorable influence on HDL cholesterol. 300 to 900 mg. daily is frequently sufficient. A few require more.

L-carnitine lowers total cholesterol and raises HDL levels, too. While it's at it, it lowers triglycerides, another blood fat. Although one of the more expensive nutrients, it's one of the most effective. 250 mg. three or four times daily usually does the job.

Iodine can effectively bring down high cholesterol. Although much less dangerous than drugs, iodine can have side effects for a few people, and should only be used on prescription, even though it's a nutrient.

Fish oil (after oat bran) has been the most widely publicized nutritional substance capable of lowering serum cholesterol. However, fish oil contains "omega-3" fatty acids, and our bodies need a "balance" of "omega-3", "omega-6" and "omega-9" fatty acids to stay healthy over time. The best balanced single oil is flaxseed (linseed). Olive oil is the best known omega-9 oil, and most other vegetable oils are sources of omega-6 fatty acids. When using unsaturated oils, remember to always use vitamin E.

We usually recommend flaxseed oil, 4 to 6 grams daily. If fish oil is used, 3 to 5 grams daily is often necessary.

Vanadium can lower total serum cholesterol. Except in combination multiples, it's currently available only on prescription at a very few places.

"Sitosterols" (a group of sterols found in plants) are effective cholesterol-lowerers. Beta-sitosterol appears to be the most effective of this group. 500 to 1000 mg. daily is useful.

(Once again, please remember that if several of the above foods and food supplements are used, the full amounts stated frequently aren't needed.)

So there we have our list: 27 foods, botanicals and nutrients (counting "unsaturated oils", lecithin and its relatives, and the sitosterols each as one item, which they really aren't) which can lower serum cholesterol and in some cases raise beneficial HDL cholesterol. And this is in addition to what we can do with strictly dietary changes!

So leave the patent medications on the drugstore shelf, and go easier on the oat bran, Wilbur. There's a world of alternatives out there!

And please remember to check with a knowledgeable health-care professional!

# REFERENCES

The references listed below are in most cases just one or two of the many available on each topic, and are selected as a "starting point". A search at a medical library will turn up much more information.

As noted, these references ARE NOT the sources for the "dosages" noted above.

SOY PROTEIN: Sirtori CR, et al. Am J Clin Nutr 1979;32:1645

CARROT: Robertson J et al. Am J Clin Nutr 1979;32:1889

YOGURT: Mann GV. Atherosclerosis 1977;26:335

GARLIC: Sharma KK et al. Indian J Nutr Diet 1976;13:7
    Barrie S et al. J Ortho Med 1987;2(1):15

YEAST: Elwood et al. J Am Coll Nutr 1982;1:253

ONIONS: Wymelenberg S. Am Health 1983(Nov/Dec):33

ALFALFA: Hastings AW. Medical Tribune 1979 Nov; 21:3
    Malinow MR. Atherosclerosis 1978;30:27

GINGER: Gujaral S. Nutr Rep Int 1978;17:183 (animal study)

PECTIN: Miettinen TA Tarpila S. Clinica Chimica Acta 1977;79:471
    Cerda J. Clin Card 1988;11:589

GUAR: Khalsa N Sharma PK. Indian J Nutr Diet 1980;17:297

ASCORBATE (VITAMIN C): Horsey J et al. J Hum Nutr 1981;35:53

LECITHIN: Greten H et al. Atherosclerosis 1980;36:81
    Adlersberg D Sobotka H. J Mt Sinai Hosp 1943;9:955

MAGNESIUM: Davis WH. Curr Ther Res 1984;36:341

CALCIUM: Bierenbaum ML et al. Lipids 1972;7:202

CHROMIUM: Abraham AS et al. Atherosclerosis 1982;42:185 (animal study)
    Wallach S. J Am Coll Nutr 1985;4:107
    Evans G. Int J Biosocial Med Res 1989;11(2):163

VITAMIN E: Hermann WJ et al. Am J Clin Pathol 1979;72:848
    Howard DR et al. Am J Clin Pathol 1982;77:86
    (these 2 studies appear to contradict each other. As is often the case, the "dose" and case selection are the keys to success)

COPPER: Allen KGD Klevay LM. Nutr Rep Int 1980;22:295
(animal study)
Klevy LM. Metabolism 1984;33:1112
CHONDROITIN: Nakazawa K Murata K. J Int Med Res
1978;6:217
PANTETHINE: Galeone F et al. Curr Ther Res 1983;34:383
Maoioli M et al. Curr ther Res 1984;35:307
CARNITINE: Abdel-Aziz MT et al. Nut Rep Int 1984;29:1071
Pola P et al. Drugs Exptl Clin Res 1983;9:925
Rossi CS Siliprandi N. Johns Hopkins Med J 1982;150:51
IODINE: Pitel NY. Fed Proc (trans) 1963;22(2)T135 (from Tera-
pevtiicheskii Arkhiv 1962;34(4):53
FISH OIL: Simons LA et al. Atherosclerosis 1985;54:75
Harris WS et al. Metabolism 1984;33:1016
Illingworth DR et al. Arteriosclerosis 1984;4:270

# Appendix C
## NUTRIENTS AND BONE HEALTH

Alan R. Gaby, M.D. and Jonathan V. Wright, M.D.

ABSTRACT: Osteoporosis is a major epidemic in the United States, responsible for at least 1.2 million fractures per year. Current management of bone loss consists primarily of estrogen therapy and calcium supplements. This approach is helpful in many cases, but its success is limited.

This review presents a new concept: that bone health depends not just on estrogen and calcium, but on a wide range of other nutrients, including vitamins B6, C, D, K, folic acid, magnesium, manganese, boron, zinc, copper, strontium and silicon. The typical Western diet, with its high content of sugar and refined foods, appears to be deficient in many of these vitamins and minerals. Furthermore, the requirement for certain nutrients may be increased by genetic factors or by metabolic changes that occur at the time of menopause. Failure to meet one or more of these nutritional needs could result in accelerated osteoporosis. On the other hand, supplementation with a balanced combination of appropriate micronutrients may prove to be a useful adjunct to calcium and estrogen therapy.

## Introduction

Nearly one-third of all American women will, during their lifetime, develop osteoporosis severe enough to cause a fracture. At least 1.2 million fractures (primarily of the hips, vertebrae or wrists) occur each year as a direct result of osteoporosis. The medical and social costs of this epidemic are estimated to be $6.1 billion annually.[1]

In women, bone mass begins to decline at 35 years of age, and then accelerates rapidly for 8 to 10 years around the time of menopause. Thereafter, bone loss continues at a slower rate.

The risk of developing fractures is closely related to bone mass. However, fracture risk is also influenced by other factors, such as 1) breakdown of the protein matrix and other supporting structures in bone and 2) accumulation of microfractures from repeated mild trauma.[2] Preventing fractures therefore requires attention to at least three factors: 1) preserving adequate mineral mass, 2) preventing loss of protein matrix and other structural elements, and 3) assuring optimal repair mechanisms to remodel damaged areas of bone.

## Current Therapy: Estrogen and Calcium

Current management of osteoporosis focuses primarily on estrogen therapy and calcium supplements. Numerous studies have shown that, although estrogen retards bone loss, it does not completely prevent it.[3] Fractures do occur, although less frequently, in estrogen-treated women. The benefit of estrogen must be weighed against its risks, particularly an increased incidence of endometrial cancer.

Calcium supplements, usually in dosages of 800-1,500 mg/day, play an important role in prevention and treatment of bone loss. However, it is becoming increasingly clear that calcium alone is not enough. There is no question that calcium deficiency can cause osteoporosis, and that some women consume less than the Recommended Dietary Allowance (RDA) for calcium. However, skeletal calcium depletion is present in only about 25% of osteoporotic women.[4] Calcium supplements were found to increase bone mass in these women, but had no effect in the other 75% who were not calcium deficient.

A number of early studies showed that calcium supplements partially prevent bone loss.[5,6,7,8] The validity of these studies is called into question, however, because of technical limitations, which restricted measurements to the forearm, metacarpal bones, and fingers. Bone mass at these sites is known to correlate poorly with that of clinically important areas, such as the hips and spine. The development of dual photon absorptiometry eventually made it possible to measure bone mass of the hip and spine.[9] Using this technique, Riis et al.[10] found that calcium supplementation to postmenopausal women (2,000 mg/day for 2 years) did not significantly reduce bone loss.

Thus although estrogen and calcium therapy have a definite place in the overall management of osteoporosis, new approaches are needed.

## Possible Role of Other Nutrients

The estrogen/calcium approach could probably be improved upon if proper attention were given to other nutrients. The evidence reviewed below suggests that supplementation with certain vitamins and minerals might be a useful adjunct to current therapy.

It is sometimes forgotten that bone is more than just a collection of calcium crystals. Bone is active, living tissue, continually remodeling itself through osteoblastic (bone forming) and osteoclastic (bone resorbing) activity, constantly participating in a wide range of biochemical reactions. Like any living tissue, bone has diverse nutritional needs. Failure to meet these needs could presumably compromise the strength and integrity of bone tissue.

The typical Western diet, with its high proportion of refined sugar, white flour, fat, and canned foods, contains far less of certain vitamins and minerals than diets consumed by our ancestors. Furthermore, the requirement for certain nutrients may be increased by genetic factors or by metabolic changes that occur at the time of menopause. Inadequate intake of any one of these nutrients could play a role in the development of osteoporosis.

Multiple deficiencies over a prolonged period of time may have even greater significance. This possibility is supported by the work of Albanese, who found that adding "all known micronutrients" to a calcium supplement reduced bone loss to a significantly greater degree than calcium alone.[11] Some of the nutrients that may play a role in bone health are discussed below.

### Vitamin K

Vitamin K is known primarily for its effect on blood clotting. However, this vitamin is also required to synthesize osteocalcin, a protein found uniquely and in large amounts in bone.[12] Osteocalcin is the protein matrix upon which calcium crystalizes. The component of osteocalcin that attracts calcium ions is a modified amino acid, gamma-carboxyglutamic acid, formed by the vitamin K-dependent carboxylation of glutamic acid. Because of its role in osteocalcin production, vitamin K is essential for bone formation, remodeling, and repair.

It is generally assumed that vitamin K deficiency is rare. However, assessment of vitamin K status is based on relatively insensitive tests, such as prothrombin time. Recent advances have made it possible to measure vitamin K levels in blood. In a series of 16 patients with osteoporosis, mean serum vitamin K concentration was only 35% that of age-matched controls.[13] If osteocalcin synthesis is sensitive to changes in serum vitamin K levels, then the low levels in osteoporotic patients may have clinical significance. That possibility was supported by a recent study in which vitamin K supplementation of a typical Western diet increased urinary excretion of gamma-carboxyglutamic acid by 23%.[14]

Vitamin K deficiency is probably more common than previously believed. Deficiency may occur in individuals whose vegetable consumption is low. Another factor that could promote deficiency is frequent use of antibiotics, which can destroy naturally occurring vitamin K-producing bacteria in the intestines.

Rats fed a vitamin K deficient diet had significantly increased urinary calcium excretion.[15] Furthermore, vitamin K supplementation accelerated the healing of experimental fractures in rabbits, even though they were already receiving "adequate" levels in their diet.[16] In a preliminary study of osteoporotic patients, treatment with vitamin K reduced urinary calcium loss by 18–50%.[17] The evidence suggests that, when accelerated bone formation is desirable, as in osteoporosis or after a fracture, a greater amount of vitamin K is required.

### Vitamin D

Vitamin D is required for intestinal calcium absorption. Reduced plasma vitamin D levels are common in elderly individuals, especially women.[18] Factors that lower vitamin D levels in the elderly include reduced exposure to sunlight, decreased dietary intake, and malabsorption.

Impaired conversion of vitamin D to its biologically active form, 1,25-dihydroxyvitamin D3, may in some cases exacerbate a marginal deficiency. Indeed, abnormal metabolism of vitamin D precursors may sometimes be a more significant problem than dietary deficiency.

Treatment of osteoporotic patients with 1,25-dihydroxyvitamin D3 increased calcium absorption, improved calcium balance,[19] and reduced bone loss[20] in some studies. However, in other trials, this treatment was without benefit.[21] Routine use of 1,25-dihydroxyvitamin D3 has been limited by its high cost and by the risk of hypercalcemia associated with long-term therapy.

Vitamin D should be supplemented in cases where dietary intake and sunlight exposure are inadequate. Measures should also be taken to enhance the conversion of vitamin D precursors to the biologically active 1,25-dihydroxyvitamin D3. This conversion may be facilitated by treatment with magnesium and boron (see below).

## Magnesium

Magnesium participates in a number of biochemical reactions that take place in bone. Alkaline phosphatase, an enzyme involved in forming new calcium crystals, is activated by magnesium.[22] The conversion of vitamin D to its biologically active form, 1,25-dihydroxyvitamin D3, also appears to require magnesium.[23] Deficiency of magnesium can produce a syndrome of "vitamin D resistance."[24]

Whole-body content and bone concentrations of magnesium were below normal in 16 of 19 osteoporotic women.[25] All sixteen women with low magnesium levels also had abnormal crystal formation in their bones, a factor which might increase the risk of fractures. The three women with normal magnesium status had normal crystal formation.

The typical American diet is often low in magnesium. Dietary surveys have shown that 80–85% of American women consume less than the RDA for this mineral.[26] Daily magnesium intake in two other studies was only about two-thirds of the RDA.[27,28] These studies suggest that magnesium deficiency is common in the United States.

## Manganese

Manganese is required for bone mineralization,[29] and for snythesis of connective tissue in cartilage and bone.[30] Rats fed a manganese deficient diet had smaller, less dense bones with less resistance to fractures than those fed adequate amounts of manganese.[29] The optimal intake of manganese is not known, but at least half of the manganese in a typical diet is lost when whole grains are replaced by refined flour.[31] Genetic factors influence the susceptibility of animals to manganese deficiency.[32] It is therefore likely that certain subsets of the human population are unusually sensitive to the effects of marginal manganese intake.

Interest in the relationship between manganese and osteoporosis was stimulated by observations on a famous professional basketball player, who had repeatedly suffered poorly healing fractures and who was found to have unexplained osteoporosis. Examination of his blood revealed no detectable manganese, as well as deficiencies of other minerals. Within six weeks of supplementing his diet with these minerals, he was back to playing basketball. These observations led to a study of osteoporotic women, in whom blood manganese levels were found to be only 25% that of controls.[33]

### Folic Acid

The importance of folic acid for bone health seems to be related to its role in homocysteine metabolism. Methionine, one of the eight essential amino acids present in food, is converted in part to homocysteine, a potentially toxic compound. The danger of homocysteine has been discovered by studying individuals with a genetic disorder in which abnormally large amounts of homocysteine accumulate. These individuals develop severe osteoporosis at an early age, possibly due to an adverse effect of homocysteine on bone.[34]

Prior to menopause, women are especially efficient at converting homocysteine to less toxic compounds. This unique metabolic efficiency may account in part for the resistance of premenopausal women to bone loss.[35]

The following study suggests that, at the time of menopause, a breakdown of homocysteine metabolism occurs, which can be partly corrected by folic acid supplementation. Serum homocysteine levels were measured in female volunteers after administration of methionine. These levels were substantially greater in post-menopausal than in pre-menopausal women, with no overlap between the two groups. Treatment with folic acid partially prevented the methionine-induced rise in serum homocysteine, even though none of the women were deficient in folic acid by standard laboratory criteria.[36] Thus, it appears that menopause is associated with an increased requirement for folic acid which, if unmet, may result in an elevation of serum homocysteine.

Folic acid deficiency is relatively common, occurring in as many as 22% of individuals 65 years of age.[37] Typical American diets often contain only half of the RDA for folic acid.[38] Tobacco smoking, drinking alcohol, and using oral contraceptives also tend to promote folic acid deficiency.

### Boron

Previously thought to be essential only for plants, boron now appears to play a role in human nutrition, particularly in relation to bone health. Postmenopausal women were fed a standard diet for 119 days, supplying about 0.25 mg of boron/day. Supplementation of this diet with boron (3 mg/day) reduced urinary calcium excretion by 44% and markedly increased serum concentrations of the estrogenic hormone, 17$\beta$-estradiol.[39,40] In fact, the levels of 17$\beta$-estradiol in boron-supplemented women were the same as in women receiving estrogen therapy. This increase in hormone concentration may be important, since 17$\beta$-estradiol is the most biologically active form of naturally occurring human estrogen.

The way in which boron acts in the body is not known. However, it seems to be required for the formation of activated (hydroxylated) forms of certain steroid hormones. Boron is known to complex with organic compounds containing hydroxyl groups. It may therefore participate in hydroxylation steps necessary for the synthesis of 17$\beta$-estradiol and 1,25-dihydroxyvitamin D3. Boron deficiency exacerbated signs of vitamin D deficiency in chicks, including abnormal bone formation and elevation of alkaline phosphatase.[41]

Based on animal studies, Nielsen has estimated the human boron requirement to be approximately 1–2 mg/day. Fruits, vegetables and nuts are the main dietary sources of boron. Diets containing inadequate amounts of these foods may be deficient in boron.

Toxicity studies in animals have shown a comfortable margin of safety for "nutritional" doses of boron (1–3 mg/day). No adverse effects were seen in dogs and rats fed chronically with 350 ppm of boron,[42] which corresponds to approximately 117 mg/day in humans. In certain parts of the world where the diet contains as much as 41 mg of boron/day,[43] no problems have been reported.

The fact that boron raised endogenous estrogen levels does not suggest that this mineral poses the same risks as estrogen therapy. The cancer-causing effect of estrogen is dose-related. Because orally administered 17β-estradiol (conjugated estrogens) is mostly converted to estrone by the gastrointestinal tract, large amounts of estrogen must be given by mouth to achieve a clinically useful serum level of 17β-estradiol. In contrast, the amount of endogenously produced 17β-estradiol required to maintain beneficial serum levels may be as little as 5% of the oral dose.[44] Thus, boron appears capable of producing an estrogenic effect without exposing the body to dangerous amounts of estrogen.

Another factor that argues against a cancer risk is the apparent participation of boron in hydroxylation reactions. Synthesis of estriol, a weak estrogen with documented anti-cancer activity, involves a hydroxylation step, which would presumably be catalyzed by boron. Increasing estriol levels (as a proportion of total estrogens) may reduce the incidence of certain types of cancer.[45] If boron does indeed increase estriol production, then it might actually help prevent cancer.

### Strontium

Strontium occurs in relatively large concentrations in bones and teeth, where it is thought to replace a small fraction of the calcium in hydroxyapatite crystals.[46] Awareness of the nutritional significance of strontium has been overshadowed by the fear of radioactive strontium, a component of nuclear fallout. Because strontium tends to accumulate in bone tissue, radioactive strontium may be particularly hazardous to vertebrates. On the other hand, non-radioactive strontium occurs naturally in food. This mineral is apparently quite safe, even with long-term administration at doses hundreds of times greater than the usual dietary intake.[47]

Several studies suggest a beneficial effect of strontium on calcified tissues. The incidence of dental caries was reduced in geographical regions with high levels of strontium in drinking water. Furthermore, addition of 0.27% strontium to the drinking water of mice reduced bone-resorbing activity by 11.3%.[48]

The effect of strontium in human osteoporosis has also been investigated. Thirty-two patients were given pharmacologic doses of strontium (1.7 g/day) for periods ranging from 3 months to 3 years (10 also received estrogen and testosterone). Twenty-seven (84%) experienced marked reduction in bone pain. Radiologic examination showed possible improvement in 78% of the strontium-treated patients.[47]

The effect of physiologic doses of strontium (several milligrams/day) has not been studied. However, chronic consumption of strontium-depleted, refined foods[49] may adversely affect bone strength.

### Silicon

High concentrations of silicon are found at calcification sites in growing bone.[50] This mineral appears to strengthen the connective tissue matrix by crosslinking collagen strands.[51] Chicks fed a silicon deficient diet developed gross abnormalities of the skull and had unusually thin leg bones. The number of trabeculae was reduced and there was evidence of impaired calcification.[51,52]

It is not known whether the typical American diet provides adequate amounts of silicon. As with other nutrients, subclinical deficiencies could result from overconsumption of refined foods. In patients with osteoporosis, where accelerated bone regeneration is desirable, silicon requirements may be increased.

## Pyridoxine (Vitamin B$_6$

Vitamin B$_6$ deficient diets produced osteoporosis in rats.[53] The effect of B$_6$ on bone health may involve several different mechanisms. This vitamin is a cofactor in the enzymatic cross-linking of collagen strands,[54] which increases the strength of connective tissue. Vitamin B$_6$ also helps break down homocysteine,[55] a methionine metabolite which is believed to promote osteoporosis (see section on folic acid).

Dietary surveys indicate that B$_6$ intake by American women is frequently less than the RDA.[56,57] Biochemical evidence of B$_6$ deficiency was found in more than half of a group of presumably healthy volunteers.[58]

## Zinc

Zinc is essential for normal bone formation.[59] This mineral also enhances the biochemical actions of vitamin D.[60] Zinc levels were low in serum and bone of elderly patients with osteoporosis.[61] Low serum zinc levels were also found in individuals with accelerated bone loss of the alveolar ridge of the mandible.[62]

The typical American diet is low in zinc. In one dietary survey, 68% of adults consumed less than two-thirds of the RDA for zinc.[63] Widespread dietary zinc deficiency has been reported in other studies.[64,65]

At present, the picolinic acid salt of zinc (zinc picolinate) appears to have a greater degree of bioavailability than other zinc supplements.[66] Picolinate is a naturally occurring metabolite of tryptophan which is believed to enhance zinc absorption and transport in humans.

## Copper

Rats fed a copper deficient diet had reduced bone mineral content and reduced bone strength.[67,68] Copper supplementation also inhibited bone resorption in vitro.[69] The mechanism of action of copper is not known. However, this mineral is a cofactor for the enzyme lysyl oxidase,[70] which strengthens connective tissue by crosslinking collagen strands.

Since a typical American diet contains only about 50% of the RDA (2 mg/day) for copper,[71] deficiency of this trace mineral may be quite common.

## Ascorbic Acid (Vitamin C)

Osteoporosis can result from vitamin C deficiency.[72] Although frank scurvy is rare in the United States, subclinical ascorbic acid deficiency may be common. Biochemical evidence of vitamin C deficiency was found in 20% of elderly women, even though they were consuming more than the RDA of 60/mg/day.[73]

## A Note on Calcium Absorption

Individuals with osteoporosis often absorb calcium poorly.[74] Impaired calcium absorption may be caused by vitamin D deficiency. Hypochlorhydria (inadequate production of gastric acid), which is relatively common in women over the age of 50,[75,76] may also reduce absorption of most forms of calcium.[77,78,79,80]

Recent studies suggest that calcium citrate is more efficiently absorbed by both achlorhydric and normal individuals than calcium carbonate.[77,81]

## Conclusion

This review has presented evidence that a wide range of nutrients affect bone health. Chronic deficiencies of one or more of these nutrients may play an important role in the etiology of osteoporosis.

# REFERENCES

1. Riggs BL, Melton LJ III. Involutional osteoporosis. N Engl J Med 1986;314:1676–1686.

2. Avioli LV. *The Osteoporotic Syndrome.* Harcourt Brace Jovanovich, New York, 1983.

3. Recker RR, Saville PD, Heaney RP. Effect of estrogens and calcium carbonate on bone loss in postmenopausal women. Ann Intern Med 1977;87:649–655.

4. Burnell JM, Baylink DJ, Chesnut CH III, Teubner EJ. The role of skeletal calcium deficiency in postmenopausal osteoporosis. Calcif Tissue Int 1986;38:187–192.

5. Albanese AA. Calcium in the prevention and management of osteoporosis. J Nutr Elderly 1984;3(3):57–65.

6. Lee CJ, Lawler GS, Johnson GH. Effects of supplementation of the diets with calcium with calcium-rich foods on bone density of elderly females with osteoporosis. Am J Clin Nutr 1981;34:819–823.

7. Nordin BEC, Horsman A, Crilly RG, Marshall DH, Simpson M. Treatment of spinal osteoporosis in postmenopausal women. Br Med J 1980;280:451–454.

8. Horsman A, Gallagher JC, Simpson M, Nordin BEC. Prospective trial of oestrogen and calcium in postmenopausal women. Br Med J 1977;2:789–792.

9. Health and Public Policy Committee, American College of Physicians. Radiologic methods to evaluate bone mineral content. Ann Intern Med 1984;100:908–11.

10. Riis B, Thomsen K, Christiansen C. Does calcium supplementation prevent postmenopausal bone loss? N Engl J Med 1987;316:173–177.

11. Albanese AA, Lorenze EJ Jr, Wein EH, Carrol L. Effects of calcium and micronutrients on bone loss of pre- and postmenopausal women. Scientific Exhibit presented to the American Medical Association in Atlanta, Georgia, January 24–26, 1981.

12. Gallop PM, Lian JB, Hauschka PV. Carboxylated calcium-binding proteins and vitamin K. N Engl J Med 1980;302:1460–1466.

13. Hart JP, Shearer MJ, Klenerman L, Catterall A, et al. Electrochemical detection of depressed circulating levels of vitamin K in osteoporosis. J Clin Endocrinol Metab 1985;60:1268–1269.

14. Suttie JW, Mummah-Schendel LL, Shah DV, Lyle BJ, Greger JL. Vitamin K deficiency from dietary vitamin K restriction in humans. Am J Clin Nutr 1988;47:475–480. (The 23% increase noted in the text was not statistically significant.)

15. Robert D, Jorgetti V, Lacour B, Leclerq M, Cournot-Witmer G. Hypercalciuria during experimental vitamin K deficiency in the rat. Calcif Tissue Int 1985;37:143–147.

16. Bouckaert JH, Said AH. Fracture healing by vitamin K. Nature 1960;185:849.

17. Tomita A. Post menopausal osteoporosis [47]Ca study with vitamin K2. Clin Endocrinol (Jpn) 1971;19:731–736.

18. Anonymous. Vitamin D supplementation in the elderly. Lancet 1987;1:306–307.

19. Gallagher JC, Riggs BL, DeLuca HF. Effect of treatment with synthetic 1,25-dihydroxyvitamin D in postmenopausal osteoporosis. Clin Res 1979;27:366A.

20. Anonymous. Two studies indicate vitamin D metabolite curbs osteoporosis. Family Pract News 1984(March 15):2.

21. Brautbar N. Osteoporosis: Is 1,25-(OH)2D3 of value in treatment? Nephron 1986;44:161–166.

22. Iseri LT, French JH. Magnesium: nature's physiologic calcium blocker. Am Heart J 1984;108:188–193.

23. Rude RK, Adams JS, Ryzen E, Endres DB, Niimi H, et al. Low serum concentrations of 1,25-dihydroxyvitamin D in human magnesium deficiency. J Clin Endocrinol Metab 1985;61:933–940.

24. Medalle R, Waterhouse C, Hahn TJ. Vitamin D resistance in magnesium deficiency. Am J Clin Nutr 1976;29:854–858.

25. Cohen L, Kitzes R. Infrared spectroscopy and magnesium content of bone mineral in osteoporotic women. Isr J Med Sci 1981;17:1123–1125.

26. Morgan KJ, Stampley GL, Zabik ME, Fischer DR. Magnesium and calcium dietary intakes of the U.S. population. J Am Coll Nutr 1985;4:195–206.

27. Lakshmanan FL, Rao RB, Kim WW, Kelsay JL. Magnesium intakes, balances, and blood levels of adults consuming self-selected diets. Am J Clin Nutr 1984;40:1380–1389.

28. Srivastava US, Nadeau MH, Gueneau L. Mineral intakes of uni-

versity students: magnesium content. Nutr Rep Int 1978;18:235–242.
29. Amdur MO, Norris LC, Heuser GF. The need for manganese in bone development by the rat. Proc Soc Exp Biol Med 1945;59:254–255.
30. Leach RM Jr, Muenster A-M. Studies on the role of manganese in bone formation. I. Effect upon the mucopolysaccharide content of chick bone. J Nutr 1962;78:51–56.
31. Wenlock RW, Buss DH, Dixon EJ. Trace nutrients. 2. Manganese in British food. Br J Nutr 1979;41:253–261.
32. Hurley LS, Bell LT. Genetic influence on response to dietary manganese deficiency in mice. J Nutr 1974;104:133–137.
33. Raloff J. Reasons for boning up on manganese. Science News 1986(Sept. 27):199.
34. Grieco AJ. Homocystinuria: pathogenetic mechanisms. Am J Med Sci 1977;273:120–132.
35. Boers GH, Smals AG, Trijbels FJ, Leermakers AI, Kloppenborg PW. Unique efficiency of methionine metabolism in premenopausal women may protect against vascular disease in the reproductive years. J Clin Invest 1983;72:1971–1976.
36. Battstrom LE, Hultberg BL, Hardebo JE. Folic acid responsive postmenopausal homocysteinemia. Metabolism 1985;34:1073–1077.
37. Infant-Rivard C, et al. Folate deficiency among institutionalized elderly. J Am Geriatr Soc 1986;34:211–214.
38. Clark AJ, Gates R. Folacin status of adolescent females. Fed Proc 1983;42:830.
39. Nielsen FH. Boron—an overlooked element of potential nutritional importance. Nutr Today 1988(Jan/Feb):4–7.
40. Nielsen FH, Hunt CD, Mullen LM, Hunt JR. Effect of dietary boron on mineral, estrogen, and testosterone metabolism in postmenopausal women. FASEBJ 1987;1:394–397.
41. Hunt CD, Nielsen FH. Interaction between boron and cholecalciferol in the chick. In Gawthorne JM, Howell JM, White CL (eds.). *Trace Element Metabolism in Man and Animals.* Springer-Verlag, Berlin, 1982, pp. 597–600.
42. Weir RJ Jr, Fisher RS. Toxicologic studies on borax and boric acid. Toxicol Appl Pharmacol 1972;23:351–364.
43. Schlettwein-Gsell D, Mommsen-Straub S. Ubersicht spurenele-

mente in lebensmitteln. IX. Bor. Int Z Vitaminforsch 1973;43:93–109.

44. Barnhart ER (Publisher). *Physician's Desk Reference*, Medical Economics Company, Inc., Oradell, N.J., 1988, p. 867.

45. Lemon HM, Wotiz HH, Parsons L, Mozden PJ. Reduced estriol excretion in patients with breast cancer prior to endocrine therapy. JAMA 1966;196:1128–1136.

46. Anonymous. Strontium and dental caries. Nutr Rev 1983;41:342–344.

47. McCaslin FE Jr, Janes JM. The effect of strontium lactate in the treatment of osteoporosis. Proc Staff Meeting Mayo Clin 1959;34:329–334.

48. Marie PJ, Hott M. Short-term effects of fluoride and strontium on bone forming and bone resorbing cells in the mouse. Calcif Tissue Int 1985;38(Suppl):S17.

49. Schroeder HA, Tipton IH, Nason AP. Trace metals in man: strontium and barium. J Chronic Dis 1972;25:491–517.

50. Carlisle EM. Silicon localization and calcification in developing bone. Fed Proc 1969;28:374.

51. Anonymous. Silicon and bone formation. Nutr Rev 1980;38:194–195.

52. Carlisle EM. Silicon an essential element for the chick. Fed Proc 1972;31:700.

53. Benke PJ, Fleshood HL, Pitot HC. Osteoporotic bone disease in the pyridoxine-deficient rat. Biochem Med 1972;6:526–535.

54. Anonymous. Vitamin B6 deficiency affects lung elastin crosslinking. Nutr Rev 1986;44:24–25.

55. Seashore MR, Durant JL, Rosenberg LE. Studies on the mechanism of pyridoxine-responsive homocystinuria. Pediatr Res 1972;6:187–196.

56. Kirksey A, Keaton K, Abernathy RP, Greger JL. Vitamin B6 nutritional status of a group of female adolescents. Am J Clin Nutr 1978;31:946–954.

57. Hampton DJ, Chrisley BM, Driskell JA. Vitamin B6 status of the elderly in Montgomery County, Va. Nutr Rep Int 1977;16:743–750.

58. Azuma J, Kishi T, Williams RH, Folkers, K. Apparent deficiency

of vitamin B6 in typical individuals who commonly serve as normal controls. Res Commun Chem Pathol Pharmacol 1976;14:343–348.

59. Calhoun NR, Smith JC Jr, Becker KL. The effects of zinc on ectopic bone formation. Oral Surg 1975;39:698–706.

60. Yamaguchi M, Sakashita T. Enhancement of vitamin D3 effect on bone metabolism in weanling rats orally administered zinc sulphate. Acta Endocrinol 1986;111:285–288.

61. Atik OS. Zinc and senile osteoporosis. J Am Geriatr Soc 1983;31:790–791.

62. Frithiof L, Lavstedt S, Eklund G, Soderberg U, Skarberg KO, et al. The relationship between marginal bone loss and serum zinc levels. Acta Med Scand 1980;207:67–70.

63. Holden JM, Wolf WR, Mertz W. Zinc and copper in self-selected diets. J Am Diet Assoc 1979;75:23–28.

64. Patterson KY, Holbrook JT, Bodner JE, Kelsay JL, Smith JC Jr, et al. Zinc, copper, and manganese intake and balance for adults consuming self-selected diets. Am J Clin Nutr 1984;40:1397–1403.

65. Greger JL, Higgins MM, Abernathy RP, Kirksey A, DeCorso MB, et. al. Nutritional status of adolescent girls in regard to zinc, copper, and iron. Am J Clin Nutr 1978;31:269–275.

66. Barrie SA, Wright JV, Pizzorno JE, Kutter E, Barron PC. Comparative absorption of zinc picolinate, zinc citrate and zinc gluconate in humans. Agents Actions 1987;21:223–228.

67. Smith RT, Smith JC, Fields M, Reiser S. Mechanical properties of bone from copper deficient rats fed starch or fructose. Fed Proc 1985;44:541.

68. Follis RH Jr, Bush JA, Cartwright GE, Wintrobe MM. Studies on copper metabolism. XVIII. Skeletal changes associated with copper deficiency in swine. Johns Hopkins Hosp Bull 1955;97:405–409.

69. Wilson T, Katz JM, Gray DH. Inhibition of active bone resorption by copper. Calcif Tissue Int 1981;33:35–39.

70. Anonymous. Activation of lysyl oxidase by copper. Nutr Rev 1979;37:330–331.

71. Wolf WR, Holden J, Greene FE. Daily intake of zinc and copper from self selected diets. Fed Proc 1977;36:1175.

72. Hyams DE, Ross EJ. Scurvy, megaloblastic anaemia and osteoporosis. Br J Clin Pract 1963;17:332–340.

73. Morgan AF, Gillum HL, Williams RI. Nutritional status of aging. III. Serum ascorbic acid and intake. J Nutr 1955;55:431–448.

74. Spencer H, Menczel J, Lewin I, Samachson J. Absorption of calcium in osteoporosis. Am J Med 1964;37:223–234.

75. Brechner J, Armstrong WD. Relation of gastric acidity to alveolar bone resorption. Proc Soc Exp Biol Med 1941;48:98.

76. Sharp GS, Fister HW. The diagnosis and treatment of achlorhydria: ten year study. J Am Geriatr Soc 1967;15:786–791.

77. Recker RR. Calcium absorption and achlorhydria. N Engl J Med 1985;313:70–73.

78. Ivanovich P, Fellows H, Rich C. The absorption of calcium carbonate. Ann Intern Med 1967;66:917–923.

79. Mahoney AW, Hendricks DG. Role of gastric acid in the utilization of dietary calcium by the rat. Nutr Metabol 1974;16:375–382.

80. Hunt JN, Johnson C. Relation between gastric secretion of acid and urinary excretion of calcium after oral supplements of calcium. Dig Dis Sci 1983;28:417–421.

81. Nicar MJ, Pak CYC. Calcium bioavailability from calcium carbonate and calcium citrate. J Clin Endocrinol Metab 1985;61:391–393.

# Appendix D
# THE "TRYPTOPHAN SCARE"

In 1989 and 1990, the Food and Drug Administration created a panic about the safety of tryptophan. It was ordered withdrawn from sale, unfortunately depriving many individuals who had depended on it for relief of problems including depression and insomnia. Contamination of tryptophan products was suspected by most practicing doctors familiar with its use; one doctor published a report of a complete cure eosinophilia-myalagia syndrome with vitamin C and quercitin (a bioflavonoid), WHILE THE AFFECTED PERSON CONTINUED TO TAKE TRYPTOPHAN.

Despite this the FDA has continued the "tryptophan ban", partly for political reasons.

The following brief article taken from the *Seattle Times* best summarizes the situation.

## Disorder linked to impurities in diet aid

EAST LANSING, Mich.—The rare blood disorder linked to the dietary supplement L-tryptophan appears to be caused by impurities found in the supplements, and immune-system weaknesses that make some individuals more susceptible to the illness, federal health officials said yesterday.

The officials said they found chemical contaminants in all of the L-tryptophan samples they studied.

About 1,550 cases of eosinophilia-myalgia syndrome, or EMF, have been reported in the United States since last November, according to the U.S. Centers for Disease Control. The disorder causes breathing difficulty, coughing, muscle pain, swelling of the extremities, fever and rash. Twenty-four deaths have been reported.

"A lot of people were taking L-tryptophan for years, but they were getting sick in 1989. This suggests there is something different about the product on the market in 1989," Dr. Leslie Swygert of the CDC said yesterday at a conference on Issues in Food Safety and Toxicology.

L-tryptophan is an amino acid, a protein essential to the body found naturally in some foods. It was also sold over the counter to combat symptoms of premenstrual syndrome, depression, stress, insomnia and hyperactivity in children.

Seattle Times, Thursday May 31, 1990, page A5

## REFERENCE

Jaffe, R.M. "Eosinophilia-Myalgia Syndrome Caused by Contaminated Tryptophan." *International Journal of Biosocial and Medical Research*, vol. 11(2), 1989, pp. 181–184.

# Appendix E

Interested in more information about healing with nutrition? There are 41 more case histories in my previous book, *Dr. Wright's Book of Nutritional Therapy*, almost all of them different from the cases you've read already, all with recommendations for nutritional treatment.

Here's the list:

1 A Case of Menstrual Upset with Acne and Depression
2 A Case of Leg-Cramp (Intermittent Claudication)
3 A Case of Dry Skin
4 A Case of Eczema
5 A Case of Acne
6 A Case of Long-Standing Depression
7 Three More Cases of Depression
8 A Case of Recurrent Infection
9 A Case of Cramps from a Low-Residue Diet
10 A Case of Colitis
11 A Case of Afternoon Fatigue
12 A Case of Heart Disease
13 A Case of Diabetes and High Blood Pressure
14 A Case of Bursitis and Dupuytren's Contracture
15 A Case of Chronic Bladder Irritation and Bowel Upset
16 A Case of Preeclampsia (Early Toxemia of Pregnancy)
17 A Case of Palpitations
18 A Complex Case of Food Allergy
19 A Case of Allergic Bed-Wetting
20 A Case of Bed-Wetting from Nerve Compression
21 A Case of Allergic Arthritis
22 A Case of Headaches, Tiredness, and Hidden Food Allergy
23 A Headache for a Chiropractor
24 A Case of B Vitamin Deficiency in a Healthy 90-Year-Old
25 A Case of $B_6$-Responsive Arthritis
26 The 'Nightshade' Elimination Diet for Arthritis
27 A Case of Degenerative Arthritis
28 A Case of Weak, Tingling Hands
29 A Case of Hepatitis
30 A Case of Kidney Stones
31 High-Dose Vitamin C and Kidney Stones
32 A Case of Prostate Enlargement
33 A Case of Calluses
34 A Case of Lead Toxicity
35 A Case of Nosebleeds
36 A Case of 'Growing Pains'
37 A Case of Sciatica
38 A Case of Severe Body Odor
39 A Case of Unexplained Tiredness
40 A Deficiency of 'Midnight Moonlight'
41 A Case of Air Ion Sensitivity

*Dr. Wright's Book of Nutritional Therapy* is available in hardcover from Tahoma Clinic, 24030 132nd Street SE, Kent, WA 98042 or from Jonathan V. Wright, M.D., PO Box 973, Maple Valley, WA 98038, for $15.00, including postage and handling.

# TAHOMA CLINIC

## FREE
## NUTRITION and ALLERGY
## HOTLINE
## 1-(800) 825-8924

Tahoma Clinic Nutrition and Allergy Hotline answers questions or problems relating to nutrition, diet, vitamins, minerals, food or environmental allergies and sensitivities, chelation therapy and mercury (dental amalgam) toxicity.

CALL US AT
1-(800) 825-8924
Between 3:00-5:00 p.m.
Monday through Thursday
and speak to one of our
physicians or nurses.

Hotline Service is free of charge.

We ask that you limit your calls to no more than ten minutes.

# INDEX

# P

Pantethine, 569
Para-aminobenzoic acid for skin problems, 9
Parathyroid hormone, 209, 210
Phosphorus and calcium, 210, 452
Photosensitivity, 516–21
Physician, how to locate a nutrition-oriented, 533–53
Platelet aggregation, 184–97
    cod-liver oil and, 192, 295
    diabetes and, 295
    garlic oil and, 190–91, 192, 294
    primrose oil and, 193
    sugar and, 193–94
    symptoms of, 184–87
Polybrominated biphenyls, *See* PBB
Potassium
    cramps and, 536
    sodium and, 350
Potassium iodide
    for erythema nodosum, 469–71
    for salivary duct stone, 553–57
Pregnancy. *See also* Birth defects
    Bendectin, 462
    dark circles beneath the eyes, 10
    folate and, 81–89, 558
    nausea in, 457–65
    toxemia and, 15
    vitamin $B_6$ and, 458, 462, 519
    vitamin K with vitamin C and, 459–61, 464
Primrose oil
    allergic symptoms alleviated by, 333
    cystic mastitis and, 276
    platelet aggregation and, 193
    poor fingernails and, 345
    prostaglandin metabolism and, 256
Prostaglandins, 251–52, 255
Prostate gland
    fatty acids for the, 374
    heartbeat irregularity and, 373–74
    lack of zinc and enlargement of the, 303–4, 314, 315, 374, 561–65
    leg ulcer and the, 303
    linseed oil and the, 374, 564–65
    pumpkin seeds and the, 374, 562
Protein
    depression and, 283
    during pregnancy, 15
    insomnia and, 283
    osteoporosis and, 443–44, 446

    tryptophan and, 283
Pumpkin seeds and prostate problems, 374

# R

Raynaud's, 532, 536
Riboflavin and cataracts, 9
Ritalin, 397, 400
Rosacea, 10, 33, 131–38

# S

Salicylate, 10, 401, 406
Sciatica, 482, 483, 485
Scleral hemorrhage, 10
Scurvy and vitamin C, 74–75
Seborrheic dermatitis, 8
Selenium, 8, 14, 202, 203, 334, 428–29, 430–31, 543–45
Senility, 472–79
Shingles, 480–88
Silicon, 582–83
Sinus problems and allergy, 489–97
Sitosterols, 570
Skin problems
    acne, 10, 21
    bumps, 11, 14
    calluses, 15
    dry, 14–15, 253–55
    eczema, 13, 16, 33
    erythema nodosum, 466–71
    itching, 417–23
    rosacea, 10, 131–38
    seborrheic dermatitis, 8
    thickening of hand tissues, 12–13
    vitamins for, 8–9, 10, 11
    yellow cast of facial skin, 10
Sodium and fluid retention, 350–352
Sodium ascorbate
    allergic conjunctivitis and, 249
    eyedrops of, 249
    ulcerated cornea and, 247–50
    viral infections and, 249
Spasms, magnesium and, 531–537
Speech problems and platelet aggregation, 185
Stomach acidity, low. *See also* Hydrochloric acid
    age and, 33
    anemia and, 155–56, 157–58, 322

cystic mastitis, case of, 260–77
edema and, 351
estrogens in, 100–102
iron levels in, 105
nutrients for, 14, 15, 255
osteoporosis and, 441–56
in pregnancy, 10, 15

# Y

Yeast infections, 142

# Z

Zinc
anemia and excess, 377
cadmium and, 202, 203
copper and, 378, 561, 564
cramps and, 258
drinking and depletion of, 311–18
for the ears, 9
eczema and, 13
fatty acids and, 271
for the fingernails, 12
irregular heartbeat and, 376
leg ulcer and, 303, 304, 307–8
macular degeneration and, 544, 545
osteoporosis and, 583
pancreatic enzymes and, 305
prostate gland and, 303–4, 314, 315, 374, 561–65
vitamin A and, 315
Wilson's disease and, 378–79